RETHINKING MENTAL HEALTH AND DISORDER

Rethinking Mental Health and Disorder

Feminist Perspectives

Edited by

MARY BALLOU
LAURA S. BROWN

THE GUILFORD PRESS
New York   London

© 2002 The Guilford Press
A Division of Guilford Publications, Inc.
72 Spring Street, New York, NY 10012
www.guilford.com

Printed in the United States of America

Library of Congress Cataloging-in-Publication Data

Rethinking mental health and disorder : feminist perspectives / edited
by Mary Ballou, Laura S. Brown.
    p.   cm.
Includes bibliographical references and index.
    ISBN 1-57230-799-4
    1. Feminist therapy. 2. Feminist psychology. 3. Women—Mental
health.   I. Ballou, Mary B., 1949–   II. Brown, Laura S.
RC489.F45 R48 2002
616.89′14082—dc21
                                                    2002007091

About the Editors

Mary Ballou, PhD, is Professor at Northeastern University and Director of the Counseling Psychology Program. Within the master's counseling psychology program she has created a curriculum that encourages students to select concentrations that are interdisciplinary; one of them, for example, is Culture, Gender, and Political Psychology. Within the doctoral program Dr. Ballou has been one of the leaders in developing an ecological model that supports structural analysis, interdisciplinarity, and paradigm change for the combined counseling and school psychology program. She also practices feminist psychology in counseling and consulting, holding the firm belief that practice helps scholarship even while scholarship facilitates practice and that understanding and action need to be wed in psychology as in politics.

Laura S. Brown, PhD, is Professor of Psychology, Washington School of Professional Psychology at Argosy University, in Seattle. She has also maintained a practice of feminist psychotherapy, forensic psychology, and consultation in Seattle since 1979. She has written extensively on issues of feminist practice, including diagnosis and assessment, feminist forensic practice, ethics and boundary issues, psychotherapy with lesbians, trauma and memory of abuse, and theory in feminist therapy. Dr. Brown has published over 120 articles and book chapters, and with this volume has edited or authored six professional books. Her numerous awards include the APA Award for Distinguished Professional Contributions to Public Service, the Sarah Haley Memorial Award for Clinical Excellence of the International Society for Traumatic Stress Studies, and the Leadership Citation of the Committee on Women in Psychology. Her 1994 book, *Subversive Dialogues* (Basic Books), won the Distinguished Publication Award of the Association for Women in Psychology. In 2000, in a departure from her usual activities, she served as the on-site psychologist for the popular reality television series *Survivor: The Australian Outback*.

Contributors

Mary Ballou, PhD (see "About the Editors")

Joan C. Chrisler, PhD, is Professor of Psychology at Connecticut College in New London. She teaches undergraduate and graduate courses on health psychology and the psychology of women, and conducts research on women's health and on gender roles. Dr. Chrisler is the author of over 75 articles and book chapters, and has edited four books, including *Lectures on the Psychology of Women* (2000, McGraw-Hill) and *Arming Athena: Career Strategies for Women in Academe* (1998, Sage). She is best known for her work on premenstrual syndrome, eating behavior, body image, and media coverage of women's health topics. A Fellow of the American Psychological Association and the American Psychological Society, she has won awards for both her scholarship and her service to the profession.

Lynn H. Collins, PhD, is Associate Professor of Psychology at La Salle University in Philadelphia. She speaks and writes about gender and psycho-pathology, including the myth of codependency and the impact of power differentials on behavior. She has worked in a variety of settings, including the anxiety disorders units of Johns Hopkins University and Yale University Schools of Medicine. Dr. Collins has also treated individuals suffering from alcohol dependence through the University of Connecticut Health Center. Dr. Collins is on the executive committees of APA Divisions 35 (Society for the Psychology of Women) and 52 (International Psychology) as well as an active member of the Association for Women in Psychology. She has served as president of the Baltimore Psychological Association, and is currently president-elect of the Philadelphia Society of Clinical Psychologists.

Susan Contratto, EdD, is a lecturer in the Psychology Department at the University of Michigan in Ann Arbor. In her teaching, she combines feminist clinical practice with independent scholarship and political action. Like all productive mergers, it continues to be a work in progress.

Linda M. Hartling, PhD, is Associate Director of the Jean Baker Miller Training Institute at the Stone Center of Wellesley College. She coordinates trainings and publications exploring the practice and applications of relational–cultural theory. Dr. Hartling's areas of expertise include the impact of humiliation, relational resilience, substance abuse prevention, and research on relational–cultural theory. She has published a scale to assess the internal experience of humiliation and is collaborating on the development of a scale to assess organizational relational health.

Ingrid Johnston-Robledo, PhD, is a social psychologist and is currently Assistant Professor in the Department of Psychology at State University of New York, College at Fredonia, where she teaches a course on the Psychology of Women, Women's Health, and Human Sexuality. Dr. Johnston-Robledo's areas of expertise are women's health, reproductive health education, and women's experiences with pregnancy, childbirth, postpartum adjustment, and motherhood. She has published on topics such as attitudes toward the menstrual cycle, low-income women's experiences with childbirth, the motherhood mystique, and postpartum depression.

Judith V. Jordan, PhD, is Codirector of the Jean Baker Miller Training Institute at the Stone Center of Wellesley College and Assistant Professor in Psychiatry at Harvard Medical School. She is coauthor of *Women's Growth in Connection* (1991, Guilford Press) and editor of *Women's Growth in Diversity* (1997, Guilford Press), and has authored numerous articles and chapters on the psychology of women, gender, and psychotherapy.

Jeanne Marecek, PhD, is Professor of Psychology and Coordinator of the Women's Studies Program at Swarthmore College. She is interested in gender and feminist theory, the development of interpretive research methods, and cultural psychology. She has been studying the shifting and multiple meanings of feminism in the daily work, clinical formulations, and professional identities of feminist therapists. Dr. Marecek has also been engaged in research in Sri Lanka for several years. There, her work concerns the social practices and symbolic meanings that surround the dramatic upsurge in suicidal acts in rural communities. She is coeditor of the series *Qualitative Studies in Psychology* for New York University Press.

Atsushi Matsumoto is a doctoral student in the Law, Policy, and Society program at Northeastern University. His interests are focused on feminist inquiry on gendered violence in intimate relationships, forced prostitution and trafficking of women and children in a global context, and making a connection among theory building, practice, and activism.

Natalie Porter, PhD, is Associate Vice President for Academic Affairs at Alliant International University (formerly the California School of Professional Psychology), where she previously served as Dean of the Clinical Psychology Programs at the San Francisco Bay campus. She has primarily concentrated on feminist, antiracist, and multicultural frameworks in psychotherapy, ethics, and supervision, particularly with children, adolescents, and women.

Margo Rivera, PhD, is Assistant Professor of Psychiatry in the Faculty of Medicine at Queen's University and Director of the Personality Disorders Service at Providence Continuing Care Centre Mental Health Services, both located in Kingston, Ontario, Canada. Dr. Rivera has worked for more than 30 years as a psychotherapist with adults and children who are survivors of childhood trauma and has published and lectured widely in Canada, the United States, and Europe on trauma, psychotherapy, personality disorders, and posttraumatic dissociation. She is the author of two books, *More Alike Than Different: Treating Severely Dissociative Trauma Survivors* (1996, University of Toronto Press) and *Fragment By Fragment: Feminist Perspectives on Memory and Child Sexual Abuse* (Gynergy Press, 1999).

Elizabeth Sparks, PhD, is Associate Professor in the Department of Counseling, Developmental, and Educational Psychology at Boston College. Prior to her academic career, she worked for 17 years as a practicing clinician. Dr. Sparks currently teaches courses in multicultural issues in counseling, psychopathology, and counseling supervision/consultation and maintains a private psychotherapy practice. Her research interests stem from her clinical career and focus on interventions for at-risk youth, mental health issues in women of color, and multicultural training and supervision.

Karen L. Suyemoto, PhD, is Assistant Professor in Psychology and Asian American Studies at the University of Massachusetts, Boston, where she teaches classes related to psychology and gender, race, and culture as well as clinical psychology undergraduate and graduate courses. Dr. Suyemoto has presented and published on multiracial identity and issues, particularly identity in multiracial Japanese Americans. Her current research interests include racial and ethnic identities in multiracial and Asian American individuals and groups, and the psychological and educational needs of Asian American urban undergraduates.

Michael Wagner, MA, is a doctoral candidate in Counseling Psychology at Northeastern University, and is in the process of writing his dissertation regarding an ecosystemic analysis of clinical work with the homeless. At Northeastern, he participated in early efforts to refine the ecological model that is used in the Counseling and School Psychology Program, and has also been involved in consultation, tutoring, neuropsychological assessment, and studying systems issues in mental health services. Mr. Wagner currently works as a clinical coordinator and consultant at the North Suffolk Mental Health Association in Chelsea, Massachusetts. His expertise continues to be sought in mental health settings for training and consultation about the role of psychology and use of the ecological model in community mental health.

Denise Webster, RN, PhD, CS, is Professor and Chair of the Division of Health Experience and Technology in the School of Nursing at the University of Colorado Health Sciences Center. She was cofounder of one of the first doctoral programs in women's health and currently coordinates the psychiatric–mental health nursing advanced practice specialty in the School of Nursing. Dr. Webster has been working with women in private practice for more than 25 years and has been published in the areas of women and mental health, feminist and solution-focused therapy, and women's self-care for poorly understood conditions. She recently coauthored *Recrafting a Life: Solutions for Chronic Pain and Illness* (2002, Brunner-Routledge).

Preface

FEMINIST APPRAISALS OF PERSONALITY
AND PSYCHOPATHOLOGY

Ten years ago we edited *Personality and Psychopathology: Feminist Reappraisals*. Although feminist therapists had been discussing and critiquing mainstream models of distress and development for almost two decades, that volume marked the first attempt to draw together, in a coherent whole, the feminist lens for psychopathology with feminist critiques of various mainstream personality theories. We believe we achieved the goal of creating a central reference for discourse on these topics, and by so doing, encouraged the growth and development of these ideas within feminist practice. We challenged, in that volume, the notion that accepted models for understanding development and distress could ever be adequate to assist feminist and other critical psychologists in their work with people's pain.

Those 10-year-old chapters continue to stand as solid analyses. Both the experiences of oppression and the sources of resilience arising from structures of gender, culture, class, race, and sexuality continue to play a part in how the "normal" and the "abnormal" are construed in the discourse of mainstream mental health professions. In the interim, both mainstream and feminist appraisals of human behavior have been altered. The past decade has seen a resurgence of funding of regressive research and theory in the service of contemporary conservative political ideologies within the behavioral sciences. Human behavior is increasingly being forced into the box of biology. Hormonal, evolutionary, and genetic models of behavior are more frequently being proposed as explanations for all human behaviors, even in the absence of strong empirical science to support such models, or in the presence of science that refutes regressive social constructions of the findings of evolutionary psychology.

The interests of feminist practice have expanded as well. In the 1990s, general knowledge of the disorders of oppression, posttraumatic, and dissociative disorders became more widespread among mental health practitioners. Even as debates raged over the reality of delayed recall for trauma, new research discovered the rich and complex biopsychosocial and cultural–structural roots of posttraumatic, postoppression phenomena in both normative and distressed human contexts. Insights that had been unique to feminist practice began to be mainstreamed in other corners of psychology.

Consequently, this new volume is a text with its own message, not a revision or a second edition. It stands as an autonomous series of new looks at developing feminist theory and at our comprehension of both normative and distressed life experiences for the diverse population of humanity. It reflects our collective engagement with questions of how human beings develop their capacities for good function, particularly in highly challenging circumstances, as well as our curiosity about the nature and parameters of distress. As is true for much of feminist practice, we use women's experiences as our central analytic location; our view of distress and disorder begins with women's experiences, although in most cases also speaks to that of men and of transgendered or intersexed persons.

In this volume, we offer a variety of emerging paradigms, each better assisting in feminist understandings of personality. We have also included chapters that look at women's distress and disorder, including diagnostic categories that were either insufficiently addressed in the earlier volume, or on which new feminist understandings have been developed in the past decade.

Feminist psychology does not stand alone at the commencement of a new era in theory building. Psychology as an enterprise has been affected by, and has begun to struggle with, a range of issues brought to it by critical theories and models of epistemology. No longer is the field of psychology confined to a quest to uncover universal laws through the application of rationality and through logical positivism. Although quantitative empiricism continues to offer useful and necessary sources of information about how human beings function, the range of ways of knowing is expanding. These new epistemologies have allowed fuller looks at the human process of construction of inner and interpersonal realities. Past is the optimistic 19th- and 20th-century view of science that in time all would be known through the scientific method held nearly sacred by Western intellectual disciplines. In the 20th century, new science and new intellectual movements—existential, civil rights, humanist, feminist, and environmental—came to the forefront of social and behavioral science knowledge claims. None of this has occurred easily; the hegemony of empiricism can be seen in, for example, what Beutler and Moleiro (2001) have described as "scientism," that is, a bias toward defining as "not science" those paradigms and data sources that do not fit easily, or at all, into positivist models of inquiry.

Now, at the beginning of the 21st century, epistemologies deriving from critical psychologies such as postmodern, multicultural, or ecological are more commonly utilized and more broadly understood. A range of scholars has embraced psychology's heritage in constructivist models. Jeanne Marecek writes a chapter in this text that reviews some of the epistemological and political tension in psychology and in the psychology of women. In the first volume we critiqued, revised, and extended feminist personality theory, as well as explored some emerging explanatory models. This book presents some of that emergent theory development for the reader. It draws from several traditions, but each chapter presents a set of explanatory notions that exists as its own potential path for the creation of enhanced understanding of human behavior.

Unlike the critiques in the earlier volume, which focused largely on problems in mainstream models, here we present theory being built from several diverse perspectives within feminist standpoints. We use the idea of standpoints as a strategy to communicate substantially different positions, including not only different aspects of person and constructs, such as relationship, identities, and multiplicities of reciprocal influences, but also, importantly, different ways of knowing. We see all of these standpoints as coming within a feminist lens; the inclusion of multiple perspectives reflects the diversity within feminist theorizing itself. One of the debates within U.S. feminist and multicultural psychology is the depth of the critical transformation. Do feminist and multicultural perspectives increase our sensitivities to diversity within the groups and content of psychology, or do they also call into question the constructs, assumptions, operations, and purposes of psychology? Are we truly getting beyond "add your favorite oppressed group and stir" as a strategy for understanding the development of a stance on human diversity? Or has the flowering of feminist theorizing simply enabled different versions of that simplistic strategy? Finally, do feminist, multicultural, liberation, and critical psychology assist us in reflective thinking and praxis as we engage our discipline and practice of psychology? In this text we strive to use a broader range of standpoints. These coalescing critical perspectives offer points to stand on in inspecting the progress and adequacy of work already accomplished, and that which is to come.

In the West, and particularly in the academy where psychology has situated itself in the past century, we are most often limited in the received ways of knowing to some combination of rationality and empiricism. So we apply logic, observe, and attempt to reason in ordinary and in complex ways. However, there are several other ways to know, about which the 20th-century academy has been largely silent, at least within psychology.

Some of these ways, including humanized systems thinking, intuition, ethical judgment, communitarian paradigms, personal experience, and phenomenological reflection, are used here to position some of our theories beyond reason and direct sensory observation. These models, in some part, eschew conferring the role of the theory-maker or expert upon the psychologist alone, looking, rather, to interactive consensus about the value of a model to the communities where it is applied. We believe these models are important in part because of our own experiences in their application. Many of our authors are practicing psychotherapists, making regular use of and trusting in our intuitions. Clinicians who apply these models know of the value of such nonexperimentally derived, albeit soundly empirical knowing. Our experiences in practice and our daily observations of interactions and patterns among multiple levels of knowing—cognitive, emotional, embodied, spiritual—are the common theme in our own and our clients' lives. Some of us have watched carefully how social groups and individuals organize, interact, and value one another and things. We see how necessary and useful it is to evaluate our models of distress and intervention based on principled ethical judgments and actions. Perhaps because we are dealing with the tensions between mainstream theory and feminist/ multicultural views, we can entertain a plethora of constructs simultaneously in the moment-to-moment demands of clinical work. Feminist therapists and theorists are both continually engaged with the mainstream, and continually questioning it, doing what works to empower and liberate people from their suffering. This capacity to hold multiple realities and ways of knowing is core in feminist theorizing (Ballou, 1990), and present in the work in this volume.

Tensions continue to exist between dependence on empiricist constructs that have yielded valuable information and those various other ways of knowing. Being-knowing, using-knowing, experiencing-knowing, reflecting-knowing, knowing as a means of ethical action, just-knowing, and other epistemologies no longer entirely silenced still compete for our intellectual space, and can be challenging to fit into academic frameworks such as the chapters in this book. By drawing on the concept of standpoint as a framework for understanding all of these meanings, our book is filled with the multiple groundings necessary to feminism, multiculturalism, and critical theory.

We hope this volume, like the first, evokes another burst of work from our colleagues in feminist, postmodern, and other critical psychologies who are thinking about personality, distress, and disorder. We also hope to invite work that moves us past the usual frameworks of psychology. Out of necessity, our book does not address a number of aspects of human experience that have been the subject of feminist experience and commentary. We have once again passed by discussions of spirituality, although we do address issues of meaning-making. Nor do we strongly address social pathology that is thrust upon the individual and buoys up geopolitical institutions, such as institutionalized racism, classism, sexism, or militarism. We also do not explore alternative criteria for making judgments about what counts as knowledge in the face of multiple knowledge claims. Nor do we reflect on psychology with interdisciplinary mirrors. Feminist, multicultural, and other critical psychologists need to build our theory and relevant constructs with such issues in our central vision, and to work across geographical and disciplinary boundaries to do so.

We also need to pay more attention to geopolitical forces and to the variety of nondominant groups. As we understand the complexities and nuances of human diversity more thoroughly, we realize that just as we can no longer speak of generic "women," we can also not speak of generic "modified women"; each group contains within it its own diversities. We need to look to multiple communities and cultural traditions to understand the organization, constructs, and strengths about which the dominant culture remains largely ignorant. If we doubt this, we need only look to the country's responses to the horrors of September 11, 2001, in order to see how stereotype and ignorance continue to dominate popular and political discourses, especially when influenced by reductionistic and conservative ideologies. We need to examine and make sense of these phenomena through modes of knowing other than those of the majority culture. Spirituality is not understood through scale development or through evolutionary theory (leaving aside for a moment arguments about specific brain regions that activate upon contemplative activity). Spirituality has been neglected by psychology precisely because it is not easily quantifiable, but rather is experienced and reflected upon at the most private levels of phenomenology. Similarly, in understanding the distress of the oppressed, we must continue to be mindful that the self-hate and/or other-hate resultant from hegemony of racism, classism, monoculturalism, and capitalism is not personality disorder, no matter how much it may resemble its DSM doppelganger.

This brings up the question of personality disorders. We have chosen not to include a chapter on this topic in this book. This decision reflects several current states of being in feminist discourses on disorder and distress. First, it is not at all clear that the concept of a personality disorder, as defined in the fourth edition of the *Diagnostic and Statistical Manual of Mental Disorders* (American Psychiatric Association, 1994), will survive into future editions of the diagnostic manual. As more sophisticated understandings of extremes of distress and dysfunction are beginning to emerge, the mainstream itself is offering more complex ways of configuring those types of distress. For example, it is more useful, and even more empirically supportable, to talk about disorders of certain capacities (e.g., emotion regulation, self-care, critical thinking, capacity for mindfulness), rather than to characterize these phenomena as distinctive disorders of personality.

Second, the role of severe childhood maltreatment in the development of these deficits in self-capacities is becoming more clear and more accepted. Issues raised largely or only by feminists two decades ago are now routinely accepted by most people studying and writing about extremes of distress and dysfunction.

Finally, feminists have ourselves not developed much by way of new insights into what is problematic about the concept of a disordered personality. We continue to assert what we did in 1990, when Brown, in our first volume, suggested that these so-called disorders needed to be reconceptualized as artifacts of oppression. That paradigm has not been challenged, but rather strengthened by mainstream work in the field of severe distress. Feminists may be more interested than mainstream theorists in what we call these phenomena, questioning whether these forms of distress are incorrectly named disorders. But it appears that the mainstream has caught up with feminist understandings, and the interest of feminists who engage with this topic has moved on.

The place of feminist and other critical psychologies is less tenuous at the beginning of this new century than it was 10 years ago. However, the insistence of feminist standpoints on the complexity of human behavior, the meanings attached to it, and the absolute necessity that all things be understood within their context continues to be in conflict with resurgent attempts to create simplistic, universal explanatory models for distress. An excellent example can be found in some iterations of evolutionary psychology. Correctly utilized, evolutionary models do not, as is claimed by some, cement social norms for gender and gendered behaviors as hard-wired in biology. In fact, as Susan Contratto (Chapter 2) helps us see, when feminist ethological observations, such as those of Hardy, are integrated into evolutionary psychological thinking, then quite radical models, supporting social change and complexity, emerge from evolutionary psychological thinking (see Silverstein, 1996; Silverstein & Auerbach, 1999). Yet these critical paradigms are themselves not central to evolutionary psychology, which has more frequently been a fellow traveler of the social status quo, a sort of postmodern social Darwinism. Consequently, the current trend in psychology toward adoption of uncritical evolutionary models challenges feminist paradigms.

What are these feminist perspectives? First, that "self," as Karen L. Suyemoto in Chapter 4 suggests, is a construct or series of constructs, and that human beings construct the self both intra- and interpersonally on a constant basis. That selves are in flux, and contextual, albeit retaining some core allegiances to temperament. That human resilience, as Judith V. Jordan and Linda M. Hartling explore in Chapter 3, is as interesting, if not more so, than human distress, and that distress may be a manifestation of attempts at resilient responses in extraordinary circumstances, rather than a failure of resilience. That relationships and the nature of relationships are central to understanding human behavior and the nature of both normal and deviant functioning; that humans exist always and only relationally, even when in apparent isolation. That social, political, spiritual, and interpersonal contexts are in constant interaction and interplay with biological and intrapsychic phenomena in the ongoing evolution of human experience within the context of multiple levels of reciprocal influence, as Mary Ballou, Atsushi Matsumoto, and Michael Wagner discuss in Chapter 5 on feminist ecological theory. And that the knowledge claims of many systems, including literature, philosophy, anthropology, and physics, to name but a few, are as essential to the development of a complex comprehension of human behavior as are those from the traditional mental health and behavioral sciences disciplines.

Each of these streams of thought represents important current trends, attempting to warn, expand, and reorient the building of theory that can be helpful in understanding the experiences of occupying nondominant positions in the social/economic matrix, be that for a moment or for a lifetime. These concepts emphasize the critically important influences of multiple factors, and they offer the reader a view of the future from the standpoints of feminist conceptualization.

As has been true throughout the development of feminist theories of personality, psychopathology, and therapy, the work in this book eschews the false construct of objectivity. Rather, we utilize and privilege multiple subjectivities, including those emerging from empirical data collection as well as those reflecting other ways of knowing. Our emphasis instead is on the development of improved theory, abstract concepts that can shape and direct our inquiry, our ideas of helping, our image of wellness, and our definitions of illness. Several of these chapters utilize theory building as a pathway to substantively new ways of conceptualizing these phenomena. Taken together, these theory chapters suggest that the conditions of theory building have changed. Contemporary theory building in feminist, multicultural, liberation, and critical theory is different not only in content but in shape as well. These chapters call for a shift in thinking and assumptions, as new paradigms must.

One of the important starting points of this theorizing is a challenge to the very notion that distress and difficulty are equivalent to disease or psychopathology. This is a very challenging subtext to make visible in the context of the mental health cultures of the 21st century. In the mainstream, the "diseasing" of distress can be profitable, with larger and larger corporate entities taking over the management and control of access to mental and physical health (normalizing) services for people in distress. With this corporate model of illness comes the discounting assumption that if one experiences distress or difficulties in coping, one is ill, broken, and unable to perform at acceptable levels consistently.

If we even glance at feminist, multicultural, liberation, or critical psychology, we see that the decision to call nonconforming thoughts, values, and actions (or even oppressive behaviors) psychopathology does two things. First, it discounts she or he who is described as such. Second, it blocks our ability to look outside the individual to see forces, dynamics, and structures that influence the development of such thinking, values, and actions. While individual problems are certainly significant, it is also significant and meaningful that individuals are enormously impacted by multiple forces and systems. For example, recent sociological study of women involved in hate groups demonstrates clearly that these are not passive, pathological persons, but rather, agentic, powerful women whose context empowers them, even while it proposes to oppress or even kill members of other groups.

The chapters in this book confirm this multiplicity. Natalie Porter's chapter on child psychopathology shows us very clearly that cultural, gender, and power issues are very relevant in understanding children's development and difficulties. In Chapter 11, Elizabeth Sparks writes clearly of culture, race, class, and gender competence as absolutely important in understanding psychosis and depression. Denise Webster's discussion of somatoform disorders in Chapter 6 portrays the level of misdiagnosis and misunderstanding within medicine that comes from not listening and not valuing women's experiences and perceptions of their own bodies. Joan C. Chrisler and Ingrid Johnston-Robledo's analysis of "raging hormones" in Chapter 7 shows a different version of the same phenomena. Here, women's unique physical experiences of predictable, cyclic, hormonal change become the source of name-calling psychopathology. Normal processes are first hidden and ignored and later exaggerated for control and profit. The discussion of addictions in Chapter 8 by Lynn H. Collins brings our awareness to the complexity of interlocking issues across both the disorders and the substances. This chapter explores how those substances that offer profits to corporations—alcohol, tobacco, selective serotonin reuptake inhibitors, anxiolytics—are socially constructed in their use as either nonpathological or less pathological, while the use of those substances that have been made illegal or lack profitability is always defined as pathology. The chapter also reminds us that gender continues to matter in human experience, and that the experience of addiction has gendered phenomenology, something already too well known to many women who have been in 12-step programs.

Finally, in Margo Rivera's chapter we are exposed to what occurs when a clinician stands with women's experiences and tries to creatively develop programs that honor and help. Her description of distress does not fit as comfortably under the rubric of "psychopathology." We see that personality disorders, posttraumatic stress disorder, anxiety, depression, and psychosis are terms that come from outside categories and are nearly irrelevant to the experience(s) of women and the mechanisms that facilitate their struggle to overcome and become liberated to choice.

Thus, this book, as did our previous volume, challenges you, the reader, as well as we, the editors and authors, to a careful examination of our own understandings of human resilience, function, distress, and dysfunction, whose experience they stem from and in whose benefit they are constructed. The challenge is also to the adequacy of single disciplines and limited epistemologies. In 1992, we were comfortable using the terms "feminist" and "psychopathology" in one place. Today, in 2002, we challenge that connection, and ask ourselves, through these authors, how we might name and understand human distress and difficulty, without requiring that we define it as disease or deficit. We also call for continued building of ideas about human nature(s) that include multiple influences, multiple disciplines, multiple ways of knowing, and flexible foundations.

When psychology split off from its parent field of philosophy over a century ago, certain ways of knowing became the focus of our discipline. When, after World War II, psychology became identified with the treatment of human distress, we began to accept, with little question, medical constructions of distress as disorder. These two trends—the narrowing of epistemologies and the focus on disorder—have characterized mainstream psychology. Feminist and other critical psychologies have had as our tasks the subversion of these trends, and the movement of psychology into a plethora of paradigms and a dis-disordering of human distress. We welcome you to join us in this continuing conversation on feminist concepts of being and disorder.

REFERENCES

American Psychiatric Association. (1994). *Diagnostic and statistical manual of mental disorders* (4th ed.). Washington, DC: Author.

Ballou, M. (1990). Approaching a feminist-principles paradigm in the construction of personality theory. In L. S. Brown & M. P. P. Root (Eds.), *Diversity and complexity in feminist therapy* (pp. 23–40). New York: Haworth Press.

Beutler, L. E., & Moleiro, C. (2001). Clinical versus reliable and significant change. *Clinical Psychology: Science and Practice, 8*, 44–59.

Silverstein, L. B. (1996). Fathering is a feminist issue. *Psychology of Women Quarterly, 20*, 3–27.

Silverstein, L. B., & Auerbach, C. F. (1999). Deconstructing the essential father. *American Psychologist, 54*, 397–407.

Contents

I. Developing Feminist Theories

II. Psychopathology

Part I

Developing Feminist Theories

Chapter 1

Unfinished Business
Postmodern Feminism
in Personality Psychology

JEANNE MARECEK

Psychologists have set about describing the true nature of
women with a certainty and a sense of their own infallibility
rarely found in the secular world. . . . Psychology has nothing
to say about what women really are like, what they need, and
what they want, essentially because psychology does not
know.
                                        —Weisstein (1971, pp. 207, 209)

Theories of feminine personality were easy targets for the ire of second-
wave feminists inside and outside psychology. Indeed, the history of psychology amply justifies Weisstein's scorn. As the first wave of feminism was
cresting, Grant Allen declared women to be "the sex sacrificed to reproductive necessities," the "passive transmitters" of the gains in human civiliza-
tion produced by men (1889, p. 258). He summed up the distinction between the sexes succinctly: "All that is distinctly human is man . . . ; all that
is truly woman . . . is merely reproductive" (p. 263).

Writing at the height of the campaign for women's suffrage, Joseph
Jastrow (1915) devoted a lengthy section to male–female differences in his
personality textbook *Character and Temperament*. In Jastrow's account,
woman was little more than a uterus surrounded by a supporting personality. He was persuaded that the "divergent anatomy and physiology of sex"

3

gave rise to a host of male–female dichotomies, including male reason and female emotion.

In contrast to claims about female personality grounded in reproductive biology, psychoanalysis offered theories based on girls' early experience. At least in theory, psychoanalysis offered possibilities for multiple developmental pathways, diverse feminine personalities, and female sexual subjectivity. But this multiplicity did not survive in the reworking of psychoanalysis in the postwar United States. Representations of feminine personality in American popular culture during the 1950s enshrined such psychoanalytic concepts as penis envy, the weeping womb, and female masochism. Writers took as inevitable the inferiority of women's character, moral fiber, and mental stability. Popular accounts of feminine personality were prescriptive as well, insisting that for women, heterosexuality, monogamy, marriage, and motherhood were essential conditions for normality, maturity, and fulfillment. A runaway best-seller of the era was *Modern Woman: The Lost Sex* by Ferdinand Lundberg and Marynia Farnham (1947). The authors claimed that wartime participation in paid work had "masculinized" women, reducing them to a "bundle of anxieties" and generating an epidemic of neurosis, delinquency, and disordered emotions throughout society.

Sexist claims about female psychology did not go unchallenged. In the early 20th century, feminist psychologists such as Helen Thompson Woolley and Leta Stetter Hollingworth spoke out forcefully against what they regarded as bogus accounts of female psychology. Woolley, for example, assailed psychologists for "flagrant personal bias, logic martyred in the cause of supporting a prejudice, unfounded assertions, and even sentimental rot and drivel" (1910, p. 340). Hollingworth argued against the Darwinian claim that women's genetic makeup made them less likely than men to be highly creative or intelligent. A pacifist, she also spoke out against the nationalistic pronatalism of World War I propaganda. Later on, psychoanalytic theories also drew sharp criticism. Karen Horney and Clara Thompson, both revisionist psychoanalysts, argued that it was cultural pressures on women that lay behind the feminine personality patterns that their colleagues had attributed to the intrapsychic residue of early childhood. These pressures included social and economic dependence on men, the suppression of women's ambition, puritanical restrictions on female sexuality, and limited opportunities for self-expression and development (Horney, 1926/ 1967; Thompson, 1942). Horney (1926/1967) courageously took issue with the notion of penis envy, pointing out that the ideas on the subject put forth by male analysts resembled the "naïve assumptions" of small boys. In doing so, she challenged Freud as well as Karl Abraham, her own analyst and teacher. Horney paid a high price for her audacity: she was ostracized from the psychoanalytic communities in Berlin and in the United States (Garrison, 1981).

The stirrings of second-wave feminism prompted *Daedalus* to devote an issue to the subject "The Woman in America" in the spring of 1964. Erik Erikson's (1964) infamous paper "Inner and Outer Space: Reflections on Womanhood" was the lead article. Erikson saw himself as a champion of women. In his eyes, his was a positive view of female difference and an antidote to both the negative Freudian view and the wrongheaded claims emerging from the nascent women's movement. For Erikson, women's "inner space"—the "somatic design" that destined them to bear offspring—created a "biological, psychological and ethical commitment" to care for human life (1964, p. 586). This inner space was the key to women's identity and psychological development, as well as to their happiness. Charging that contemporary feminists were "moralistic," "volatile," and "sharp," Erikson dismissed calls for equality of the sexes. In his opinion, the clamor to expand women's presence in public life was a response to deep-seated anxieties about nuclear annihilation. Such a feminine presence could bring to public life ethical restraint, a commitment to peace, devotion to healing, and the nurturing values associated with home and family.[1]

Second-wave feminists took issue with all these characterizations of women's psychology. By the mid-1970s, several volumes of collected papers challenged psychoanalytic claims about personality, psychopathology, and psychotherapy (Franks & Burtle, 1974; Miller, 1973; Strouse, 1974). This critical work gained momentum from the broad-based political movement behind it. Moreover, a cohort of feminist academics and practitioners stood ready to build upon it. At least to some extent, the organized presence of feminists staved off the professional isolation and ostracism that earlier feminists had endured. Indeed, these second-wave feminists took on the task of reforming the practice of psychotherapy and counseling more generally. They formulated sets of guidelines for curbing sexism in clinical practice that were promulgated by the American Psychological Association and by the Division of Counseling Psychology.

Feminist scholars of the 1970s also made signal conceptual and methodological advances. Anne Constantinople (1973), for example, pointed out that standard psychological tests had been constructed with masculinity and femininity as a single, bipolar continuum, making them mutually exclusive. Test takers were therefore forced to disavow masculinity in order to be categorized as feminine and vice versa. Building on Constantinople's

critique, Sandra Bem (1974) devised a measure of masculinity and femininity (the Bem Sex Role Inventory) that permitted respondents to endorse
mixtures of masculine and feminine attributes. Feminist researchers en-
deavored to reform knowledge-producing practices in psychology more
generally. They drew up numerous guidelines for eliminating sexist biases
in the design, execution, and interpretation of studies of male–female differences, as well as guidelines for eliminating sexist language.

The publication of *Personality and Psychopathology: Feminist Reappraisals* (Brown & Ballou, 1992) carried the feminist critical project further,
with its contributors scrutinizing a variety of theoretical approaches to personality and psychopathology. The papers collected in that volume made it
clear that psychoanalysis was not unique in incorporating biases against
women. (Nor indeed were psychoanalytic theories always and necessarily
incompatible with feminism.) Moreover, by 1992, diverging points of view
had emerged within feminist scholarship. Various theories of feminine personality had both their champions and their opponents, as did various approaches to therapy, various methods of producing knowledge, and varying
ideologies of feminism. Feminist personality theory had become—and remains—an arena for vibrant, sometimes fierce, critical interchange and rigorous debate.

POSTMODERNISM AND FEMINIST PSYCHOLOGY

In this chapter, I describe developments in postmodern psychology and
critical psychology. These movements offer feminists additional critical
tools to rethink gender, personality, and psychopathology. Postmodernists
are skeptical of received truths and taken-for-granted frames of reference.
In the postmodern view, knowledge is never innocent, but always value-
laden and predicated on specific sociopolitical conditions that it serves to
legitimize. Postmodern inquiry points up the power of discourse—
utterances, interactions, and practices—to produce consensual reality and
a shared arena of public conduct. Discourse both regulates and constitutes
consciousness. It constitutes what we know to be the body, conscious and
unconscious mind, and emotional life (Weedon, 1987). The dynamics of
power in everyday social life are another site of postmodern inquiry. This
power "from the bottom" is ubiquitous and far-reaching. Indeed, what
Foucault referred to as "Power/Knowledge" complicates our ideas of freedom. Whether or not we are subject to relations of force ("power from
above"), we are implicated in the webs of power circulating through lan-

guage. The critical psychology movement turns its eye on psychology as a cultural institution, studying how cultural knowledge flows into psychology and how psychological knowledge circulates back through culture, shoring up the status quo and legitimating prevailing power structures (Fox & Prilleltensky, 1997).

For many feminists, postmodernism and critical psychology have been important allies. They have provided valuable resources for continuing the tradition of critique that originated with first-wave feminists like Helen Thompson Woolley. But by and large, in the United States, feminist psychologists have been wary of (and often hostile to) these movements, hurling brickbats like "jargon mongers," "number-phobics," and "antiscience types." The *Psychology of Women Quarterly* (*PWQ*), our flagship journal, has maintained an official stance that is resolutely opposed to postmodernism. In 1995, the incoming editor set the journal's policy on an exclusionary course: "As a scientific journal, *PWQ* provides a voice for a side of feminist psychology that we want to preserve in this age of postmodernism. . . . *PWQ* is a research journal with an empirical, scientific tradition that is centered in the discipline of psychology" (Russo, 1995, pp. 1, 2).

In 2000, the policy statement of the new editor, entitled "*PWQ*: Feminist Empiricism for the New Millennium," renewed and hardened this stance: "Nancy Russo argued rightly that *PWQ* is the scientific voice in feminist psychology. As feminists, the new Editorial Board remains committed to the idea that '*PWQ* is a research journal with an empirical, scientific tradition that is centered in the discipline of psychology' " (White, 2000, p. 1).

How odd that a journal's editors would proudly announce their aim of keeping out innovation! How odd that preserving a single mode of producing knowledge for a full decade would be elevated to a feminist ideal. The later editorial policy goes on to invite "diversity" in journal submissions, but the examples of diversity it gives are quite staid: "articles with male participants, articles using older data bases, and articles using qualitative methods" (White, 2000, p. 1).

The description of *PWQ* as a journal of "feminist empiricism" suggests that its resistance to postmodern psychology stems not only from resistance to innovation, but also from an unexamined residue of a timeworn tradition in psychology. Empiricism is the epistemological stance that all knowledge originates in experience and observation, without the aid of theory or received knowledge.[2] From early on, American psychology was dominated by an empiricist bias toward data gathering to the exclusion of introspection, theory, and reflection. James McKeen Cattell, who championed experimentalism, connected the production of "hard" data in the laboratory to the ideals of masculine "hardness," muscularity, vigor, and physical exertion embodied in the "New Man" movement; in contrast, he viewed reflection, contemplation, and theory building as passive and therefore associated with femininity and even effeminacy. It is ironic to find Cattell's sexist dichotomy unwittingly echoed by prominent feminist psychologists (e.g., Hyde, 1995; Weisstein, 1993). The latter, for example, has dismissed postmodernism as a "swamp of self-referential passivity" and a "cult of high retreat" (Weisstein, 1993, p. 244).

In short, postmodern ideas have had only limited circulation in U.S. feminist psychology, even while they have flowered in women's studies, in other social sciences, and in feminist psychology in other national contexts. Moreover, these ideas have often been seen through the distorting lens of positivism. The editors of this volume, Mary Ballou and Laura Brown, asked me to discuss "postpostmodernism," that is, the directions that feminist psychology might take after postmodernity. In pondering their charge, I came to believe that we in this country have only scratched the surface of what feminist postmodernism can offer to the study of personality and psychopathology. Much of this chapter, therefore, takes up the unfinished business of postmodern personality theory.

FEMINISM, POSTMODERNISM, AND PERSONALITY PSYCHOLOGY: UNFINISHED BUSINESS

Postmodern psychology has encompassed a broad array of initiatives and ideas. I describe those that seem especially fruitful for feminists working in personality psychology and psychopathology.

Interrogating Psychology's Constructs

Evelyn Fox Keller (1995) has described gender as "a silent organizer of discursive maps of the social and natural world . . . even of those worlds women never enter." We can pose two questions about how gender silently organizes the discursive map of psychology:

- How does gender, in concert with other categories of social hierarchy, organize the discourse of psychology?
- How do the resulting psychological constructs serve to distribute power and resources unequally across the social landscape?

Feminists have shown that many personality constructs have been conceptualized in gender-biased ways. They include attachment, passivity, aggression, field dependence, codependency, attractiveness, emotion, self-esteem, autonomy, and humor. Stephanie Shields (1995, 2002) poses some questions that a postmodern exploration of emotion might address: How and when is emotion explicitly labeled in everyday situations? What does it mean to say that someone "got emotional"? What counts and does not count as "an emotion" in psychological theory? What kinds of emotional displays are associated with low-status groups (e.g., women, men of color, and gay men)? How do these displays impact on perceived authority, credibility, and power?

Recently feminists and other cultural critics have used the tools of postmodern analysis to reconsider the constructs of trauma, stress, and posttraumatic stress disorder (PTSD). These constructs have been important in feminists' struggle for public recognition of the seriousness of gender-linked violence, as well as in practitioners' efforts to develop therapeutic approaches for victims. Critiques of constructs that some trauma theorists have put forward are not meant to deny the suffering connected to traumatic events or to impugn the goodwill or good intentions of theorists or therapists. Indeed, the concern of the critics is that the conceptual apparatus of trauma theory has come to have unforeseen negative consequences for sufferers. When gender-linked violence is inserted into the medicalized framework of psychiatric diagnosis, the sociopolitical nature of the violence is expunged (Kleinman, 1995). Moreover, if diverse instances of violence, atrocity, betrayal, and sexual invasion are simply lumped together as "trauma," their psychic meanings, their interpersonal significance, and possibly even their moral import are lost to view. Little effort is made to understand how the lifeworlds and identities of the sufferer and those around her have been altered. Instead, the focus comes to rest on routine procedures of symptom removal. That eye movement desensitization and reprocessing (EMDR) could be proposed as a treatment both for the survivors of the World Trade Center attack and for a young girl repeatedly molested by her father seems less a testimony to the efficacy of EMDR than a reminder of the narrowed outlook of the medicalized perspective.

Other prominent meanings associated with psychological trauma concern the status of victims. One meaning is that victims inevitably and uniformly suffer lasting, even permanent, psychological damage, a meaning that is double-edged (Haaken, 1998; Lamb, 1999). Also, as Dana Becker (2000) has persuasively argued, the category PTSD has become part of a "caste system of diagnosis and treatment": women with PTSD are "good girls" and women with borderline personality disorder are "bad girls." Many feminist therapists have favored the diagnosis of PTSD because, in their view, it announces to a woman that "she is normal," that is, she is having a "normal" response to an abnormal situation (Marecek, 1999a). However, PTSD, as part of a medicalized and technocratic diagnostic system, represents a further embrace of the medicalization of women's problems, not an escape from it.

I briefly mention two additional constructs that have received recent attention in the psychological literature. One is forgiveness, a construct promoted heavily by the so-called positive psychology movement. From a feminist perspective, we can raise many important questions about the meaningfulness and ethics of conceptualizing forgiveness as a state to be inculcated by cognitive-behavioral techniques: Can we theorize forgiveness apart from specific contexts of harm? Is forgiveness *always* a moral good? Does it *always* promote the psychological well-being of the forgiver, as its proponents claim? Embedding forgiveness in its relational context raises further questions: What harm is to be forgiven? What is the relationship between the injured party and the harm-doer? What was the intent of doing harm? Should the harm-doer be asked to acknowledge responsibility, show remorse, and make restitution as a condition for being forgiven? We must also question why there has been a rush to devise therapies that will inculcate forgiveness, but no companion efforts to devise therapies that inculcate remorse. To make forgiveness a moral imperative while disregarding the moral status of the harm-doer is one-sided at best and ethically repugnant at worst.

Forgiveness is overtly a gender-neutral construct. Yet it is hard to ignore the fact that forgiveness emerged as a research topic promoted by the positive psychology movement and as a therapeutic goal in a time of intense public and professional discussion of the sexual abuse of children and intimate violence against women. As a construct abstracted from ongoing experience, forgiveness appears neutral. This masks the relations of power involved in gender-linked violations, forgiving, remorse, and restitution. Moreover, laboratory studies of forgiveness in which one stranger inflicts trivial harm (e.g., the loss of 25 cents) on another are unlikely to contribute meaningful knowledge about social relations. In fact, by further shunting aside the complex power dynamics of real life, such studies can only obfuscate our understanding.

Resilience, another emerging construct in mainstream psychology, has been extolled by some feminist psychologists. They see it as celebrating women's efforts to cope and prevail despite hardship, discrimination, and life crises. But resilience has another side. As McKinley (2001) has noted, resilience too often refers to "a woman's ability to adapt to risk in a manner that is consistent with life trajectories valued by the middle and upper middle class" (p. 85). Moreover, the search to identify women and girls who are "resilient" can be a quest for heroines who overcome adversity by personal effort or inner strength. In this way, the quest to identify the qualities of resilient women seems parallel to the search for the personal and familial characteristics of "notable" women and "successful" women that occupied feminist psychology in the early 1970s. (See, e.g., the inaugural issue of *Psychology of Women Quarterly* [1976] for several examples of this quest.) The "Resilient Woman" (or "Girl") can easily be the other side of the coin of what Mary Crawford and I called the "Woman-As-Problem" (Crawford & Marecek, 1989). Like the Woman-As-Problem, the Resilient Woman stifles social critique; her image replaces a focus on social and economic injustices with a focus on individual triumph through personal will. Moreover, when resilience is construed as a product of personal effort, it suggests that those who do not thrive are responsible for their plight. The slide from there to victim blaming seems nearly inevitable.

Historicizing the Psychology of Personality

Like volcanic eruptions, debates about the true differences (and similarities) between women and men have boiled up at intervals since the beginning of U.S. psychology. As early as 1910, Helen Thompson Woolley warned that the observational design of sex-difference studies made it impossible to draw firm conclusions about the origins of such differences. She noted that it was impossible to draw comparable samples of men and women because the social circumstances of their lives were so different. Similar caveats about sex-difference research have been reiterated repeatedly over the subsequent 90-odd years. More recently, research on male–female difference has also been criticized for its essentialism and false universalism (Hare-Mustin & Marecek, 1994). That is, studies assume that there are inherent (essential) qualities of womanhood; furthermore, they make spurious generalizations about all women based on observations of a limited subgroup of women (usually those who are white, middle class, and living in industrialized Western countries). Yet despite these fundamental critiques, studies of male–female differences—by feminists, antifeminists, and others—continue to be churned out. By 2000, at least 18,700 such studies had been published in English-language psychology journals.

A postmodern feminist might approach the literature on male–female differences not as a scientific record, but as a historical archive of cultural trends in the discipline and in the larger society (Marecek, 1995). What is revealed about cultural change and continuity when we observe the trends in the record? What are the shifting ideological purposes that have driven the research? Over the past 30 years, the focus of psychologists' attention has shifted from sex differences in cognitive abilities to sex differences in emotional capacities to sex differences in mating and reproductive strategies. Research in the 1970s focused on reevaluating claims of male–female difference and associated notions of women's inferior intellectual abilities. In the 1980s, the ground shifted to assessments of male–female differences in morality, empathy, and care of others, with women touted as superior to men. This emphasis on difference took a different and less celebratory turn in mass-market psychology, where celebrity gender experts like Deborah Tannen, John Gray, and Michael Gurian argued that the sexes were so different that failures of communication, mismatched motives, and incommensurable interests were inevitable. In the 1990s, it was evolutionary psychologists who grabbed the microphone (or perhaps we should say megaphone). They too claimed universal and profound differences, differences that served to legitimate and naturalize male privilege, male sexual dominance, and even violent predation of women by men. Close analysis of these shifts could tell us a great deal about the changing preoccupations, anxieties, and vested interests of researchers and funders, as well as the culture at large.

Psychologists often presume that the objects of psychological knowledge are fixed and stable, like those of physics and chemistry. But there are no brute data of the social world comparable to those of the natural world. Instead, the terms by which we understand our social relations and ourselves fluctuate as the social world changes. The meanings of psychological constructs—for example, self-esteem, depression, assertiveness, masculinity, femininity, and premenstrual distress—are local, time-bound, and matters of social negotiation. Consider, for example, the construct of assertiveness. Popularized by behavior therapists in the 1960s, assertiveness was at that time contrasted with passivity and self-effacement. By the mid-1970s, however, lack of assertiveness had become identified as a "woman's problem," with an assortment of psychotherapies, training workshops, professional development seminars, and self-help books to help women become assertive. As a woman's problem, assertiveness gained an additional layer of meaning. Learning to be assertive was prescribed as an antidote not just for passivity but also for aggression. Indeed, a best-selling self-help book of the time was called *How to Be an Assertive (Not Aggressive) Woman* (Baer, 1976).

Another example is premenstrual difficulties. Premenstrual difficulties were earlier called *premenstrual tension*-(PMT). PMT was said to involve feeling nervous or "keyed up." When premenstrual distress reemerged as *premenstrual syndrome* (PMS) during the 1980s, the central psychological feature shifted from tension to irritability, "bitchiness," or rage. Moreover, its name change (from "tension" to "syndrome") elevated its severity and presaged its eventual certification as a psychiatric condition. As psychological constructs, assertiveness and PMS have several things in common. Both shifted in meaning as the second wave of feminism took hold. Both were widely discussed in self-help culture. Both identified women's anger as a psychological problem in need of remedy. This latter view was in sharp contrast to the views of feminists of the 1970s, for whom anger could be invigorating, righteous, and even therapeutic. Seventies feminists (including some feminist therapists) hoped to instigate women's anger, not to quell it. They saw anger as a spur to take action and to struggle against unfair conditions.[3] Seen against this background, both PMS and assertiveness seem like early portents of the backlash against feminism that was to mount over the next decade.

For a postmodern psychologist, examining the history of constructs serves as a reminder of their indeterminacy. Our constructs are not faithful representations of a reality "out there"; instead, their meanings shift in accord with meaning shifts in the surrounding culture. Negotiation over the status of certain scientific constructs can be contentious. Parlee (1994), for example, documents the struggle among feminist social scientists, gynecologists, and psychiatrists for control over the meanings of premenstrual distress. Scott (1990) describes a different political struggle—this one involving Vietnam veterans—over the definition and medicalization of PTSD.

Rethinking Sex and Gender

By and large, feminist psychologists have challenged biological explanations for gender difference. Nonetheless, U.S. feminist psychology retains strong undercurrents of biological foundationalism, as does U.S. psychology and culture. Consider the syllogism that sex is to gender as nature is to nurture. That is, sex pertains to what is biological or "natural," gender to what is learned or cultural. Rhoda Unger (1979) put forward this formulation in the *American Psychologist* over 20 years ago. She defined gender as "those characteristics and traits socio-culturally considered appropriate to males and females." Her formulation was intended to set apart social aspects of maleness and femaleness from biological mechanisms, so the former could be submitted to scientific scrutiny. The sex/gender dichotomy was a significant conceptual advance in its time, but a reformulation of both "sex" and "gender" in her model is now long overdue.

Unger's conceptualization of gender advanced an individual difference model. Feminist theorists have since articulated other meanings of gender. Some view gender as a socially prescribed set of relations. Some see gender as a complex set of principles—a meaning system—that organizes male–female relations in a particular social group or culture (Hare-Mustin & Marecek, 1990). Some see gender as social processes by which status, hierarchy, and social power are distributed. Some conceive gender in terms of social practices that produce masculinity and femininity in mundane interactions and in social institutions (Bohan, 1993; West & Zimmerman, 1987). These meanings focus on processes and practices, not static traits, on relations and social transactions, not private minds. By and large, U.S. feminist psychologists have yet to make full use of these alternative meanings of gender. Most remain mired in Unger's view of gender as individual difference and as little more than the cultural elaboration of sex. With such a view, not only is our sense of gendered possibilities limited, we cannot readily theorize the emergent gender categories put forward by transgendered, transsexual, intersexed individuals (Fausto-Sterling, 2000; Parlee, 1998). Nor can we make use of the provocative theoretical resources put forward by queer theorists.

The conception of biological sex in Unger's sex/gender dichotomy is also outdated. In that dichotomy, sex stands as some immutable bedrock that remains after gender is stripped away. But a large and fascinating body of work in critical science studies, social history, cultural studies, anthropology, and feminist critical psychology points out that sex, biology, and "the" body are not pretheoretical, ahistorical, and prediscursive "givens" (e.g., Fausto-Sterling, 2000; Laqueur, 1990). What any cultural group takes to be "natural" does not exist outside the realm of interpretation and language. Biological "facts" are lodged within webs of assumptions that shift from one cultural setting to another and from one epoch to another within the same culture. Feminist psychologists who have shaken loose from biological foundationalism have been able to pursue a variety of questions about embodied practices. An early example is Suzanne Kessler and Wendy McKenna's *Gender: An Ethnomethodological Approach* (1978). More recent examples are the collection edited by Kathy Davis (1997) and Kessler's (1998) study of intersexed children. Leonore Tiefer (1995, 2001) has mounted powerful and persuasive critiques of the discourse of sexology, including the human sexual response cycle, conceptions of sexual dysfunction, Viagra culture, and, more recently, the emerging diagnostic category female sexual dysfunction.

Cultural Determinism, the Person, and Psychic Life

Feminist psychologists have compiled an impressive corpus of empirical knowledge about how social contexts structure women's lives and gender relations. Slowly but surely, that corpus of information is coming to encompass women and girls from diverse backgrounds and social locations. But the emphasis on the power of the social context to shape women's lives often slides into cultural determinism. In describing the results of empirical studies, we slide too easily from statistical generalizations (typically showing modest effects and considerable variability) to overgeneralizations to universal claims. Such universal claims imply that extrapersonal forces fully determine human action; the person is robbed of any agency whatsoever. A streak of cultural determinism also runs through postmodern psychology. Feminists in psychology who "took the discursive turn" emphasized the power of language to structure subjective experience. In our analyses of the linguistic categories and dominant discourses authorized by the culture, those categories often were granted a determining influence over psychic life. In short, the slide into cultural determinism has been an easy one for psychologists, no matter where they start.

Why should we bemoan the disappearance of agency from theories in feminist psychology? What do we gain from formulating theories of personality and adult development that go beyond figuring people as automatons responding to social conditioning or hapless victims of gender (as phrases like "gender effects" imply)? There are many answers to this question. Most of us have a philosophical commitment to view women as agents. If our theories and research methods do not make space for psychic life, intention, and subjectivity, we cannot examine resistance and agency. We need such theoretical space to study how some people rebel, chafe at restrictions, and produce change. As feminists, many of us are "socialization failures," as Nancy Datan (1989) put it: we were not automatons who absorbed the cultural dictates of our time. We have made different political investments than the norm, we interpret the world in a skewed way, we may have chosen to live nonnormative or unconventional lives, and we engage in oppositional politics, speaking unpopular truths as to power. As Datan asserted, our theories should enable us to examine and explain our own lives.

The challenge is to devise what Nancy Chodorow (1999) has called "both–and" theories. Such theories see people as *both* constrained by their circumstances *and* "doers," as *both* socially constituted *and* causal agents. Such theories must offer an account of how people invest in certain identities and projects, while resisting or rejecting other ones. Such investments are both rational and emotional, both conscious and not conscious. People sometimes espouse identities and pursue courses of action that go against their self-interest or their conscious desires. Thus far, efforts by psychologists to theorize agency and resistance have drawn upon versions of psychoanalytic theory (see, e.g., Henriques, Hollway, Urwin, Venn, & Walkerdine, 1984/1998) or on the work of the Soviet theorists Vygotsky and Bakhtin (1935/1981). Contemporary cultural anthropologists such as Catherine Lutz, Sherry Ortner, and Dorothy Holland—all of whom have interests in gender—have developed a particular rich set of resources for theorizing selves, identities, feelings, agency, and resistance (cf. Holland, Lachicotte, Skinner, & Cain, 1998).

Psychology of Women and History

Concern with real-life contexts sets feminist work apart from much of mainstream psychology. In the mainstream, social context is seen as a source of nuisance variance to be eliminated by laboratory controls; college students (presumed to be stand-ins for generic human beings) are often the population under study. In contrast, the corpus of research in feminist psychology encompasses a range of respondents and acknowledges their particularity. Feminist psychology has focused on social contexts as sites of injustice and domination: school classrooms, peer groups, marriages and romantic partnerships, dating relationships, and therapy relationships. By and large, however, our concern for context has been confined to such microsocial contexts. It is time for us to turn our gaze farther outward, to interrogate the larger frameworks of history, society, and culture in which personal relations are nested.

Some feminist psychologists have shown us the way toward linking women's lives to larger political, social, and economic structures. Abigail Stewart and her students and colleagues, for example, have addressed the impact of historical events on the identities and life trajectories of women involved in them. These events include the feminist movement, the civil rights movement, and World War II (see, e.g., Franz & Stewart, 1994, and Romero & Stewart, 1999). Brinton Lykes and her colleagues (e.g., Lykes, Brabeck, Ferns, & Radan, 1993) have worked with Guatemalan women living under conditions of civil upheaval, state-sponsored terrorism, and guerilla warfare. Walkerdine, Lucey, and Melody (2001) have noted the demand for cheap, mobile female labor created by global capitalism: factory workers, domestic service workers, sex workers, childcare workers. Walkerdine and colleagues' work takes up the ways that schools and other social settings prepare poor and working-class British girls (especially girls of color) to become part of this labor pool.

MORE UNFINISHED BUSINESS:
CHALLENGING METHODOLOGICAL IMPERATIVES

Michelle Fine has urged feminist psychologists to set aside laboratory studies, surveys, and interviews. She implores: "Watch me with women friends, my son, his father, my niece, or my mother, and you will see what feels most authentic to me. These very moments, which construct who I am when I am most me, remain remote from psychological studies of individuals or even groups" (Fine & Gordon, 1993, p. 16).

Many feminist psychologists have made a commitment to research that addresses women's lived experience. But, as Michelle Fine says, the methodological norms of the discipline keep us from doing so. One such norm is the preference for standardized instruments. This preference rests on the assumption that there exist universal, fixed attributes that can be assessed in a uniform way across locales and social groups. The apparent ease of using "canned" instruments holds great appeal, especially when the professional milieu demands high-speed productivity. But such instruments can lead to suppression of local variations and "what feels most authentic" when their meanings do not square with those of respondents. Drawing on his own research in Puerto Rico, Lloyd Rogler (1999) described how items on a standardized scale for measuring stress made no sense in the respondents' life situations. A study by Hope Landrine and her colleagues (Landrine, Klonoff, & Brown-Collins, 1992) offers a powerful refutation of the assumption of uniformity across cultural backgrounds. They asked U.S. women from different ethnic groups to rate themselves on a set of items assessing gender-stereotypic traits. Overall, the groups did not differ in their ratings. Yet when the women were asked to interpret the response categories for the items, ethnic differences emerged for several items. The researchers argued that effectively, women did not complete the "same" questionnaire because the words and phrases carried different meanings depending on a woman's ethnic/cultural background. Calling for a revision in methodology, they noted that "what we take to be the voice of data is the voice of the researcher's interpretation of them" (p. 161).

Another methodological norm that postmodern psychologists have criticized is categoricalism. By "categoricalism," I mean the practice of dividing people into categories (e.g., white/African American/Latino; heterosexual/lesbian/bisexual) and searching for the personal traits and attributes that distinguish one group from the other. This has been a standard approach to producing knowledge in psychology, including feminist psychology. The following statements, for instance, are taken verbatim from a psychology of women textbook: "Lesbians had significantly higher self-esteem than college women"; "Black women reported a lower level of functioning than Black men, White women, and White men." A moment's reflection on these statements reveals how porous the boundaries of such categories are. "Lesbians" and "college women" are hardly mutually exclusive categories. Neither are black and Latina or white and Latina. Moreover, statements like these take categories of race/ethnicity, class, sexual orientation, and the like as a priori givens. We might better see them as historically specific ideologies. Instead of regarding gender, class, race/ethnicity, and sexual orientation as ontological categories, we could investigate them as provisional markers of identity and status. Another possibility would be to study class, gender, and race as markers that set in motion relations of privilege, power, subordination, and rebellion.

For postmodern psychology, any account of reality—including a scientific account—is a redescription. All accounts are organized within particular assumptive frameworks and embed certain interests. Alternate accounts that represent social reality in other ways are always possible. Psychological constructs such as personality traits and psychiatric diagnoses are accounts of reality that have certain features and that embed certain power relations. For example, they redescribe social experiences as internal qualities. They assume that those experiences (e.g., math anxiety, aggression, or depression) are similar for everyone and can be measured in the abstract, apart from ongoing experience. In the clinical domain, diagnostic classifications have become the dominant way of accounting for suffering. Diagnostic categories redescribe psychic distress in a particular way. For example, diagnostic categories redescribe psychic suffering as a discrete disorder, an "it." They reduce distressing experience to a collection of symptoms lodged within a person. Eliminating or reducing those symptoms becomes the goal of treatment. This redescription is cloaked in the twin mantles of scientific objectivity and benevolent medicine. Feminist critics have often asked which diagnostic categories are good and which are bad, but they have paid less attention to the consequences of the category system per se.

One alternative to diagnostic categories is to construe psychological symptoms as idioms for expressing suffering. Such idioms are culture-specific, taking forms and conveying meanings that are intelligible to other members of the culture. Thus, for example, "ants crawling in the head" is a common idiom of emotional distress in Nigeria, while cold hands is an idiom of distress in Cambodia. Idioms of distress can also be thought of as relational practices that accomplish certain interpersonal goals. Consider recent reports of a dramatic rise in suicides among young women in the People's Republic of China. Based on ethnographic work on recent deaths and their knowledge of the cultural tradition of protest suicides, Lee and Kleinman (2000) have interpreted these self-inflicted deaths as means of registering protests against arranged marriages and other obstacles women face when they try to improve their social status.

Studying Subjectivity

The questions that postmodern psychologists ask call for methods of investigation that go beyond canonical psychology research methods. Rather than measuring people or categorizing them, postmodern psychologists prefer to listen to them. Attending to people's own words brings us closer to their psychological reality than having them check boxes or circle numbers. The goal of this listening is to retain the rich texture and multiple layers of people's experience, not to reduce it to a set of unidimensional codes.

A number of feminist projects have developed sophisticated strategies for analyzing unstructured talk. Some examples include *The Male in the Head* (Holland, Ramazanoglu, Sharpe, & Thomson, 1998), *Raising Their Voices* (Brown, 1998), *Flirting with Danger* (Phillips, 2000), and *Young Masculinities* (Frosh, Phoenix, & Pattman, 2001). But the question of how to interpret others' talk brings us face to face with a prior question: Who should have authority over interpretation and meaning? This is an ethical question as well as an epistemological one. An extreme position would restrict the researcher's task to bringing forward the voices of her participants without any analysis or interpretation. In this view, any interpretation involves a kind of psychological imperialism: it appropriates participants' words for researchers' purposes and imposes researchers' meanings on them. Some feminists have experimented with ways of acknowledging different truths, negotiating the different positions of researcher and respondent, and representing conflicting interpretations. For instance, Glenda Russell (2000) deliberately constructed an interpretive team with a disparate mix of members, so that multiple investments and multiple ways of seeing would be in play during the process of data analysis. Judith Stacey (1990) requested the participants in her study of Silicon Valley families to provide a gloss on her ethnography, granting them, as she put it, "the right to control its closing words" (p. 273).

Objectivity

The discipline of psychology has long held that adequate controls can prevent the social identity of researchers from influencing the research process. But philosophers of social science (some influenced by postmodernism, some not) have long challenged this notion of knowledge uninfluenced by values and personal commitments. Researchers do not have what Donna Haraway has called "the god's-eye-view" of the world: objective, disinterested, all-seeing. Our value commitments and social identities inevitably influence choices we make regarding the topics we study, as well as our theoretical frameworks, research procedures, and interpretations of the data. Value-free research is a myth akin to the myth of value-free psychotherapy. Critics who challenged the notion of value-free therapy pointed out that often therapy seems value-free because it upholds the values prevailing in the culture. Fish do not recognize that they are swimming in water. A parallel claim might be made about research: research that appears to be objective or value-free might appear so only because the pretheoretical assumptions hovering over it are those of the culture and thus remain unseen.

Rethinking Ethical Responsibilities

The research approaches that I have been describing demand that we rethink our ethical responsibilities and move beyond the Ethical Principles of Psychologists. The ethical principles of research seem designed with the prototypical psychology study in mind: an encounter that takes place in a clearly demarcated time and place (e.g., a laboratory session) in which both the experimenter's and the participant's everyday identities are bracketed. Furthermore, the ethical code pertains in large measure to atomistic individuals who are regarded as generic "human subjects." What happens when data collection is not so clearly delimited? For example, field data may include casual remarks passed in everyday conversations or interchanges between strangers that are accidentally overheard. Moreover, the prescribed procedures for assuring confidentiality and anonymity often are not sufficient when we work with respondents' own words and when our studies are embedded in a particular place and time, rather than in the ahistorical laboratory.

When we study individuals embedded in particular social groups or contexts (neighborhoods, ethnic communities, cultures, or schools), the ethical questions compound. The ethical code, however, deals primarily with individual respondents: their privacy rights, their physical safety, and their psychological welfare. But what about those who are spoken *about*, such as siblings, spouses, parents, and bosses? Do they have privacy rights? Furthermore, should any protections be extended to the groups or communities that respondents represent? Are these collective entities entitled to privacy, consent, or protection from harm (including harm to their reputations)? Nancy Scheper-Hughes (2001), returning to the site of her fieldwork on mental illness in rural Ireland after 25 years, found that her work, a classic of anthropology, was regarded as slander and traitorous by the villagers: "You wrote a book to please yourself at our expense. You ran us down, girl. You ran us down" (p. 311). Scheper-Hughes beat a midnight retreat out of the village under threat of physical harm.

Lisa Fontes (1998) has noted that the question "How can researchers best understand, interpret, and present findings?" is a question with ethical dimensions as well as scientific ones. Many critics (e.g., Crawford & Marecek, 1989) have noted that the person-centered interpretations that psychologists typically put forward locate the origins of behavior in the individual. This places the onus of change on the individual; in some situations, it is only a short step away from blaming the victim. Other critics, like Michelle Fine (1992), remind us that the material and social privileges that psychologists as members of the middle class have are not available to working and poor people, especially if they are not white. We psychologists are prone to underestimate the constraints that such individuals face and thus we may wrongly see them as passive, self-defeating, unresourceful, and so on. The possibilities for self-efficacy, empowerment, and self-actualization are sharply curtailed in circumstances of injustice, domination, and oppression.

NEW BUSINESS: POSTMODERNISM, POSTFEMINISM, AND THE BACKLASH

A significant and vocal backlash against feminism has emerged in popular culture (Faludi, 1991). The term *feminism* has come to be disparaged, even vilified, by the mass media. Legal gains such as affirmative action and reproductive rights have eroded; state support for poor women and their children has been severely curtailed by the welfare reforms of 1996. The backlash against feminism is also palpable in psychology as a discipline and a profession. Feminism and other progressive approaches to knowledge have been nudged aside in favor of new approaches that are more politically conservative. These include an emphasis on the biological bases of behavior, the so-called positive psychology movement, and evolutionary psychology. Conservative pressures have mounted for the field of psychology to assume a public profile more agreeable to conservative political leaders, to recruit individuals with right-wing values to the discipline, and to tone down its social activism (Redding, 2001). Feminist clinicians are faced with additional conservative pressures from managed care companies, drug companies, and the biologically oriented psychiatric establishment. Together, they compose a broad-based movement that redefines psychological difficulties as biological aberrations best controlled by medication. Feminist therapists are not necessarily opposed to medication. However, biomedical perspectives can squeeze out attention to social context. Relieving symptoms with drugs does not address the more difficult process of making necessary changes in one's life situation.

All feminists face the backlash to some degree. I have been engaged in a project involving interviews with feminist therapists (Marecek, 1999a; Marecek & Kravetz, 1998). These practitioners spoke vehemently about the antifeminist attitudes they encountered in their work; they had heard feminists characterized as angry, man-hating, "ball-busting," abrasive, home-wreckers. For some, the backlash altered what they could safely say to clients and colleagues. We feminists outside clinical settings too find ourselves making adjustments in our speech and actions in order to survive in surroundings that have become inhospitable.

Neither scientific evidence nor postmodern critique is likely to dismantle the backlash. Nonetheless, postmodernism offers some tools for understanding the ideology of the backlash. Critical discourse analysis, the study of how language figures in social processes, is one such tool. Critical discourse analysis aims to uncover the nonobvious ways in which language operates in social relations of domination and power and in ideology (Fairclough, 2001). One important function it can perform is to alert us to the ways in which the terms and forms of the backlash enter into our own language practices.

Let me return to the research on feminist therapists that I described earlier to give an example (Marecek, 1999b). In one portion of the research interview, respondents briefly narrated their development as feminist therapists. In many of the narratives, anger was a prominent element; redemption from anger was a recurrent theme. Many therapists described themselves as having been too angry when they were younger women or inexperienced therapists; at the time of the interview, they remarked that their anger had been tempered.[4] Here are some examples from the interview transcripts:

Th. 103: I think in the earlier years of my practice, I was—the anger that I had with men and with patriarchy and with institutions that were male-dominated would come through more.

Th. 53: Well, I think I'm pretty typical and part of it is age. And wisdom, which comes with age, which is nice. Because you don't have to be so angry.

Th. 225: I'd say 10 or 15 years ago, I was very outspoken. I would probably say anything I wanted to say anywhere to anybody. I was probably very angry with myself and you feel depressed. What I've done now is I have more understanding.

Th. 150: When I was younger, I was more strident [in therapy]. The factors that have affected that are experience, living in the world longer. [Int.: What specifically made that change?] I wasn't having the same level of overflow of my own issues into my work. I matured in the heart sense.

These accounts place anger in opposition to maturity, wisdom, reason, and understanding. Like the backlash's characterizations of feminists as abrasive and ball-busting, the accounts leave little room for the possibility that a feminist's anger might be legitimate or reasonable. Accounting for anger as a developmental stage of immaturity (akin perhaps to adolescent rebellion) serves to discredit it. Such accounts deflect attention from the legitimate reasons women might have for being angry. We cannot, of course, demonstrate a direct connection between the backlash ideology and the presence of these themes in feminists' narratives of their own personal development. However, the language and meanings circulating in the culture furnish the material available for crafting personal accounts and personal identities. We feminists may resist and reshape the meanings that the cultural backlash has given to feminism, but we cannot lift ourselves out from the culture.

CONCLUSION

It would be rash to predict what twists and turns lie ahead for feminism, postmodernism, psychology, and possible combinations of them. Nor can I predict what twists and turns lie in the future for the strained relation between mainstream culture and feminism. Yet there are a few predictions that are safe to make. What lies ahead will not be a return to the past. Certain claims of postmodernism have transformed intellectual inquiry in most humanities and social science disciplines throughout much of the world. The discipline of psychology in the United States is one of the few sites to remain largely ignorant of these transformations (see the essays collected by Marecek, in press). The claims of postmodernism seem unlikely to disappear in a swing back to brute realism. Three such claims seem central: that there can be no prediscursive knowledge that is free from the values and assumptions of its social setting; that knowledge is always situated and any knower has access only to partial truth; and that a researcher's social identity inevitably shapes the research process. Feminism too has had a transformative effect on most academic disciplines, though its effect on academic psychology in the United States has been muted. Feminist psychologists have argued that social life is gendered in profound ways, as is intellectual life. They have exposed gender-linked power relations, calling attention to experiences of violence, intimidation, and abuse of power in intimate relations and domestic life. Feminists have set off storms of controversy and embarked on novel forms of social action. Whatever new possibilities feminist psychologists invent to theorize gender, personality, and psychopathology, we must continue our tradition of disrupting the taken-for-granted, speaking truth to power, and taking leaps into the unknown.

NOTES

1. Note how closely Erikson's line of thought parallels that of Jean Baker Miller in *Toward a New Psychology of Women* (1976). Feminists of the sixties vilified Erikson, while Baker Miller's version of women's difference became a touchstone for many feminists of the eighties.
2. Empiricism originally referred to the practice of medicine based purely on observation; two synonyms are "quackery" and "charlatanism."
3. For example, a review of a book on women and madness was titled "Now That We're Angry, We're No Longer Mad."
4. Neither a therapist's actual age or the length of time she had been doing therapy was related to her use of this developmental narrative.

REFERENCES

Allen, G. (1889). Woman's place in nature. *Forum, 7*, 258–263.

Baer, J. (1976). *How to be an assertive (not aggressive) woman in life, in love, and on the job: The total guide to self-assertiveness.* New York: New American Liberty.

Bakhtin, M. (1981). *The dialogic imagination: Four essays* (C. Emerson & M. Holmquist, Trans.; M. Holmquist, Ed.). Austin: University of Texas Press. (Original work published 1935)

Becker, D. (2000). When she was bad: Borderline personality disorder in a posttraumatic age. *American Journal of Orthopsychiatry, 70*, 422–432.

Bem, S. L. (1974). The measurement of psychological androgyny. *Journal of Consulting and Clinical Psychology, 42*, 155–162

Bohan, J. S. (1993). Regarding gender: Essentialism, constructionism, and feminist psychology. *Psychology of Women Quarterly, 17*, 5–21.

Brown, L. M. (1998). *Raising their voices: The politics of girls' anger.* Cambridge, MA: Harvard University Press.

Brown, L. S., & Ballou, M. (Eds.). (1992). *Personality and psychopathology: Feminist reappraisals.* New York: Guilford Press.

Chodorow, N. J. (1999). *The power of feelings: Personal meaning in psychoanalysis, gender, and culture.* New Haven, CT: Yale University Press.

Constantinople, A. (1973). Masculinity–femininity: An exception to a famous dictum? *Psychological Bulletin, 80*, 389–407.

Crawford, M., & Marecek, J. (1989). Psychology reconstructs the female, 1968–1988. *Psychology of Women Quarterly, 13*, 147–166.

Datan, N. (1989). Illness and imagery. In M. Crawford & M. Gentry (Eds.), *Gender and thought: Psychological perspectives* (pp. 175–187). New York: Springer-Verlag.

Davis, K. (Ed.). (1997). *Embodied practices: Feminist perspectives on the body.* London: Sage.

Erikson, E. H. (1964, Spring). Inner and outer space: Reflections on womanhood. *Daedalus*, pp. 582–601.

Fairclough, N. (2001). The discourse of New Labor: Critical discourse analysis. In M. Wetherell, S. Taylor, & S. J. Yates (Eds.), *Discourse as data: A guide for analysis* (pp. 229–268). Milton Keynes, UK: Open University Press.

Faludi, S. (1991). *Backlash: The undeclared war against American women.* New York: Crown.

Fausto-Sterling, A. (2000). *Sexing the body: Gender politics and the construction of sexuality.* New York: Basic Books.

Fine, M. (1992). Coping with rape: Critical perspectives on consciousness. In M. Fine, *Disruptive voices: The possibilities of feminist research* (pp. 61–76). Ann Arbor: University of Michigan Press.

Fine, M., & Gordon, S. M. (1992). Feminist transformations of/despite psychology. In M. Fine, *Disruptive voices: The possibilities of feminist research* (pp. 1–25). Ann Arbor: University of Michigan Press.

Fontes, L. A. (1998). Ethics in family violence research: Cross-cultural issues. *Family Relations, 47*, 53–61.

Fox, D., & Prilleltensky, I. (Eds.). (1997). *Critical psychology: An introduction.* London: Sage.

Franks, V., & Burtle, V. (Eds.). (1974). *Women and therapy.* New York: Brunner/Mazel.

Franz, C. E., & Stewart, A. J. (Eds.). (1994). *Women creating lives: Identities, resilience, resistance.* Boulder, CO: Westview Press.

Frosh, S., Phoenix, A., & Pattman, R. (2000). *Young masculinities.* Unpublished manuscript, University of London.

Garrison, D. (1981). Karen Horney and feminism. *Signs, 6*, 672–691.

Haaken, J. (1998). *Pillar of salt: Gender, memory and the perils of looking back.* New Brunswick, NJ: Rutgers University Press.

Hare-Mustin, R. T., & Marecek, J. (1990). *Making a difference: Psychology and the construction of gender.* New Haven, CT: Yale University Press.

Hare-Mustin, R. T., & Marecek, J. (1994). Asking the right questions: Feminist psychology and sex differences. *Feminism and Psychology, 4*, 531–537.

Henriques, J., Hollway, W., Urwin, C., Venn, C., & Walkerdine, V. (1998). *Changing the subject: Psychology, social regulation, and subjectivity.* London: Routledge. (Original work published 1984)

Holland, D., Lachicotte, W., Skinner, D., & Cain, C. (1998). *Identity and agency in cultural worlds.* Cambridge, MA: Harvard University Press.

Holland, J., Ramazanoglu, C., Sharpe, S., & Thomson, R. (1998). *The male in the head: Young people, heterosexuality, and power.* London: Tufnell Press.

Horney, K. (1967). *Feminine psychology.* New York: Norton. (Original work published 1926)

Hyde, J. S. (1995). Women and maternity leave: Empirical data and public policy [Presidential address]. *Psychology of Women Quarterly, 19*, 299–313.

Jastrow, J. (1915). *Character and temperament.* New York: Appleton.

Keller, E. F. (1995). *Changing the subject of science and psychoanalysis: Problems of agency and authority in a post-modern world.* Unpublished manuscript, Department of Science, Technology, and Society, Massachusetts Institute of Technology, Cambridge, MA.

Kessler, S. J. (1998). *Lessons from the intersexed.* New Brunswick, NJ: Rutgers University Press.

Kessler, S. J., & McKenna, W. (1978). *Gender: An ethnomethodological approach.* New York: Wiley.

Kleinman, A. (1995). *Writing at the margin: Discourse between anthropology and medicine.* Berkeley and Los Angeles: University of California Press.

Lamb, S. (1999). *New versions of victims: Feminists struggle with the concept.* New York: New York University Press.

Landrine, H., Klonoff, E. A., & Brown-Collins, A. (1992). Cultural diversity and methodology in feminist psychology. *Psychology of Women Quarterly, 16*, 145–163.

Laqueur, T. (1990). *Making sex: Body and gender from the Greeks to Freud.* Cambridge, MA: Harvard University Press.

Lee, S., & Kleinman, A. (2000). Suicide as resistance in Chinese society. In E. J. Perry & M. Selden (Eds.), *Chinese society: Change, conflict and resistance* (pp. 189–210). London: Routledge.

Lundberg, F., & Farnham, M. F. (1947). *Modern woman: The lost sex.* New York: Grosset & Dunlap.

Lykes, M. B., Brabeck, M. M., Ferns, T., & Radan, A. (1993). Human rights and mental health among Latin American women in situations of state-sponsored violence. *Psychology of Women Quarterly, 17*, 525–544.

Marecek, J. (1995). Gender, politics, and psychology's ways of knowing. *American Psychologist, 50*, 162–163.

Marecek, J. (1999a). Trauma talk in feminist clinical practice. In S. Lamb (Ed.), *New versions of victims: Feminists struggle with the construct.* New York: New York University Press.

Marecek, J. (1999b, June). *Feminist identities in the '90s: Necessity is the mother of (re)invention.* Paper presented at the Seventh Women's Congress, Tromsø, Norway.

Marecek, J. (in press). The subject in question: A re-appraisal of *Changing the subject: Psychology, social regulation and subjectivity*. *Feminism and Psychology*.

Marecek, J., & Kravetz, D. (1998). Putting politics into practice: Feminist therapy as feminist praxis. *Women and Therapy, 21*(2), 17–36.

McKinley, N. M. (2001). A feminist look at adolescent girls. *Feminism and Psychology, 25*, 84–85.

Miller, J. B. (1973). *Psychoanalysis and women*. New York: Brunner/Mazel.

Miller, J. B. (1976). *Toward a new psychology of women*. Boston: Beacon Press.

Parlee, M. B. (1994). The social construction of premenstrual syndrome: A case study in scientific discourse as cultural contestation. In M. G. Winkler & L. B. Cole (Eds.), *The good body: Asceticism in contemporary culture* (pp. 91–107). New Haven, CT: Yale University Press.

Parlee, M. B. (1998). Situated knowledges of personal embodiment: Transgender activists' and psychological theorists' perspectives on "sex" and "gender." In H. J. Stam (Ed.), *The body and psychology* (pp. 120–140). London: Sage.

Phillips, L. M. (2000). *Flirting with danger: Young women's reflections on sexuality and domination*. New York: New York University Press.

Redding, R. (2001). Sociopolitical diversity in psychology: The case for pluralism. *American Psychologist, 56*, 205–215.

Rogler, L. (1999). Methodological sources of cultural insensitivity in mental health research. *American Psychologist, 54*, 424–433.

Romero, M., & Stewart, A. J. (Eds.). (1999). *Women's untold lives: Breaking silence, talking back, voicing complexity*. New York: Routledge.

Russell, G. M. (2000). *Voted out: The psychological consequences of anti-gay politics*. New York: New York University Press.

Russo, N. F. (1995). PWQ: A scientific voice in feminist psychology [Editorial]. *Psychology of Women Quarterly, 19*, 1–3.

Scheper-Hughes, N. (2001). *Saints, scholars, and schizophrenics: Mental illness in rural Ireland*. Berkeley and Los Angeles: University of California Press.

Scott, W. (1990). PTSD in DSM-III: A case in the politics of diagnosis. *Social Problems, 37*, 294–310.

Shields, S. A. (1995). The role of emotion beliefs and values in gender development. In N. Eisenberg (Ed.), *Review of personality and social psychology* (Vol. 15, pp. 212–232). Thousand Oaks, CA: Sage.

Shields, S. (2002). *Speaking from the heart: Gender and the social meaning of emotion*. New York: Cambridge University Press.

Stacey, J. (1990). *Brave new families: Stories of domestic upheaval in late twentieth century America*. New York: Basic Books.

Strouse, J. (1974). *Women and analysis*. New York: Grossman.

Thompson, C. (1942). Cultural pressures in the psychology of women. *Psychiatry, 5*, 331–339.

Tiefer, L. (1995). *Sex is not a natural act and other essays*. Boulder, CO: Westview Press.

Tiefer, L. (2001). A new view of women's sexual problems: Why new? Why now? *Journal of Sex Research, 38*, 89–96.

Unger, R. K. (1979). Toward a redefinition of sex and gender. *American Psychologist, 34*, 1085–1094.

Walkerdine, V., Lucey, H., & Melody, J. (2000). *Growing up girl: Psychosocial explorations of gender and class.* New York: New York University Press.

Weedon, C. (1987). *Feminist practice and poststructuralist theory.* Oxford, UK: Basil Blackwell.

Weisstein, N. (1971). Psychology constructs the female. In V. Gornick & B. K. Moran (Eds.), *Woman in sexist society* (pp. 207–224). New York: Basic Books.

Weisstein, N. (1993). Power, resistance, and science: A call for a revitalized feminist psychology. *Feminism and Psychology, 3,* 239–245.

West, C., & Zimmerman, D. H. (1987). Doing gender. *Gender and Society, 1,* 125–151.

White, J. W. (2000). *PWQ:* Feminist empiricism for the new millennium. *Psychology of Women Quarterly, 24,* 1–3.

Woolley, H. T. (1910). Psychological literature: A review of the recent literature on the psychology of sex. *Psychological Bulletin, 7,* 335–342.

Chapter 2

A Feminist Critique
of Attachment Theory
and Evolutionary Psychology

SUSAN CONTRATTO

This chapter offers an overview of attachment theory (an early case of evolutionary psychology), a discussion of some recent papers in evolutionary psychology, and a feminist critique of these. Both theories have been enormously popular in recent years. I give some suggestions as to why I think that is the case. They are of interest to feminist psychology not necessarily because they are correct (they are theories, after all, not facts), or provocative and interesting—which some of them certainly are—but because they can be put to profoundly conservative uses. It is not that the writers of the theories are themselves conservative (though some, such as Bowlby, were), but "scientific" theories that claim to describe universals of the human condition are often used to justify, as well as to explain, the status quo. It is relatively easy both to understand attachment theory and to critique it. It is harder to grasp evolutionary psychology, and therefore all the more important to struggle with it. If a theory can be used against women, as this one can, it is critical to debate from within it, to try to understand it, and to ask the unsettling questions. While I certainly don't claim to understand all of evolutionary psychology, I have come to the point, I believe, where I can ask a number of such questions.

ATTACHMENT THEORY AND CRITIQUE

John Bowlby, who had a background in ethnology and psychoanalysis, first proposed in the late 1960s the fundamentals of a theory that would lead to a cottage industry of theorizing, research, and practice. He argued that the human infant was preprogrammed to seek and stay close to her mother, forming a powerful emotional bond (Bowlby, 1969). To develop the theory he relied heavily on the work of Harry Harlow with primates (Harlow, 1965). Later, Mary Ainsworth (1967; Ainsworth & Wittig, 1969) and her colleagues developed the "Strange Situation," a laboratory observation of mother, toddler, and stranger, that is still the most common means of measuring attachment. Using Bowlby's theory and language, Ainsworth argued that what they were seeing were securely and insecurely attached children. She further argued that within the insecurely attached group, there were two types of children, insecure/ambivalent children and insecure/avoidant children—classifications that continue to form the basis of research on attachment today.

Bowlby theorized that internalized models of these types of attachment persisted into adulthood (though they might shift and undergo transformations), that they affected attachments in adulthood and that they influenced how one parented (Rholes, Simpson, & Stevens, 1998). Furthermore, Bowlby (1988) theorized that these relationships with early caregivers would become the basis of childhood and later adult psychopathology.

Bowlby proposed that good mothering ability was a psychological inheritance: mothers who themselves had secure attachments with their own mothers would be unambivalent about the hard work of mothering. A good mother's needs would converge with her infant's needs.

Bowlby's theory and Ainsworth's way of classifying attachment have become a dominant intellectual thread in mainstream psychology. A recent book edited by Simpson and Rholes (1998b) provides an excellent overview of the state of this research, highlighting advances as well as controversies and disagreements. A number of chapters in this book (Simpson & Rholes, 1998a; Brennan, Clark, & Shaver, 1998; George, Kaplan, & Main, 1985, cited in Simpson & Rholes, 1998a) describe in meticulous detail measurement concerns and differences, including the usefulness of and problems with adult self-report of what they imagine their attachments to have been like. Others describe a range of applications, including how a person with a particular attachment style, measured mostly through self-report, copes with stressful life events (Mikulincer & Florian, 1998) and the clinical implications of attachment theory (Dozier & Tyrrell, 1998).

While careful researchers and theoreticians are cautious about attachment theory, citing its methodological questions, its uneven empirical results (Simpson & Rholes, 1998a, pp. 16–17), and whether, in Bowlby's own evolutionary terms, attachment between infants and mothers is the same internal model as mating attachment (see Kirkpatrick, 1998), there has been an explosion of work in this area. Just recently, there were three articles on attachment in the *Journal of Counseling Psychology* (Lopez & Brennan, 2000; O'Brien, Friedman, Tipton, & Linn, 2000; Vivona, 2000). They demonstrate the range of work in this area as well as some current theorists' grandiose claims. Lopez and Brennan (2000) review the literature on adult attachment as it relates to cognitive processes, affect self-regulation, and relationship behaviors. They argue that attachment theory provides the basis for understanding what a healthy and effective person is. They state: "We believe that attachment theory offers an integrative perspective on the healthy and effective self, one capable of illuminating the interplay of cognitive, affective, and relational behavior process. . . . Beginning with one's earliest interactions with primary caregivers, the experience of attachment security enables the development and deployment of adaptive cognitive processing, affect regulation, and relationship problem-solving processes" (p. 292). In essence, they argue that the evidence is in: Bowlby's developmental *theory* has moved into the realm of *fact*.

As a feminist psychologist, theorist, and clinician, I see a number of problems with the wholesale adoption of this theory. These include well-documented measurement problems (see Birns, 1999; Kagan, 1998, pp. 98–105; Simpson & Rholes, 1998a, for a discussion of these), an assumption of the importance of early development, a privileging of mother–child interaction that ignores work on temperament and resilience, a neglect of environmental stressors, and documented ethnic biases.

A fundamental premise of the theory is its assumption that what happens within the first 2 years of life creates the foundation for later development, a belief that the development psychologist Jerome Kagan (1998) calls *infant determinism*. He argues that though the faith placed in this theory is high, it is simply faith and not fact. Evidence from studies of different childrearing practices and later adoption do not support this deterministic position (pp. 107–108).

Kagan suggests that it is not what happens within this early period between mother and child that is critical for problematic development but the consistent and repetitive stressors the child experiences throughout her childhood. He describes a longitudinal study of over 600 children on Kauai, Hawaii, who were followed by researchers from birth until they were over age 30: "The best predictor of later psychological problems . . . was continued residence in a family of poverty, combined with prematurity or other biological stress surrounding birth" (p. 111). But even this combination of factors was not strongly predictive. He quotes the researchers: "As we watched these children grow from babyhood to adulthood, we could not help but respect the self-righting tendencies within them that produced normal development under all but the most persistently adverse circumstances" (Werner & Smith, 1982, p. 159, quoted in Kagan, 1998, p. 111). Other studies he describes follow children who lived in depriving, institutional settings. He argues that their healthy or symptomatic development is dependent on their life circumstances after 2 years of age (pp. 111–112).

This study joins a number of others that document the remarkable resiliency of children (see, e.g., Bernard, 1996; Burger, 1994)—an entirely different perspective on childhood than the fragile, vulnerable one that emerges from attachment theory. This notion of both infant determinism and infant psychological fragility has dominated women's experience of mothering from the early 20th century to the present (Chodorow & Contratto, 1981; Contratto, 1984). It has contributed enormously to women's stress and guilt about doing well by their children. Also, it underlies political debates over childcare, women's work force participation, school outcomes, "cycles" of poverty, gun control, and drug use. There is always the assumption that if parents (read "mothers") were doing their jobs well, we would live in a happier, safer, healthier world. It is a function of the ongoing subtle sexism in mainstream psychology that it continues to marginalize the growing literature on resilience in children.

Kagan (1998) makes the point, ignored by the attachment researchers, that temperament and life experiences have a major impact on how children respond in the Strange Situation. Some 15–20% of children are by nature somewhat fearful. These children would very likely be described as "insecurely attached," reflecting a problem in the mother–toddler relationship, rather than temperamentally fearful if they were evaluated by an attachment researcher. Kagan also notes that a child who was used to multiple caretakers, for example in a daycare setting, would respond differently to the Strange Situation than a child whose world revolved solely around mother and home.

Attachment theory is embedded in Western, middle-class assumptions. This is apparent when researchers look closely at attachment outcomes in other countries. Kagan (1998) describes an area in northern Germany where there is particular concern that children grow up to become self-reliant. To foster this trait, mothers typically do not go into the bedroom to soothe a crying infant and will leave their infants alone for an hour or two when they go shopping—this is an acceptable community practice. These infants learn to self-soothe when mother disappears for a short period of time, and so they are not fearful. When evaluated in the Strange Situation, their lack of fearfulness leads researchers to classify many of these children as "insecurely attached/avoidant" and therefore at psychological risk.

A recent article by Rothbaum and his colleagues (Rothbaum, Weisz, Pott, Miyake, & Morelli, 2000) uses data from Japan to demonstrate the cultural bias of the fundamental assumptions of attachment theory and measurement. They summarize:

> Youngsters of many cultures use the secure base with the attachment figure to gain the support they need to adapt to the outside world, but cultural differences abound in the behavioral system to which attachment is most closely linked, as well as in the meaning of adaptation. In the United States, the major link is with exploration, and adaptation primarily refers to individuation and autonomous mastery of the environment. In Japan, the major link is with dependence, and adaptation primarily refers to accommodation, avoidance of loss, fitting in with others, and ultimately loyalty and interdependence. (p. 1100)

These researchers conclude by arguing that the Western bias in both assessment and interpretation not only leads to cultural misunderstanding but also to culturally and ethnically insensitive and therefore meaningless interventions (pp. 1100–1101). Kagan's conclusion is even stronger: "The claim that insecurely attached children are at psychological risk because they do not have sensitive mothers is an ethical judgment as to which maternal behaviors and infant reactions to parental absence are considered the most virtuous" (1998, p. 101). Certainly a feminist analysis would argue, as does Kagan, that it is not only culturally insensitive but also unethical to impose one group's standards of what constitutes emotional health and well-being on another group. In the German case, it would be the child who was fearful when left by her mother who would be perceived by the community as having difficulties. Likewise, the Japanese toddler who explored too much, was too independent, and too demonstrative wouldn't fit in. Attachment theory does not honor the important cultural differences that continue to influence childrearing practices.

Lopez and Brennan (2000) argue that attachment theory provides meaningful criteria for what constitutes an emotionally healthy life. One can imagine a time when adults walk into a therapy office and are administered an AAI (Adult Attachment Interview) that would give them a diagnosis and then generate a treatment plan. The person is labeled with pathology that is both internal to the individual and supposedly arose from failures in her mothering.

What a familiar mother-blaming scenario—one that has a long history in psychology starting from the initial institutionalization of the discipline and continuing to the present! And, I imagine that it is a scenario that would appeal to an HMO: simple, to the point, one-size-fits-all, and hopefully responsive to an inexpensive drug! This story presumes infant determinism, the accuracy of the instrument, and the universality of the theory. All of these are false assumptions. And it once again minimizes the multiple situational life experiences that are hard to change but can profoundly influence individuals' development. Kagan talks at some length about the impact of poverty on development. Others have documented the impact of trauma on emotional health (Herman, 1992; Jacobs, 1994). And we know that living with racism is bad for psychological and physical health and, like homophobia, can lead to injury, death, and incarceration. But if we place the problem on early development and blame mothers, we can ignore our political responsibility for social change.

EVOLUTIONARY PSYCHOLOGY AND CRITIQUE

Reviewing and assessing evolutionary psychology is a taunting assignment. The vocabulary is new, the theory is (often) complex, and some of its claims are grandiose—for example, that this is the unifying theory for psychology. While Bowlby's original theory was grounded in evolutionary theory, psychology has appropriated it without referring to or evaluating its origins. When discussing attachment theory, psychologists wear blinders concerning the intense debates about the fine points of theory within evolutionary biology and consequently don't worry about the foundation of the theory. But that the foundation itself may be flawed becomes clear in debates about evolutionary psychology.

In their landmark publication *The Adapted Mind*, Barkow, Cosmides, and Tooby (1992) define evolutionary psychology as follows: "Evolutionary psychology is simply psychology that is informed by the additional knowledge that evolutionary biology has to offer, in the expectation that understanding the process that designed the human mind will advance the discovery of its architecture. It unites modern evolutionary biology with the cognitive revolution in a way that has the potential to draw together all of the disparate branches of psychology into a single organized system of knowledge" (p. 3). They argue that culture as we know it "is generated in rich and intricate ways by information-processing mechanisms situated in human minds" and that "these mechanisms are, in turn, the elaborated sculpted product of the evolutionary past" (p. 3).

The three foundational premises of their work are: First, "that there is a universal human nature, but that this universality exists primarily at the level of evolved psychological mechanisms, not of expressed cultural behaviors." Second, "that these evolved psychological mechanisms are adaptations, constructed by natural selection over evolutionary time." And third, "that the evolved structure of the human mind is adapted to the way of life of Pleistocene hunter–gathers, and not necessarily to our modern circumstances" (p. 5).

In his popular and extremely well-written book *How the Mind Works*, Steven Pinker (1997) provides an overview of the subject matter of evolutionary psychology. These range from mechanisms for avoiding predators, eating the right food, forming alliances and friendships, providing help to children and other relatives, recognizing what is on someone else's mind, communicating with other people, and selecting mates. For a fairly comprehensive overview of the field, which is well beyond the scope of this chapter, I would strongly recommend Pinker's book.

There has been an explosion of literature in this field within the last 30 years. I have chosen to use two articles by David Buss (1995, 2000) as a jumping-off place for a critical discussion of the field. Both of these appeared in the *American Psychologist*, the journal sent to all members of the American Psychological Association regardless of their area of specialization. As such, the articles purport to represent the most interesting work of a particular subfield within psychology, presented to the field as a whole in accessible, scholarly form.

David Buss (1995) argues that evolutionary theory accounts for fairly consistent sex differences in statements about preferred mate, which he and other researchers have found. He claims that evolutionary psychology would predict no or minimal sex differences between men and women except in those areas in which they have faced substantially different adaptive problems. Key for men is uncertainty over paternity. Therefore, "all people descend from a long line of ancestral men whose adaptations [i.e., psychological mechanisms] led them to behave in ways that increased their likelihood of paternity and decreased the odds of investing in children who were putatively theirs but whose genetic fathers were other men" (p. 164).

Unique to women was the need to find a mate who could provide resources (food and supplies) during her periods of pregnancy and lactation. "All people are descendants of a long and unbroken line of women who successfully solved this adaptive challenge—for example, by preferring mates who showed the ability to accrue resources and the willingness to provide them for particular women" (p. 165). Buss notes that "to an evolutionary psychologist, the likelihood that the sexes are psychologically identical in domains in which they have recurrently confronted different adaptive problems over the long expanse of human evolutionary history is essentially zero" (p. 165).

Buss (1995) goes on to argue that evolutionary psychology would predict the documented differences in attitudes between men and women: for example, men are much more likely to enjoy and engage in casual sex than women, women are more concerned than men with finding a mate with financial resources and protection abilities, and (documented in the earlier study [1992]) men were more likely to seek younger partners with the symmetrical features that signal reproductive ability and good health.

Buss reassures the reader that the theory is not proscriptive, simply descriptive, that the differences are not intractable, and that to deny the origin of the differences would, in fact, be a handicap to changing them. As he notes, "Knowledge is power, and attempts to intervene in the absence of knowledge may resemble a surgeon operating blindfolded—there may be more bloodshed than healing" (1995, p. 168).

As Buss argued that an evolutionary psychology offered the best hope of understanding sex difference, so he applies the same overarching theory to happiness (Buss, 2000). He describes three barriers to happiness: first, the discrepancies between modern and ancestral environments; second, adaptations that cause subjective distress; and third, adaptations designed for competition.

Buss describes the ancestral environment as one of small groups (50–100), which included all sorts of extended kin and a dozen or two dozen potential mates. They relied on friends and relatives to "seek justice, to correct social wrongs, to deal with violence" (2000, p. 16). Modern humans he characterizes as living in a massive urban metropolis, "surrounded by thousands of potential mates," relying on complex systems for justice.

According to Buss, adaptations themselves can cause distress and are meant to. These include varieties of anxieties and specific forms of anger and upset. He uses jealously as an example: jealousy is an emotion that has evolved to be triggered when there is a threat to mate retention. Though it is a highly unpleasant feeling, he argues that "it exists today in modern humans because those in the evolutionary past who were indifferent to the sexual contact that their mates had with others lost the evolutionary contest to those who became jealous" (2000, p. 19). He lists other negative emotions, which, if they did not exist, would have caused "fitness failure."

Buss (2000) argues that there are adaptations that arise from the competition inherent to evolution by selection: "Humans have evolved psychological mechanisms designed to inflict costs on others, to gain advantage at the expense of others, to delight in the downfall of others, and to envy those who are more successful at achieving the goals toward which they aspire" (p. 19). In addition to this leading to hierarchy, envy, success for some, failure for others, and constant self-evaluation, there are particular mechanisms that cause conflict between the sexes. "Men's evolved desire for sexual variety, for example, sometimes prompts sexual overtures that are sooner, more persistent, and more aggressive than women want" (p. 19). Men find women's need for a longer courtship and a need for emotional involvement frustrating. And both sexes deceive each other in evolutionarily predictable ways.

The second half of Buss's (2000) paper suggests a variety of ways in which people might lead happier lives. These include finding ways of bridging the gap between modern and ancestral conditions, such as increasing ties with extended kin, developing deep friendships, and increasing social cooperation (he lists six strategies). He suggests three ways of reducing subjective distress: selecting a mate who is similar to oneself; using extended kin as a way of reducing incest, child abuse, and spousal battering; and being educated about evolved psychological sex differences. Managing competitive mechanisms involves promoting cooperation through teaching reciprocity, promoting equity, and enlarging the shadow of the future.

In conclusion, Buss argues that "raising human happiness involves exploiting knowledge of evolved desires" (2000, p. 24). These include having health, achieving professional success, achieving intimacy, feeling confident about success, enjoying high-quality food, feeling safe, and having the resources to attain all these. Fulfillment in marriage is high on the list, as is enjoyment of aesthetic pleasure: "Appreciating the beauty of a blossom, the loveliness of a lilac, or the grace of a gazelle are all ways in which people can, in some small measure, fill their daily lives with evolutionarily inspired epiphanies of pleasure" (p. 25). Though Buss acknowledges issues he has neglected or merely mentioned in passing, and others that have yet to be investigated by the theory, he remains confident about evolutionary psychology: "Through this knowledge, people can take a few halting steps toward fulfilling the human desire for happiness" (p. 25).

There are major problems with the scientific underpinnings of the version of evolutionary theory used by evolutionary psychologists. Furthermore, there are critiques, which emerge from standards that psychologists typically apply to their work.

Patricia Adair Gowaty (2001) reviews the problems with evolutionary psychology from a sociobiological perspective. She reminds us that sociobiologists look at behavior and that via their studies of plants and animals can evaluate selection pressures and outcomes through experimental procedures. Evolutionary psychologists, on the other hand, speculate about the development of (theorized) mental modules in response to assumed adaptational pressures. The story of the past that evolutionary psychologists call the *environment of evolutionary adaptedness* (EEA) is unknowable according to her and other scientists. Stephen Jay Gould writes:

> But how can we possibly know in detail what small bands of hunter gatherers did in Africa two million years ago? . . . How can we possibly obtain the key information that would be required to show the validity of adaptive tales about an EEA: relations of kinship, social structures and sizes of groups, different activities of males and females, the roles of religion, storytelling, and a hundred other central aspects of human life that cannot be traced in fossils? We do not even know the original environment of our ancestors—did ancestral humans stay in one region or move about? How did environments vary through years and centuries? (1997b, p. 51)

This is not a trivial concern. Cosmides, Tooby and Barkow argue that "in considering issues of functionality, behavioral scientists need to be familiar with how foraging people lived" (1992, p. 5). Gould argues that that is effectively impossible. He is supported in this by Hrdy:

> So let's be clear: humans today are an amalgam of past selection pressures on ancestors who were mammals, primates, and, most recently, hominids, who lived as foragers in a range of ecological and social settings. Like baboons, langurs, and other particularly adaptable primates, humans are found in a broad range of climates, at different altitudes, over a broad array of habitats. Humans readily adapt to different habitats as other "weedy" species do; but being culture-bearing, technologically clever primates, they have even more scope to change their environment to suit their needs. (1999, p. 101)

Undaunted by this lack of information, Buss (2000) tells a specific story of how our ancestors lived (in small groups, with a dozen or so potential mates, surrounded by genetic relatives, friends and their relatives, effectively solving social problems). Buss goes on to suggest that the purported increase in depression in the modern world is in part due to the contrast between his assumed ancestral environment and the modern environment: "An increase in depression invokes the fact that modern living conditions of relative anonymity and isolated nuclear families deprive people of the intimate social support that would have characterized ancestral social conditions" (p. 18). Not only does he claim to know the environment of our ancestors, he claims to know their social and emotional experience!

Gowaty (2001) lists a number of other general criticisms of evolutionary psychology, as does Gould (1997a, 1997b). She goes on to enumerate the criticisms of Buss's original study, which formed the basis of his 1995 article. These include "incorrect use of essential evolutionary concepts and methods . . . incorrect interpretation of crucial evolutionary ideas and subsequent inappropriate predictions and test . . . flawed sampling . . . and incorrect statistical analyses" (p. 58). She concludes by saying "that any one of these four criticisms would have kept this paper from publication in mainstream evolution journals" (p. 59).

Evolutionary psychology does not play by the same research rules as the rest of psychology. Evolutionary psychologists have appropriated a theory without fully appreciating its complexity. They have created a story as to what might have happened and then have sought data to confirm their hypotheses. But what about controls, hypothesis testing, replication, having a research design where the primary investigator can't affect the outcome of the research, and so forth? And the mind units that supposedly are the result of evolution, the mental modules, can't be looked at, described, or evaluated. They are similar, in a way, to Freud's original formulation of the ego, id, superego, libido, and unconscious. They are a closetful of mental apparatus, which may even make intuitive sense to some but are at this time purely speculative notions.

Even with all the flaws of Buss's original study, Eagly and Wood (1999) propose that many of his reported sex differences can equally well be explained by social structural theory: "Because men and women tend to occupy different social roles, they become psychologically different in ways that adjust to these roles" (p. 408). They argue that, overall, men are the primary wage earners and, though they may be secondary wage earners, women are primarily responsible for household maintenance. They reanalyze the Buss 37 cultures data to document their argument. They found that men valued "good cook and housekeeper" just as highly as "attractiveness" and "youth" in women (the sex preferences emphasized by the evolutionary psychologists). Furthermore, they found that as there was greater equality for men and women. These sex differences diminished, confirming another hypothesis generated by social structural theory.

Addressing the same study, Louise Silverstein (1998) argues that Buss overemphasizes biology and underemphasizes environment, that he focuses on fixity rather than fluidity, and that his particular emphasis "privileges heterosexual sexual behavior and the traditional, two-parent family; and renders same-sex behavior and alternate family structures invisible" (p. 375). She argues that a complex array of variables among chimpanzees, including "biological sex, resource availability, age, social context and stage within the estrus cycle" (p. 377), all effect mating patterns. She shows that when male dominance is reduced, attitudes toward casual sex change. Among the bonobo (a close relative to chimpanzees), males and females are codominant; sexual behaviors for both males and females is same-sex, opposite-sex, and frequent; and "is used to make friends, get food, calm a tense individual and reconcile after aggression" (p. 378). In fact, she sites some researchers who study this group as claiming that the female bond formed by clitoral–clitoral encounters increases female coalitions and decreases male violence. Finally, she points out that both Madonna and Roseanne, women who certainly don't need men for resources, have chosen to have babies by younger, physically fit men.

In his 2000 paper "The Evolution of Happiness," Buss does not have any data—it is all story. He describes an idyllic past and a present that we are ill-equipped for. He neglects to define major emotional terms (e.g., happiness, intimacy, depression) and his suggestions are pop psychology or worse. For example, his conclusions include the concept of "evolved desires." I am stymied as to how we could have evolved a desire for professional success—certainly a very recent notion. Others, such as intimacy (undefined), money, and feeling safe have some commonsense validity. But I was hard-pressed to find a place for "satisfying the taste for high-quality food" since so many relatively affluent people eat what we call for good reason "junk food."

But along with satisfying these "evolved desires" when possible, there are other suggestions ranging from "phone a friend" to decreasing competition, and understanding the purported evolved sex differences as a way of minimizing miscommunication. Many of these techniques are the standard fare of advice books and group work. They may work for some people. But they have minimal impact when people live in poverty, experience violence of all kinds, and are victims of trauma (often from those very family members Buss would have us reach out to). His analysis begins with a metatheory and ends with solutions that put the responsibility for happiness on the individual. It is profoundly conservative. The practitioners of evolutionary psychology profess over and over again that their stance is scientific—not moral, or political, or value-laden. But in this paper Buss makes a choice. If he believes that science shows that certain things are necessary for happiness, he could call for an end to poverty, racism, violence, and environmental destruction. He doesn't. Rather, he ignores the millions of people who can't possible, even within his own framework, attain happiness because of the conditions of their lives.

Why, then, if evolutionary psychology is fundamentally flawed as theory and as research, does it have such appeal to psychology? And why is it dangerous for feminist psychology? I believe that the answers are overlapping. It appeals to psychology because it sounds like "real" science. It is taken up by psychology and is dangerous to feminism because it is used to justify and therefore maintain the status quo as well as to render invisible differences between people and the environmental impacts on the quality of their lives.

Evolutionary psychology makes a self-conscious attempt to attach itself to science. Tooby and Cosmides (1992) begin their article by proposing evolutionary psychology as a unifying psychological theory by evoking the "hard" sciences: "Disciplines such as astronomy, chemistry, physics, geology, and biology have developed a robust combination of logical coherence, causal description, explanatory power, and testability, and have become examples of how reliable and deeply satisfying human knowledge can become" (p. 19). They go on to state that:"It is now possible to understand for the first time what humankind is and why we have the characteristics that we do" (p. 20). No wonder evolutionary psychology appeals to psychology, which has often labored under the stigma of being a "soft" science.

But just because something calls itself science and even is databased, it is not necessarily true or accurate. As Lewontin says, "The problem of the power to discern truth lies precisely in knowing how to evaluate, even roughly, the ambiguous knowledge of the world that is produced by so much of science" (1997, p. 51). Feminist scholars have argued that science has historically and up to the present been used to maintain the sexual status quo and is skewed by sexist biases (Bleir, 1984; Hubbard, 1992; Keller, 1985). Michael Carroll (1998) provides an interesting illustration of how this bias still operates. He looks at several studies that purport to show that there is a higher incidence of a particular fingerprint quality among women and homosexual males. The bias that is operating here is that gay men are effeminate, which reinforces gender stereotypes. He argues that some of the key findings are the result of methodological errors. He concludes that not only are reputable journals more willing to suspend scrutiny of those findings that confirm stereotypes, but that these kinds of studies, including those of evolutionary psychology, are increasing. It is entirely possible that he is describing the process by which the two Buss articles found their way into the *American Psychologist*. The reviewers may have been blinded to the flaws because they confirmed deeply held, sexist, and racist stereotypes.

Feminist psychology has been concerned with demonstrating the social construction and privileging of heterosexuality at the expense of other sexualities. Evolutionary psychology has an internally contradictory stance toward homosexuality and ignores the social context in which sexuality develops. Cosmides and Tooby state that homosexuality is "an evolutionary dysfunction in . . . gender modularity systems" (1999, p. 461). Yet Symons studied homosexual sexual frequency to determine heterosexual desire because "homosexual relations offer a clear window of the desires of each sex. Every heterosexual relationship is a compromise between the wants of a man and the wants of a woman, so differences between the sexes tend to be minimized" (Pinker, 1997, p. 473).

Symons completely ignores the social learning aspect of sexuality that was first documented by Kinsey, is seen in Masters and Johnson's work, and continues to this day in studies of college students' sexuality. How can the sexuality of a group who are a stigmatized minority, who are denied legal rights because of their sexuality, and who are more subject to violence because of it be "a clear window" into sexuality. Such a claim is simply naive; it ignores the complicated cultural messages we all receive about our sexuality and that of others, as well as taking as the "norm" sexual behaviors that the majority culture thinks of as deviant.

Scholars using an evolutionary perspective have similar contradictory positions on parents' impact on their children. As described above, Bowlby proposed that what happened with a mother during the first 2 years of life was of profound developmental and psychological influence for a child's later mental health. Sarah Hrdy (1999), a feminist sociobiologist and primatologist, amends Bowlby's position. She claims that maternal ambivalence is normal, that infants actively invoke maternal feelings, that all mothers are essential in most cultures, and that fathers can be an active part of nurturing. She is not specific about the development of pathology but clearly privileges a stable, loving family unit with assorted help from allomothers as optimal for development. Pinker (1997) claims that "the biggest influence that parents have on their children is at the moment of conception" (p. 449). The argument moves from mothering (nurture) to genetic (nature) with a more complex middle ground claimed by Hrdy. Within one developing area in a relatively short period of time each pole of the nature/nurture dichotomy is simultaneously claimed.

Feminist scholarship has shown that diagnosis is a profoundly political process, however much its proponents claim neutrality (Caplan, 1992; Liburd & Rothblum, 1995). There is massive documentation that the circumstances of women's lives can contribute to or cause emotional problems. Landrine, Klonoff, Gibbs, Manning, and Lund (1995) and Klonoff, Landrine, and Campbell (2000) show how the experience of sexist discrimination accounts for variance in women's physical and psychiatric problems. The emotional toll of childbirth, childcare, and work responsibilities for U.S. women has been studied and reported (Hyde, 1995; Ozer, 1995). Having less power can lead to depression, a sense of helplessness, poor self-esteem, and increased anxiety (Collins, 1998). And, finally, there is extensive research on the impact of childhood and adult trauma on people's lives (Bart & Moran, 1993; Cole, Rothblum, & Espin, 1992; Contratto & Gutfreund, 1996; Herman, 1992; Jacobs, 1994). The kind of taxonomy of disorders that evolutionary psychologists are proposing (see Cosmides & Tooby, 1999; Kirmayer & Young, 1999; Wakefield, 1999) renders invisible all those well-documented environmental stressors—poverty, violence, racism, and sexism—that require political change and not simply treatment.

Feminist psychology is about understanding and respecting differences, looking at ways in which power and circumstance have had an effect on individuals and groups, and empowering individuals and groups to change. The theory and practice of evolutionary psychology is antithetical to change and renders invisible both differences and environmental impacts. Evolutionary psychology and feminist psychology have no common ground.

But that is not to say that all biology and sociobiology is irrelevant to the development of feminist psychology. The work of biologist Anne Fausto Sterling (1985, 2000), for example, has made significant contributions to understanding sexualities. And Sarah Hrdy's (1999) recent book on mothering makes contributions to feminist psychology. She describes the enormous variability of maternal behaviors over time and context, putting the lie to simple essentialist positions as well as foregrounding maternal ambivalence. Of particular interest to me are her discussions of the erotic tie between mother and infant, which, I believe, might have psychological implications for female sexuality.

In conclusion, I would encourage feminists to be interested in both attachment theory and evolutionary psychology and to be skeptical of both their large and some of their smaller claims. To dismiss them out of hand is to relinquish a voice in an important intellectual conversation. Further, some of the writers present complicated and nuanced presentations, which can lead to the possibility of enhanced understanding. All conversation, however, is political and for us to believe that Science = Truth is, to use a favorite idea of the evolutionary psychologists, as erroneous as equating "natural" or "genetic" with "good."

REFERENCES

Ainsworth, M. D. (1967). *Infancy in Uganda: Infant care and the growth of love.* Baltimore: John Hopkins University Press.

Ainsworth, M. D., & Wittig, B. A. (1969). Attachment and exploratory behavior of one-year-olds in a strange situation. In B. M. Foss (Ed.), *Determinants of infant behaviour* (Vol. 4, pp. 111–136). London: Methuen.

Barkow, J. H., Cosmides, L., & Tooby, J. (Eds.). (1992). *The adapted mind: Evolutionary psychology and the generation of culture.* New York: Oxford University Press.

Bart, P., & Moran, E. G. (Eds.). (1993). *Violence against women: The bloody footprints.* Thousand Oaks, CA: Sage.

Bernard, B. (1996). From research to practice: The foundation of the resiliency paradigm. *Resiliency in Action, 1*(1), 4–9.

Birns, B. (1999). Attachment theory revisited: Challenging conceptual and methodological sacred cows. *Feminism and Psychology, 9*(1), 10–21.

Bleir, R. (1984). *Science and gender: A critique of biology and its theories on women.* New York: Pergamon Press.

Bowlby, J. (1969). *Attachment and loss: Vol. 1. Attachment.* New York: Basic Books.

Bowlby, J. (1988). *A secure base: Parent–child attachment and healthy human development.* New York: Basic Books.

Brennan, K. A., Clark, C. L., & Shaver, P. R. (1998). Self-report measurement of adult attachment: An integrative overview. In J. A. Simpson & W. S. Rholes (Eds.), *Attachment theory and close relationships* (pp. 46–76). New York: Guilford Press.

Burger, J. V. (1994, Summer). Keys to survival: Highlights in resilience research. *Journal of Emotional and Behavioral Problems,* pp. 6–10.

Buss, D. M. (1992). Mate preference mechanisms: Consequences for partner choice and intrasexual competition. In J. H. Barkow, L. Cosmides, & J. Tooby (Eds), *The adapted mind: Evolutionary psychology and the generation of culture* (pp. 249–265). New York: Oxford University Press.

Buss, D. M. (1995). Psychological sex differences: Origins through sexual selection. *American Psychologist, 50*(3), 164–168.

Buss, D. M. (2000). The evolution of happiness. *American Psychologist, 55*(1), 15–23.

Caplan, P. J. (1992). Gender issues in the diagnosis of mental disorder. *Women and Therapy, 12*(4), 71–79.

Carroll, M. P (1998). But fingerprints don't lie, eh?: Prevailing gender ideologies and scientific knowledge. *Psychology of Women Quarterly, 22*(4), 739–750.

Chodorow, N., & Contratto, S. (1981). The fantasy of the perfect mother. In B. Thorne (Ed.), *Rethinking the family: Some feminist questions* (pp. 54–75). New York: Longmans.

Cole, E., & Rothblum, E. (Eds.), & Espin, O. (Guest Ed.). (1992). Refugee women and their mental health: Shattered societies, shattered lives [Special issue]. *Women and Therapy, 13*(1–2).

Collins, L. H. (1998). Illustrating feminist theory: Power and psychopathology. *Psychology of Women Quarterly, 22*(1), 97–112.

Contratto, S. (1984). Mother: Social sculptor and trustee of the faith. In M. Lewin (Ed.), *In the shadow of the past: Psychology portrays the sexes* (pp. 226–255). New York: Columbia University Press.

Contratto, S., & Gutfreund, M. J. (Eds.). (1996). *A feminist clinician's guide to the memory debate.* New York: Haworth Press.

Cosmides, L., & Tooby, J. (1999). Toward an evolutionary taxonomy of treatable conditions. *Journal of Abnormal Psychology, 108*(3), 453–464.

Cosmides, L., Tooby, J., & Barkow, J. H. (1992). Introduction: Evolutionary psychology and conceptual integration. In J. H. Barkow, L. Cosmides, & J. Tooby (Eds.), *The adapted mind: Evolutionary psychology and the generation of culture* (pp. 3–15). New York: Oxford University Press.

Dozier, M., & Tyrrell, C. (1998). The role of attachment in therapeutic relationships. In J. A. Simpson & W. S. Rholes (Eds.), *Attachment theory and close relationships* (pp. 221–248). New York: Guilford Press.

Eagly, A. H., & Wood, W. (1999). The origins of sex differences in human behavior: Evolved dispositions versus social roles. *American Psychologist, 54*(6), 408–423.

George, C., Kaplan, N., & Main, M. (1985). *An adult attachment interview: Interview protocol.* Unpublished manuscript, University of California at Berkeley, Department of Psychology.

Gould, S. J. (1997a). The Darwinian fundamentalists. *New York Review of Books, 44*(10), 34–37.

Gould, S. J. (1997b). Evolution: The pleasures of pluralism. *New York Review of Books, 44*(11), 47–52.

Gowaty, P. A. (2001). Women, psychology and evolution. In R. K. Unger (Ed.), *Handbook of the psychology of women and gender* (pp. 53–65). New York: Wiley.

Harlow, H. F. (1965). Sexual behavior in the rhesus monkey. In F. A. Beach (Ed.), *Sex and behavior* (pp. 234–265). New York: Wiley.

Herman, J. L. (1992). *Trauma and recovery.* New York: Basic Books.

Hrdy, S. B. (1999). *Mother nature: A history of mothers, infants, and natural selection.* New York: Pantheon Books.

Hubbard, R. (1992). *The politics of women's biology.* New Brunswick, NJ: Rutgers University Press.

Hyde, J. S. (1995). Women and maternity leave: Empirical data and public policy [Presidential address]. *Psychology of Women Quarterly, 19*(3), 299–314.

Jacobs, J. L. (1994). *Victimized daughters: Incest and the development of the female self.* New York: Routledge.

Kagan, J. (1998). *Three seductive ideas.* Cambridge, MA: Harvard University Press.

Keller, E. F. (1985). *Reflections on gender and science.* New Haven, CT: Yale University Press.

Kirkpatrick, L. A. (1998). Evolution, pair-bonding, and reproductive strategies: A reconceptualization of adult attachment. In J. A. Simpson & W. S. Rholes (Eds.), *Attachment theory and close relationships* (pp. 353–393). New York: Guilford Press.

Kirmayer, L. J., & Young, A. (1999). Culture and context in the evolutional concept of mental disorder. *Journal of Abnormal Psychology, 108*(3), 446–452.

Klonoff, E. A., Landrine, H., & Campbell, R. (2000). Sexist discrimination may account for well-known gender differences in psychiatric symptoms. *Psychology of Women Quarterly, 24*(1), 93–99.

Landrine, H., Klonoff, E. A., Gibbs, J., Manning, V., & Lund, M. (1995). Physical and psychiatric correlates of gender discrimination: An application of the Schedule of Sexist Events. *Psychology of Women Quarterly, 19*(4), 473–492.

Lewontin, R. C. (1997). Reply [Letter]. *New York Review of Books, 44*(4), 51–52.

Liburd, R., & Rothblum, E. (1995). The medical model. In E. J. Rave & C. C. Larsen (Eds.), *Ethical decision making in therapy: Feminist perspectives* (pp. 177–201). New York: Guilford Press.

Lopez, F., & Brennan, K. (2000). Dynamic processes underlying adult attachment organization: Toward an attachment theoretical perspective on the healthy and effective self. *Journal of Counseling Psychology, 47,* 283–300.

Mikulincer, M., & Florian, V. (1998). The relationship between adult attachment styles and emotional and cognitive reactions to stressful events. In J. A. Simpson & W. S. Rholes (Eds.), *Attachment theory and close relationships* (pp. 143–165). New York: Guilford Press.

O'Brien, K. M., Friedman, S. M., Tipton, L. C., & Linn, S. G. (2000). Attachment, separation and women's vocational development: A longitudinal analysis. *Journal of Counseling Psychology, 47*(3), 301–315.

Ozer, E. M. (1995). The impact of childcare responsibility and self-efficacy on the psychological health of professional working mothers. *Psychology of Women Quarterly, 19*(3), 315–336.

Pinker, S. (1997). *How the mind works.* New York: Norton.

Rholes, W. S., Simpson, J. A., & Stevens, J. G. (1998). Attachment orientations, social support, and conflict resolution in close relationships. In J. A. Simpson & W. S. Rholes (Eds.), *Attachment theory and close relationships* (pp. 166–188). New York: Guilford Press.

Rothbaum, F., Weisz, J., Pott, M., Miyake, K., & Morelli, G. (2000). Attachment and culture: Security in the United States and Japan. *American Psychologist, 55,* 1093–1104.

Silverstein, L. B. (1998). New directions for evolutionary psychology. *Feminism and Psychology, 8*(3), 375–382.

Simpson, J. A., & Rholes, W. S. (1998a). Attachment in adulthood. In J. A. Simpson and W. S. Rholes (Eds.), *Attachment theory and close relationships* (pp. 3–31). New York: Guilford Press.

Simpson, J. A., & Rholes, W. S. (Eds.). (1998b). *Attachment theory and close relationships.* New York: Guilford Press.

Sterling, A. F. (1985). *Myths of gender: Biological theories about women and men.* New York: Basic Books.

Sterling, A. F. (2000). *Sexing the body: Gender politics and the construction of sexuality.* New York: Basic Books.

Tooby, J., & Cosmides, L. (1992). The psychological foundations of culture. In J. H. Barkow, L. Cosmides, & J. Tooby (Eds.), *The adapted mind: Evolutionary psychology and the generation of culture* (pp. 19–136). New York: Oxford University Press.

Vivona, J. M. (2000). Parental attachment styles of late adolescents: Qualities of attachment relationships and consequences for adjustment. *Journal of Counseling Psychology, 47*(3), 316–329.

Wakefield, J. C. (1999). Evolutionary versus prototype analyses of the concept of disorder, *Journal of Abnormal Psychology, 108,* 374–399.

Werner, E. E., & Smith, R. S. (1982). *Vulnerable but invincible: A longitudinal study of resilient children and youth.* New York: McGraw-Hill.

Chapter 3

New Developments in Relational–Cultural Theory

JUDITH V. JORDAN
LINDA M. HARTLING

THE BIRTH OF A THEORY

The Relational–Cultural Theory of women's development is rooted in the groundbreaking work of Jean Baker Miller, who proposed a new understanding of women's development in her book *Toward a New Psychology of Women* (Miller, 1976). In 1978, Miller, a psychoanalyst, along with three psychologists, Judith Jordan, Irene Stiver, and Janet Surrey, began meeting informally to reexamine developmental psychology and clinical practice as it pertains to women (Jordan, Kaplan, Miller, Stiver, & Surrey, 1991). Their twice-a-month meetings were the beginning of a collaborative theory-building group that led to the birth of a revolutionary approach to understanding psychological development.

In 1981, Miller was appointed as the first director of the Stone Center at Wellesley College and the theory-building group found an institutional home, allied with the Stone Center's mission to study psychological development and the prevention of psychological problems. At the Stone Center, the theory group initiated a series of colloquia in which they, along with other scholars and researchers, explored the complexities of women's development. Over the last 20 years, the proceedings from these colloquia and other presentations have been documented and published as over 100

48

"works in progress." These works became the core writings that describe the fundamental concepts of the theory that has become known as Relational–Cultural Theory (RCT).

Today, many of the core ideas underlying RCT are articulated in several books (Jordan, 1997; Jordan, Kaplan, Miller, Stiver, & Surrey, 1991; Miller & Stiver, 1997). These ideas suggest that all growth occurs in connection, that all people yearn for connection, and that growth-fostering relationships are created through mutual empathy and mutual empowerment. In particular, Miller (1986) described "five good things" that characterize a growth-fostering relationship: (1) increased zest (vitality), (2) increased ability to take action (empowerment), (3) increased clarity (a clearer picture of one's self, the other, and the relationship), (4) increased sense of worth, and (5) a desire for relationships beyond that particular relationship. These *five good things* describe the outcomes of growth-fostering relationships, that is, the outcomes when growth occurs through mutual empowerment and mutual empathy: we grow not toward separation, but toward greater mutuality and empathic possibility.

In addition to describing the benefits of growth-fostering relationships, that is, connection, RCT explores the impact of disconnection, recognizing that disconnection is an inevitable part of being in relationship (caused by empathic failures, relational violations, injuries, etc.). When, in response to a disconnection, the injured (especially the less powerful) person is able to represent her feelings and the other person is able to respond empathically, experiences of disconnection can lead to a strengthened relationship and an increased sense of *relational competence*, that is, being able to effect change and feeling effective in connections (Jordan, 1999). However, when the injured or less powerful person is unable to represent herself or her feelings in a relationship, or when she receives a response of indifference, additional injury, or denial of her experience, she will begin to keep aspects of herself out of relationship in order to keep the relationship. In RCT, this is referred to as the *central relational paradox* (Miller & Stiver, 1997). In these situations, the individual will use a variety of strategies— known as *strategies of disconnection* or *survival*—to twist herself to fit into the relationships available, becoming less and less authentic in the process (Miller, 1988). This is similar to the pathway that Carol Gilligan traces for adolescent girls who keep more and more of themselves out of relationship in order to stay in relationship (Gilligan, 1982; Gilligan, Lyons, & Hanmer, 1990). This pathway leads to failures in growth-fostering relationships, accompanied by diminished zest, empowerment, clarity, worth, and desire for connection. Within this context, one's natural yearning for connection becomes a signal of danger; the individual comes to dread the vulnerability necessary to fully engage in growth-fostering relationships.

Therapy based on RCT involves the ability to work authentically with the client's disconnections, to rework relational images (images that shape our expectations of relationship), to bring people out of their sense of isolation or shame and help them move back into healthy connection. This therapeutic process requires creating awareness of relational patterns and disconnections, helping clients to transform strategies of disconnection, which are blocking their ability to participate in healing relationships.

While RCT was initially developed to understand women's psychological experience, it is increasingly being used to gain a better understanding of all human experience, including men's experience. Special attention is being paid to examining the importance of difference, particularly difference informed by imbalances in power and privilege. RCT is the foundation for a growing body of research on depression, trauma, eating disorders, substance abuse, chronic illness, mother–daughter relationships, and lesbian relationships, as well as issues of racism, sexism, heterosexism, classism, and a multitude of other psychological and social problems (Hartling & Ly, 2000).

TOWARD A RELATIONAL PARADIGM OF DEVELOPMENT

Traditional theories of development were constructed around a core belief in the ascendancy of individualism and separation. From its inception, the field of psychology attempted to emulate the "hard" science of Newtonian physics that proclaimed the salience of material, separate objects (the atom or molecule) secondarily coming into relationship (Jordan, 1997). Ironically, Newtonian physics, which has shaped much of the thinking in science and psychology, has been challenged and replaced by modern physics, which emphasizes the primacy of relationships. Nevertheless, individualistic, "separate-self" models of development—modeled after Newtonian physics—continue to dominate the field of psychology and are perpetuated by Western and U.S. values of autonomy, separation, individualism, boundedness, and self-sufficiency (Cushman, 1996).

The Stone Center theory group, which has grown in size and diversity, continues to question separate-self models of development, especially for women. In particular, they recognize that the traditional psychological notion of the "self" is a highly spatial metaphor, connoting separation, boundedness, protection from a threatening context or milieu (Jordan,

1997). By holding up the separate-self standards of independence and autonomy as endpoints of development, women and others are frequently judged as deficient or inadequate. In the field of mental health, this has often led to pathologizing women's behavior and development (e.g., women are too needy, too emotional, too dependent).

Looking beyond the bias in psychological models that privilege independence and self-sufficiency, RCT focuses on the process of growth and differentiation within relationship, the expansion and elaboration of connection, as well as the movement toward increasing mutuality in relationship. Dominant theories have tended to emphasize the formation of intrapsychic structure as the foundation of well-being, suggesting that healthy development is the capacity to function independently. These theories often imply that the individual is an empty vessel to be filled by a "good mother" or others, leading to the ultimate outcome of being able to "stand on one's own two feet." In contrast, RCT suggests healthy development occurs when both people are growing and changing in relationship. When individuals are engaged in a mutually empathic, mutually empowering relationship, both people are becoming more responsive in fostering the well-being of the other and of the relationship itself; both people are growing through connection. RCT proposes a shift away from a one-way, individualist model of development to a relational model of mutual development.

RCT THERAPY AND PRACTICE

RCT emphasizes health, growth, and courage, and points to a new understanding of human and individual strength: strength in relationship, not strength in isolation. Isolation is seen as the source of most suffering, while the process of creating mutual empathy and mutual empowerment in relationship is seen as the route out of isolation. In therapy, mutual empathy and mutual empowerment evolve out of the client seeing, knowing, and feeling her or his impact on the therapist, on the relationship. Unlike traditional approaches that extol the practice of nonresponsiveness, neutrality, and nongratification, RCT suggests that it is important for clients to learn about their impact on others, which begins with learning about their impact on the therapy relationship. If we accept the premise that a client's sense of isolation and strategies of disconnection arise in the context of nonresponsive, nonmutual, disempowering relationships, then healing occurs in the context of a respectful, safe relationship characterized by empathic responsiveness.

Mutual empathy lies at the core of this healing connection. This is not reciprocal empathy; it involves the client seeing, knowing, and feeling that she has moved the therapist. The client has had an impact: she has learned that she matters and that she is relationally effective. This is a relationally corrective and restorative experience for the individual who suffers from a history of chronic disconnection or nonresponsiveness from important caregivers.

The responsive engagement of the therapist is crucial to the healing process in therapy. This engagement is not the same as therapist reactivity; it is therapeutic authenticity, which involves *modulated responsiveness*, not knee-jerk reactivity. Modulated responsiveness is informed by *anticipatory empathy*, anticipating the possible impact one has on another and *caring* about that impact. As all clinicians know, therapists and clients have different responsibilities in the therapy relationship. A therapist assumes the greatest responsibility in a therapy relationship by performing a role that carries with it the obligation to uphold professional ethical and legal guidelines. These guidelines inform the therapist's practice of modulated responsiveness, anticipatory empathy, and authenticity.

Authenticity in a therapeutic relationship is not about total spontaneity or unmitigated self-disclosure (Miller et al., 1999). It involves trying to bring more and more of one's experience into connection, with constant awareness of the possible impact on the other person. For example, being authentic in any relationship, especially a therapeutic relationship, involves clearly stating one's limits (e.g., "I'm not comfortable with that way of interacting. I'm sorry if that is hard for you but you need to know my limits"). Authenticity requires a person to take responsibility for describing the conditions in which one can meet the other person in relationship. This is different from suggesting that the other person is somehow deficient, needs limits imposed upon her, or that her request for a certain type of interaction is necessarily indicative of pathology.

The concept of *boundaries* is pertinent to the discussion of authenticity and mutuality. Often people misinterpret authenticity and mutuality, suggesting that the relational–cultural model espouses self-disclosure or gives permission for total spontaneity. Rather, RCT questions the seemingly innocuous concept of boundaries because it arises within, supports, and reinforces the model of a separate self, which suggests that one must protect oneself from relationships, that safety and well-being ensue from constantly armoring oneself with invisible barriers. Traditional conceptualizations of boundaries carry implications of the self always existing within a dangerous environment, a self that needs protection from, rather than good connection with, others.

Another way to think about boundaries is as places of meeting, exchange, and maximal growth. Instead of fortifying boundaries, the emphasis in RCT is on (1) clarity in relationship (e.g., this is your experience; this is mine), (2) the right to say "no" and to exercise choice in deciding what one will share or do, (3) the importance of stating limits (e.g., "I can't do this in our relationship because it makes me uncomfortable"), and (4) redefining boundaries as places of meeting and exchange, rather than as walls of protection against others. By observing these four conditions of engaging in relationship, we essentially honor growth and safety through connection, not through separation or imposing power over others. Moreover, RCT concepts—such as authenticity or mutuality—are practiced within a context of relational clarity, a context in which boundaries are places where people meet to grow through connection.

Social/Cultural Disconnections

Another key component of therapy based on RCT is the recognition that disconnections as well as opportunities for growth occur not only on the individual or familial level, but also at the sociocultural level. Societal practices of categorizing, stereotyping, and stratifying individuals have an enormous impact on peoples' sense of connection and disconnection (Walker, 1999, 2001; Walker & Miller, 2001). Racism, sexism, heterosexism, and classism impede all individuals' ability to engage and participate in growth-fostering relationships. RCT suggests that therapists must be aware that different forms of unearned advantage and power accrue to different categories of identity. For example, being middle class, white, or heterosexual carries with it all sorts of unearned privilege in a society that values these characteristics over others. bell hooks's notion of "margin" captures some of the dynamics of this distribution of privilege and advantage (hooks, 1984). Those at the center hold the power of naming reality, the power of naming deviance and norms, and often hold the power to eliminate the possibility of open conflict with or challenge from those who are forced to the margins. The exercise of dominance and privilege suppresses authenticity and mutuality in relationships, limiting and interfering with the formation of growth-fostering relationships. These sociocultural dynamics inflict disconnection, silence, shame, and isolation on marginalized groups. These issues must be in the forefront of the therapist's work with a client.

Thus, the central tenet of RCT in therapy is that people develop through and toward relationship, which occurs within and is influenced by a cultural context. Above all, RCT asserts that people need to be in connection in order to change, to open up, to shift, to transform, to heal, and to grow.

GROWING PAINS AND POSSIBILITIES: RESPONDING TO CRITIQUES

An important part of developing a robust theory is exploring and responding to questions and criticisms. Criticisms offer theory builders the opportunity to clarify, adjust, and ultimately strengthen their work. One criticism of RCT is that it offers an essentialist portrayal of development. This argument implies that one's biological sex determines fundamental, internal, individual attributes (e.g., "women are naturally more relational"). The theory builders have never intended to suggest that women are "by nature" more relational, empathic, or nurturing. Jean Baker Miller's (1976) original work clearly delineates the power of context and the power of a patriarchal culture, which has assigned women the primary responsibility for supporting and maintaining the relationships necessary for everyone's growth. Her work is profoundly sociopolitical and social constructivist. Miller's book clearly describes gender as a socially constructed variable, largely framed by power dynamics. She states:

> A dominant group, inevitably, has the greatest influence in determining the culture's overall outlook—its philosophy, morality, social theory, and even its science. The dominant group, thus, legitimates the unequal relationship and incorporates it into society's guiding concepts. . . . In the case of women, for example, despite overwhelming evidence to the contrary, the notion persists that women are meant to be passive, submissive, docile, secondary. (p. 8)

RCT explicitly elaborates on the role of power in the development of social identity and articulates the ways in which sociopolitical/cultural factors lead to disconnection, disempowerment, and isolation (Walker, 2001; Walker & Miller, 2001).

Another criticism of RCT is that it reflects the biases of the initial group of theory builders, who were white, middle-class, heterosexual, educated women. Recognizing that their perspective was limited by centrist privilege, since the mid-1980s the original members of the theory group have been committed to bringing diverse voices into the center of theory building and to being as conscious as possible of their own biases and privilege, as well as the extent to which they participate in the dominant culture. Now, through the collaboration of an expanded group of theory builders (e.g., Jenkins, 1993a, 1993b, 1998; Rosen, 1992; Sparks, 1999; Walker, 1999, 2001), RCT has grown and offers an enlarged understanding of the diversities and commonalities among women from a wide range of backgrounds and experiences. There is not one psychology of women nor one voice, but many. Voices traditionally marginalized are now at the center of the theory-building group and the challenging dialogues on race, sexual orientation, and other issues of difference are shifting our understandings of connection and disconnection. While class is acknowledged as a crucial force in creating connection and disconnection, it remains one of the most difficult to address.

Those who have followed RCT over the last 20 years will note that enriching the dialogue has transformed the theory. For example, the theory was initially known as "self-in-relation" theory; however, ongoing conversations with collaborating scholars suggested that the original name continued to overemphasize an individualist, separate-self perspective. Consequently, the theory was renamed Relational–Cultural Theory. This is only one example of how the collaborative process through which RCT emerged requires that theory development remain open and responsive to new ideas, new research, and new voices.

APPLYING RCT: THE CASE OF M

M was an 18-year-old woman who had been seen in many treatments prior to her current treatment. She had been diagnosed by other clinicians as borderline, paranoid, and depressed. Previous treatments had ended with her firing therapists when empathic impasses developed, or they ended with therapists impatiently terminating with her because of her persistent self-mutilating and sometimes suicidal behavior. In the course of treatment, it became clear that a stepfather had sexually abused her. Her history was filled with episodes of an eating disorder, some substance abuse, and other self-destructive behaviors.

In the beginning of therapy she was very cautious; she had come to the RCT-based therapist because she had heard that the therapist was more "human" and "present" than other therapists were. But she soon found fault with the therapist, who seemed too distant as well. She had great diffi-culty trusting the RCT-based therapist and would often become quite scared and/or rageful when the therapist "screwed up" by not understand-ing her completely. These disconnections were abrupt and painful. Her his-tory was replete with abuse, lack of protection from caregivers, and viola-tions of her sense of integrity. A supposedly trustworthy adult had abused her behind closed doors, and she had been silenced about her experience.

Therapeutic failures or mistakes emphasized to her that her new thera-pist was not 100% trustworthy, that is, the therapist might disappoint her, and, in response, her terror might catapult her into major strategies of dis-connection and self-protection. The therapy situation itself felt triggering to her, inviting her to a place of psychological vulnerability with a supposedly trustworthy but powerful figure, all held behind closed doors. She fre-quently threatened to quit therapy and called other therapists to complain about her current therapist. Her substance abuse got worse when she felt threatened, as did her self-destructive behavior. Although she was on medi-cation, a selective serotonin reuptake inhibitor, to stabilize her depression and to deal with some of her symptoms of posttraumatic stress disorder, psychobiological factors appeared to be contributing to her reactivity, which led her into feelings of greater disconnection (Banks, 2001).

In response to her client's struggles, the RCT-based therapist, very slowly, began to rework each empathic failure that had occurred in her rela-tionship with the client. This meant that the therapist acknowledged her own relational imperfections and limits. And the therapist began engaging with the client to repair the relationship by examining the ways in which both people contributed to disconnections. Further, they explored the ways the client's reactivity to the therapist's limitations led to her isolation and her feeling that she was even more endangered. In other words, the thera-pist and the client began to rework the client's central relational paradox: the therapist honored the client's strategies of disconnection (recognizing that these behaviors had been essential to her survival) and at the same time held and facilitated the overall movement toward connection. The cli-ent was not forced to relinquish her strategies of disconnection before she was ready to or before she felt safe enough to risk the vulnerability neces-sary to enter into greater connection. The original wisdom and usefulness of these strategies for survival were also honored (she had to move into protective inauthenticity as a child in order to stay alive in an abusive situa-tion). But, gently, slowly, the therapist invited the client to look at the patterns of her behavior that now led her to feel more frightened in her isolation than she might have been if she had been moving into more connection. Working with mutual empathy, the therapist opened herself to being impacted and affected by the client (e.g., at one point the therapist felt tears well up when the client was crying about her helplessness and pain; in another instance, when the therapist empathically failed the client, the therapist let her client see that she was pained by her own mistake and apologized). As the client sees her impact on the therapist, she slowly begins to regain a sense of relational competence, a feeling that she matters to the therapist. It is with this attitude of respect and mutuality, joining with the client in empathic resonance, that the therapist supports movement out of isolation and back into connection.

In addition to facilitating her movement toward greater connection in therapy, the therapist encouraged her client to develop other relationships to help her regulate her fear of becoming too dependent on the therapist. Furthermore, the client was encouraged to voice her dissatisfaction and discomfort with the therapist whenever these issues arose, and she was encouraged to find ways to ground herself when her biological reactivity threatened to contribute to disconnections in relationship with others. In this way, the therapist and the client began to build authentic connection and what RCT refers to as *relational resilience*, which involves movement toward empathic mutuality, relational awareness, and relational confidence, the belief in one's ability to create growth-enhancing relationships (Jordan, 1992). Rather than something that resides within the individual, RCT suggests that resilience is relational and contextual. This conceptualization of resilience dramatically alters our understanding of strength, healing, and growth.

EMERGING RESEARCH: A RELATIONAL–CULTURAL REFRAMING OF RESILIENCE

As the literature, research, and applications of RCT continue to grow and expand (Hartling & Ly, 2000), one of the most promising and compelling areas of inquiry is the study of resilience. Although many investigations are grounded in individualist theories of development, much of the research on resilience points in a relational direction, suggesting that *resilience grows through connection* (Jordan, 1992). The following section begins a discussion of the research and offers a relational reframing of characteristics associated with resilience.

Resilience: Beginning with a Feminist Framework

Jean Baker Miller (1976) and other feminist scholars urge us to critically examine the theories and assumptions underlying many areas of research (Keller, 1985; McIntosh, 1988, 1989; Minnich, 1990; Stewart, 1994). These scholars highlight the effects of privilege, power, and biased perspectives (e.g., sexism, racism, classism, heterosexism, homophobia, etc.) that can distort the study of a wide range of human behavior, including the experience of resilience. When research is designed, developed, conducted, and interpreted primarily by members of a dominant group, these individuals will tend to define themselves and their values as the norm or ideal, concomitantly implying that members of subordinate groups are deficient or abnormal. Many years ago, Jean Baker Miller named this problem when she said that "the close study of an oppressed group reveals that a dominant group inevitably describes the subordinate group falsely in terms derived from its own systems of thought" (p. xix). With regard to the study of resilience, the strengths of women and marginalized men may be misconstrued or completely overlooked by research that covertly or overtly emphasizes the values and norms of the dominant group.

For example, in the 1970s, Kobasa (1979; Kobasa & Puccetti, 1983) described the construct of "hardiness" as an individual characteristic associated with resistance to stress, a form of resilience. Based on initial research, hardiness was defined as an internal characteristic comprised of three factors: (1) commitment: the ability to easily commit to what one is doing; (2) control: a general belief that one can control events; and (3) challenge: the ability to perceive change as a challenge rather than a threat. Over the years, hardiness has been used as a standard of stress resilience in men *and women*. However, today we realize that Kobasa's research had serious limitations that were not deemed significant in the past. The subjects of investigation in Kobasa's original study were white, male, middle- to upper-level business executives. While the qualities of commitment, control, and challenge (i.e., hardiness) may accurately describe stress resilience in this particular sample, these characteristics may not be the most useful indicators of stress resilience in women or others not represented in the study.

In other words, if women from a broad range of backgrounds had been the subjects of investigation, the researchers might have identified different characteristics associated with stress resilience. For instance, in her study of African American mothers on welfare, Elizabeth Sparks (1999) described relational practices (e.g., connection, collaboration, and community action) used by a marginalized group of women to overcome the corrosive effects of poverty, racism, and being stigmatized as social scapegoats. By broadening the research population and taking a relational perspective—rather than restricting the population and focusing on individual, internal qualities or traits—researchers can make visible some of the relational, collaborative characteristics that may contribute to the resilience of many populations (Genero, 1995).

In response to the implicit limitations of much of the research, Abigail Stewart (1994) offers specific strategies for studying resilience in the lives of women, that may be helpful for examining the experience of other marginalized groups. She recommends that researchers utilize the following strategies to gain a more accurate understanding of the strengths exhibited by women:

1. Look for what's been left out.
2. Analyze your own role or position as it affects your understanding and the research process.
3. Identify women's agency in the midst of social constraint.
4. Use the concept of "gender" as an analytic tool.
5. Explore the precise ways in which gender defines power relationships and in which power relationships are gendered.
6. Identify other significant aspects of an individual's social position and explore the implications of that position.
7. Avoid the search for a unified or coherent self. (pp. 13–30)

Stewart's suggestions remind us to embrace the complexities of women's experience and begin identifying the features of women's lives that have allowed them to be resilient despite the social constraints imposed upon them. Her strategies offer us a feminist framework for exploring the research on the resilience of women and, possibly, the resilience of other subordinate groups.

A Relational Conceptualization of Resilience

The literature on resilience typically describes resilience in three ways: (1) good outcomes—the absence of deviant or antisocial behavior—after experiencing adverse conditions; (2) maintaining competence under conditions of threat; and (3) recovery from traumatic experiences (Masten, Best, & Garmezy, 1990). These definitions, combined with traditional models of development, tend to reinforce a focus on internal, individual personality traits associated with surviving adversity or trauma. Enlarging the discourse, RCT encourages researchers to examine the social, cultural, and interpersonal factors that impede or enhance one's ability to withstand or overcome hardships. An RCT view of resilience requires an analysis of the relational conditions that foster growth in the lives of those who have suffered severe disruptions, the conditions that allow people to thrive despite exposure to many forms of adversity. Hence, RCT expands and transforms conceptualizations of resilience to include understanding the dynamics of finding and moving toward mutually empathic, mutually empowering relationships in the face of adversity, trauma, or alienating social/cultural pressures—that is, the ability to connect, reconnect, and resist disconnection.

By shifting the focus beyond the individual, RCT promotes a broader perspective, which requires investigating the relational–cultural factors that influence one's ability to be resilient and to grow despite adversities. In particular, RCT attends to the influence of power in dominant–subordinate relationships and the experience of marginalized populations to determine how social/cultural systems of advantage or disadvantage may privilege or oppress an individual's ability to be resilient. Thus, an RCT-based conceptualization of resilience promotes a broader, richer, deeper inquiry into this complex experience.

Exploring Resilience: Individual and Relational Considerations

Over the years, researchers have identified numerous characteristics associated with individuals who have successfully overcome adversity or traumatic experiences (Barnard, 1994; Masten, 1994, 2001; Masten, Best, & Garmezy, 1990). While many of these characteristics are viewed as internal traits, these traits are clearly influenced by relational–cultural conditions and dynamics. Reexamining and rethinking the relational aspects of the characteristics associated with resilience moves us toward a new understanding of this phenomenon. The following discussion offers a relational analysis of six characteristics associated with resilience.

A Relational View of Temperament

Temperament is described as an internal, relatively stable, individual characteristic frequently noted in the research on resilience (Rutter, 1978; Werner & Smith, 1982). A well-known study of multi- and mixed-racial children living in adverse conditions on the Hawaiian island of Kauai suggested that "good-natured" boys and "cuddly" girls were more resilient than other children (Werner & Smith, 1982). But what are the relational–

cultural aspects of temperament? Rutter (1978) observed that children with adverse temperaments (i.e., temperaments characterized by "low regularity, low malleability, negative mood, and low fastidiousness" [p. 51]) were twice as likely to be the targets of parental criticism. He concluded that a child's temperament has a significant impact on the *parent–child relationship*, either protecting the child or putting the child at risk. In other words, temperament affects an individual's ability to participate in relationships that promote resilience.

Based on the Kauai study and Rutter's observations, one might conclude that children with adverse temperaments would always be less resilient because their temperaments would negatively affect their ability to attract, engage in, and sustain relationships. However, RCT requires that we also consider the cultural context in which a child's temperament is expressed. A study of East African Masai children found that those with difficult temperaments were more likely to survive extreme drought conditions (de Vries, 1984). The researchers theorized that these children were able to assert their need for (relational) support within a culture that values assertiveness. A relational–cultural view helps us understand that temperament has an impact on a child's opportunities to connect and gain access to resources that are necessary to facilitate her or his ability to be resilient.

Intellectual Development and Connection

Intelligence is another individual trait cited in the research on resilience. Although it is largely considered an internal, stable characteristic, Ann Masten and her colleagues (Masten, 1994, 2001; Masten, Best, & Garmezy, 1990) describe some of the contextual and relational factors that may explain the connection between intellectual development and resilience, including economic or educational advantages or having skilled parents. Analyzing the influence of relationships on intelligence, Daniel Siegel (1999) emphasizes that brain development is an "experience-dependent" process and that interpersonal relationships are the central source of experience that influences how the brain develops. Opportunities provided to children through relationships activate certain neural pathways in the brain, either "strengthening existing connections or creating new connections" (p. 13). According to Siegel, "Human connections create neuronal connections" (p. 85).

The brain is a dynamic living system, open to experiences primarily facilitated by relationships and constantly in a state of change. Although Siegel focuses on early brain development facilitated by the parent–child relationship, his analysis begins to describe the interactive dynamic of mutual influence among individuals engaged in relationships that contributes to healthy brain development and function throughout our lives. Siegel's observations suggest that researchers should continue to explore the relational–cultural factors that foster intellectual development and healthy brain function, both of which contribute to one's ability to be resilient.

Self-Esteem and Social Esteem

Self-esteem is a generally accepted personality characteristic associated with resilience (Dumont & Provost, 1999); however, RCT brings to our attention some questions about this characteristic. Judith Jordan (1994) observes that self-esteem in Western culture is primarily constructed on a separate-self, hyperindividualistic model of development, which valorizes self-sufficiency and individual achievement over collaboration and connection. Further, traditional conceptualizations of self-esteem are often built on hierarchical comparisons in which one's esteem depends on feeling superior to someone else. Consequently, the process of building self-esteem can become an exercise in individual, competitive achievement. Within this context, those who subscribe to more collaborative and collective models of achievement may be viewed as lacking in self-esteem.

Traditional, individualistic constructs of self-esteem may have limited relevance to people of color. Yvonne Jenkins (1993b) offers a group-centered, relational conceptualization of esteem, which she calls *social esteem*. She suggests that *"for collective societies, group esteem is practically synonymous with the anglocentric conceptualizations of self-esteem"* (p. 55, original emphasis). Social esteem implies a group-related identity that values "interdependence, affiliation, and collaterality" (p. 55). For diverse populations in which the unit of operation is the family, the group, or collective society, social esteem is an essential part of healthy psychosocial development, and it may enhance one's ability to cope with adversity—that is, one's ability to be resilient. As with the characteristics mentioned thus far, RCT encourages researchers to take a relational view of esteem.

Internal Locus of Control or Mutual Empowerment

Internal locus of control (ILOC) is another individual characteristic associated with resilience, in particular resilience in the form of competence under stress (Masten, Best, & Garmezy, 1990; Werner & Smith, 1982). What is ILOC? According to Roediger, Capaldi, Paris, and Polivy (1991),

"Children who take responsibility for their own successes and failures are said to have an internal locus of control" (p. 352). This definition seems to decontextualize the issues of control and fails to recognize the realities of racism, sexism, heterosexism, or other forms of discrimination that affect one's ability to feel an internal sense of control. In fact, it would appear to be advantageous for the dominant group to persuade the subordinate group that they *should* have an ILOC, they *should* feel responsible for their lack of success and their failures. Obviously, it is easier to have an ILOC when one is a member of, and exhibits the characteristics of, the dominant, privileged social group.

A 1999 study challenged thinking about ILOC (Magnus, Cowen, Wyman, Fagen, & Work, 1999). The researchers compared stress-resilient (SR) white and black children to stress-affected (SA) white and black children and found a significant difference in the ILOC between the SR white children and the SA white children, but not between the black children. Based on their results, the researchers theorized that white families may emphasize individual control while black families do not because it might promote a false belief that one can control adversities such as racism and other forms of discrimination.

From an RCT perspective, it might be helpful to move away from the individualist language of internal control and move toward a more relational language of *mutual empowerment* or *mutual influence*. A sense of control comes from feeling as though one can influence his or her environment or experience; she or he has the power to take action on behalf of her- or himself and others, creating possibilities for change. Rather than seeking to achieve an internal sense of control over experience, perhaps individuals are more resilient when they are engaged in relationships that are mutually empathic, open, and responsive. For example, research suggests that responsiveness and mutual influence are essential features of successful marriages (Gottman & DeClaire, 2001) and that couples who engage in mutual support are more resilient when faced with economic pressures (Conger, Reuter, & Elder, 1999).

The Meaning of Mastery

Mastery is a term frequently used to describe the sense of competence associated with being a resilient person. Of all the concepts discussed thus far, the term *mastery* has some dubious connotations. According to dictionary definitions, Judith Jordan (1999) notes, " 'to master' is to reduce to subjection, to get the better of, to break, to tame" (pp. 1–2). She states that the "mastery implicit in most models of competence creates enormous conflict for many people, especially women and other marginalized groups, people who have not traditionally been 'the masters' " (p. 2). Jordan's observations suggest that researchers might want to consider an alternative term and conceptualization of this quality. Nevertheless, how do people develop a sense of mastery or competence? In her research on resilience in children, Ann Masten and her colleagues (1990) identified three forms of activity parents can practice to develop competence or mastery in their children: "model effective action, provide opportunities to experience mastery, and verbally persuade children of their own effectiveness" (p. 432). Not surprisingly, these are relational activities, suggesting that mastery and competence grow through participation in supportive relationships. Once again, relationships are key in developing a sense of competence or mastery.

From Social Support to Connection

Obviously, social support is one of the most relational constructs identified in the research on resilience. The benefits of social support have been well documented in psychological and health research (Atkins, Kaplan, & Toshima, 1991; Belle, 1987; Ganellen & Blaney, 1984; Ornish, 1997). Yet social support, as it is defined in the research (Fiore, Becker, & Coppel, 1983), tends to represent a *one-way* form of relating, something that one gets from others. This is extremely different from the *two-way*, mutually empathic, mutually empowering, growth-fostering form of relating described in RCT as *connection* (Jordan, 1992). However, researchers have described some specific forms of social support that imply that these relationships foster connection.

Renée Spencer (2000) discusses a number of studies that suggest that a relationship with one supportive adult is associated with good outcomes when children are faced with various adverse conditions, including parental mental illness (Rutter, 1979), separation from a parent (Rutter, 1971), marital discord (Rutter, 1971), divorcing parents (Wallerstein & Kelly, 1980), poverty (Garmezy, 1991), maltreatment (Cicchetti, 1989), and multifaceted or a combination of risk factors (Seifer et al., 1996). In a study of over 12,000 adolescents, Michael Resnick and his colleagues (1997) determined that *connection* to parents, family members, or other adults is the most important factor associated with a reduced risk of substance abuse, violence, depression, suicidal behavior, and early sexual activity, regardless of an adolescent's race, ethnicity, socioeconomic status, or family structure. This seems to draw into question the traditional view that healthy development requires progressive separation and independence from relationships or requires "standing on one's own two feet." Furthermore, although the research in Spencer's paper clearly articulates the importance of supportive relationships, these studies continue to reflect a one-way perspective, the effects of connection on one person (the child) in the relationship rather than the effects on both people in the relationship.

Engaging in relational behaviors to cope with adverse conditions may be especially true for women. Challenging the generally accepted theory that people exhibit a *fight-or-flight* response to stress, a recent analysis by Shelley Taylor and her colleagues (2000) suggests that women may utilize a *tend-and-befriend* response to stress. Women will engage in caretaking activities or the creation of a network of associations to protect themselves and others (e.g., children) from a threat—women exhibit a relational response to stress. Taylor et al. postulate that the fight/flight response may be inhibited in women by brain chemistry that reduces fearfulness, decreases sympathetic nervous system activity, and promotes maternal caretaking and affiliative behavior. Taylor and colleagues' analysis is supported by studies that show that women are more likely to mobilize social support in times of stress, they maintain more same-sex close relationships, they turn to female friends more often, and they are more engaged in social networks than men (Belle, 1987).

The tend-and-befriend theory provides us with a relational perspective on women's responses to stress yet it simultaneously raises some serious concerns. It is troubling to think that this new theory might be used to justify patterns of discrimination and social oppression of women, offering an overly simplistic biological explanation of women's behavior, akin to suggesting that women are by nature relational—that is, an essentialist understanding of women's behavior. It is troubling because, historically, biological explanations have been used as evidence of women's inferiority (Tavris, 1992). In response to some of these concerns, Taylor and her colleagues state:

> Our analysis should not be construed to imply that women should be mothers, will be good mothers, or will be better parents than men by virtue of these mechanisms. Similarly, this analysis should not be construed as evidence that women are naturally more social than men or that they should shoulder disproportionate responsibility for the ties and activities that create and maintain the social fabric. . . . Biology is not so much destiny as it is a central tendency, but a central tendency that influences and interacts with social, cultural, cognitive, and emotional factors, resulting in substantial

behavioral flexibility. . . . some aspects of the tend-and-befriend model may characterize male responses under some conditions as well. (2000, p. 423)

These researchers acknowledge the limitations of their analysis and existing studies. They recognize that women have been the subjects of investigation in virtually all research exploring affiliation under stress. The lack of data about male subjects makes it impossible to know whether or not the tend-and-befriend model might apply to some aspects of male behavior. Although this theory offers some new possibilities for understanding a biological factor that may contribute to relational behavior, RCT suggests that relationships are highly complex, involving the interaction of numerous social, cultural, psychological, and biological factors that have yet to be explored (e.g., Banks, 2001).

Overall, studies of social support indicate that receiving support contributes significantly to one's ability to be resilient. Yet these studies predominantly focus on the experience of one individual in the relationship, exploring the one-way benefits of relating, such as assessing supportive parent–child relationships only from the child's perspective. In a recent paper, Ann Masten observes that many research models "do not accommodate the bidirectional nature of influence in living systems" (Masten, 2001, p. 230; see also Masten, 1999). She notes, for example, that "one study that found parenting to predict child competence, resilience, and change in child competence over time, also found that child competence predicted changes in the parenting quality over time" (Masten, 2001, pp. 230–231; Masten et al., 1999). RCT proposes that relationships that enhance resilience and growth are characterized by a bidirectional or two-way experience of *connection*, which involves mutual empathy, mutual empowerment, and movement toward mutuality, benefiting all people engaged in the relationship (Genero, Miller, & Surrey, 1992). By extending studies to include the outcomes for both or all people in relationship, researchers can begin to investigate how resilience grows through the dynamic of connection (Jordan, 1992; Liang et al., 1998).

THE CONTINUING GROWTH OF RCT

The study of resilience discussed in this chapter provides us with one example of the recent developments in RCT and illustrates how this theory can expand our understanding of the diversity and complexity of human experience. Through the collaborative process of theory building established in the early years of its development, RCT continues to evolve and grow, offering new insights and new possibilities for research and therapy.

In 1995, the Jean Baker Miller Training Institute (JBMTI) was established at the Stone Center at Wellesley College. The institute was formed to provide greater opportunities for clinicians, scholars, students, researchers, and others—from around the country and around the world—to meet, discuss, and deepen their understanding of the many applications of RCT. Since its inception, the JBMTI has hosted intensive training institutes, workshops, courses, and seminars exploring the clinical, business, and community applications of RCT. In addition, the JBMTI works in alliance with a network of researchers who are utilizing RCT in various investigations of human experience. To date, the JBMTI, along with the Stone Center, has published over 100 papers and books that describe fundamental concepts, new developments, and wide-ranging applications of RCT.

REFERENCES

Atkins, C. J., Kaplan, R. M., & Toshima, M. T. (1991). Close relationships in the epidemiology of cardiovascular disease. *Advances in Personal Relationships, 3*, 207–231.

Banks, A. (2001). *PTSD: Brain chemistry and relationships* (Project Report No. 8). Wellesley, MA: Stone Center Working Paper Series.

Barnard, C. P. (1994). Resiliency: A shift in our perception? *American Journal of Family Therapy, 22*(2), 135–144.

Belle, D. (1987). Gender differences in the social moderators of stress. In D. Belle (Ed.), *Gender and stress* (pp. 257–277). New York: Free Press.

Cicchetti, D. (1989). How research on child maltreatment has informed the study of child development: Perspectives from developmental psychopathology. In D. Cicchetti & V. Carlson (Eds.), *Child maltreatment: Theory and research on the cause and consequences of child abuse and neglect* (pp. 377–431). New York: Cambridge University Press.

Conger, R. D., Reuter, M. A., & Elder, G. H. (1999). Couple resilience to economic pressure. *Journal of Personality and Social Psychology, 76*(1), 54–71.

Cushman, P. (1996). *Constructing the self, constructing America: A cultural history of psychotherapy*. Reading, MA: Addison-Wesley Longman.

de Vries, M. W. (1984). Temperament and infant mortality among the Masai of East Africa. *American Journal of Psychiatry, 141*, 1189–1194.

Dumont, M., & Provost, M. A. (1999). Resilience in adolescents: Protective role of social support, coping strategies, self-esteem, and social activities on experience of stress and depression. *Journal of Youth and Adolescents, 28*(3), 343–363.

Fiore, J., Becker, J., & Copple, D. B. (1983). Social network interactions: A buffer or a stress? *American Journal of Community Psychology, 11*(4), 423–439.

Ganellen, R. J., & Blaney, R. H. (1984). Hardiness and social support as moderators

68   DEVELOPING FEMINIST THEORIES

of the effects of stress. *Journal of Personality and Social Psychology, 47*(1), 156–163.

Garmezy, N. (1991). Resiliency and vulnerability to adverse developmental outcomes associated with poverty. *American Behavioral Scientist, 34*(4), 416–430.

Genero, N. (1995). Culture, resiliency, and mutual psychological development. In H. I. McCubbin, E. A. Thompson, A. I. Thompson, & J. A. Futrell (Eds.), *Resiliency in ethnic minority families: African-American families* (pp. 1–18). Madison: University of Wisconsin Press.

Genero, N., Miller, J. B., & Surrey, J. (1992). *The Mutual Psychological Development Questionnaire* (Project Report No. 1). Wellesley, MA: Stone Center Working Paper Series.

Gilligan, C. (1982). *In a different voice: Psychological theory and women's development.* Cambridge, MA: Harvard University Press.

Gilligan, C., Lyons, N. P., & Hanmer, T. J. (Eds.). (1990). *Making connections: The relational worlds of adolescent girls at Emma Willard School.* Cambridge, MA: Harvard University Press.

Gottman, J. M., & DeClaire, J. (2001). *The relationship cure: A five-step guide for building better connections with family, friends, and lovers.* New York: Crown.

Hartling, L. M., & Ly, J. (2000). *Relational references: A selected bibliography of theory, research, and applications* (Project Report, No. 7). Wellesley, MA: Stone Center Working Paper Series.

hooks, b. (1984). *Feminist theory from margin to center.* Boston: South End Press.

Jenkins, Y. M. (1993a). African-American women: Ethnocultural variables and dissonant expectations. In J. L. Chin, V. De La Cancela, & Y. M. Jenkins (Eds.), *Diversity in psychotherapy: The politics of race, ethnicity, and gender* (pp. 117–136). Westport, CT: Praeger.

Jenkins, Y. M. (1993b). Diversity and social esteem. In J. L. Chin, V. De La Cancela, & Y. M. Jenkins (Eds.), *Diversity in psychotherapy: The politics of race, ethnicity, and gender* (pp. 45–63). Westport, CT: Praeger.

Jenkins, Y. M. (Ed.). (1998). *Diversity in college settings: Directives for helping professionals.* New York: Routledge.

Jordan, J. V. (1992). *Relational resilience* (Work in Progress, No. 57). Wellesley, MA: Stone Center Working Paper Series.

Jordan, J. V. (1994). *A relational perspective on self esteem* (Work in Progress, No. 70). Wellesley, MA: Stone Center Working Paper Series.

Jordan, J. V. (Ed.). (1997). *Women's growth in diversity: More writings from the Stone Center.* New York: Guilford Press.

Jordan, J. V. (1999). *Toward connection and competence* (Work in Progress, No. 83). Wellesley, MA: Stone Center Working Paper Series.

Jordan, J. V., Kaplan, A. G., Miller, J. B., Stiver, I. P., & Surrey, J. L. (1991). *Women's growth in connection: Writings from the Stone Center.* New York: Guilford Press.

Liang, B., Taylor, C., Williams, L. M., Tracy, A., Jordan, J., & Miller, J. B. (1998). *The Relational Health Indices* (Work in Progress, No. 292). Wellesley, MA: Stone Center Working Paper Series.

Keller, E. F. (1985). *Reflections on gender and science.* New Haven, CT: Yale University Press.

Kobasa, S. C. (1979). Stressful life events, personality and health: An inquiry into hardiness. *Journal of Personality and Social Psychology, 37*, 1–11.

Kobasa, S. C., & Puccetti, M. C. (1983). Personality and social resources in stress resistance. *Journal of Personality and Social Psychology, 45*(4), 839–850.

Magnus, K. B., Cowen, E. L., Wyman, P. A., Fagen, D. B., & Work, W. C. (1999). Correlates of resilient outcomes among highly stressed African-American and white urban children. *Journal of Community Psychology, 27*(4), 473–488.

Masten, A. S. (1994). Resilience in individual development: Successful adaptation despite risk. In M. C. Wang & E. W. Gordon (Eds.), *Educational resilience in inner-city America: Challenges and prospects* (pp. 3–25). Hillsdale, NJ: Erlbaum.

Masten, A. S. (1999). Resilience comes of age: Reflections on the past and outlook for the next generation of research. In M. D. Glantz, J. Johnson, & L. Huffman (Eds.), *Resilience and development: Positive life adaptations* (pp. 282–296). New York: Plenum Press.

Masten, A. S. (2001). Ordinary magic: Resilience processes in development. *American Psychologist, 56*(3), 227–238.

Masten, A. S., Best, K. M., & Garmezy, N. (1990). Resilience and development: Contributions from the study of children who overcome adversity. *Development and Psychopathology, 2*, 425–444.

McIntosh, P. (1988). *White privilege and male privilege: A personal account of coming to see correspondences through work in women's studies* (Working Paper, No. 189). Wellesley, MA: Center for Research on Women.

McIntosh, P. (1989, July/August). White privilege: Unpacking the invisible knapsack. *Peace and Freedom*, pp. 10–12.

Miller, J. B. (1976). *Toward a new psychology of women.* Boston: Beacon Press.

Miller, J. B. (1986). *What do we mean by relationships?* (Work in Progress, No. 70). Wellesley, MA: Stone Center Working Paper Series.

Miller, J. B. (1988). *Connections, disconnections, and violations* (Work in Progress, No. 33). Wellesley, MA: Stone Center Working Paper Series.

Miller, J. B., Jordan, J. V., Stiver, I. P., Walker, M., Surrey, J., & Eldridge, N. (1999). *Therapists' authenticity* (Work in Progress, No. 82). Wellesley, MA: Stone Center Working Paper Series.

Miller, J. B., & Stiver, I. P. (1997). *The healing connection: How women form relationships in therapy and in life.* Boston: Beacon Press.

Minnich, E. K. (1990). *Transforming knowledge.* Philadelphia: Temple University Press.

Ornish, D. (1997). *Love and survival: The scientific basis of the healing power of intimacy.* New York: HarperCollins.

Resnick, M., Bearman, P., Blum, R., Bauman, K., Harris, K., Jones, J., Tabor, J., Beuhring, R., Sieving, R., Shew, M., Ireland, M., Bearinger, L., & Ury, J. R. (1997). Protecting adolescents from harm: Findings from the National Longitudinal Study on Adolescent Health. *Journal of the American Medical Association, 278*(10), 823–832.

Roediger, H. L., Capaldi, E. D., Paris, S. G., & Polivy, J. (1991). *Psychology.* New York: HarperCollins.

Rosen, W. B. (1992). *On the integration of sexuality: Lesbians and their mothers* (Work in Progress, No. 56). Wellesley, MA: Stone Center Working Paper Series.

Rutter, M. (1971). Parent–child separation: Psychological effects on the children. *Journal of Child Psychology and Psychiatry, 12*, 233–260.

70   DEVELOPING FEMINIST THEORIES

Rutter, M. (1978). Early sources of security and competence. In J. S. Bruner & A. Garton (Eds.), *Human growth and development* (pp. 33–61). Oxford, UK: Clarendon Press.

Rutter, M. (1979). Protective factors in children's responses to stress and disadvantage. In M. W. Kent & J. E. Rolf (Eds.), *Primary prevention of psychopathology: Vol. 3. Social competence in children* (pp. 49–74). Hanover, NH: University Press of New England.

Rutter, M. (1989). Temperament: Conceptual issues and clinical implications. In G. A. Kohnstamm, J. E. Bates, & M. K. Rothbart (Eds.), *Temperament in childhood* (pp. 463–479). Chichester, UK: Wiley.

Seifer, R., Sameroff, A. J., Dickstein, S., Keitner, G., Miller, I., Rasmussen, S., & Hayden, L. C. (1996). Parental psychopathology, multiple contextual risks, and one-year outcomes in children. *Journal of Clinical Child Psychiatry, 25*(4), 423–435.

Siegel, D. J. (1999). *The developing mind: Toward a neurobiology of interpersonal experience.* New York: Guilford Press.

Sparks, E. (1999). *Against the odds: Resistance and resilience in African American welfare mothers* (Work in Progress, No. 81). Wellesley, MA: Stone Center Working Paper Series.

Spencer, R. (2000). *A comparison of relational psychologies* (Project Report No. 6). Wellesley, MA: Stone Center Working Paper Series.

Stewart, A. (1994). Toward a feminist strategy for studying women's lives. In C. E. Franz & A. J. Stewart (Eds.), *Women creating lives: Identities, resilience, and resistance* (pp. 11–36). Boulder, CO: Westview Press.

Tavris, C. (1992). *The mismeasure of woman.* New York: Simon & Schuster.

Taylor, S. E., Klein, L. C., Lewis, B. P., Gruenewald, T. L., Gurung, R. A. R., & Updegraff, J. A. (2000). Biobehavioral responses to stress in females: Tend-and-befriend, not fight-or-flight. *Psychological Review, 107*(3), 411–429.

Walker, M. (1999). *Race, self, and society: Relational challenges in a culture of disconnection* (Work in Progress, No. 85). Wellesley, MA: Stone Center Working Paper Series.

Walker, M. (2001). *When racism gets personal* (Work in Progress, No. 93). Wellesley, MA: Stone Center Working Paper Series.

Walker, M., & Miller, J. B. (2001). *Racial images and relational possibilities* (Talking Paper, No. 2). Wellesley, MA: Stone Center Working Paper Series.

Wallerstein, J. S., & Kelly, J. B. (1980). *Surviving the breakup: How children and parents cope with divorce.* New York: Basic Books.

Werner, E. E., & Smith, R. S. (1982). *Vulnerable, but invincible: A study of resilient children.* New York: McGraw-Hill.

Chapter 4

Constructing Identities
A Feminist, Culturally Contextualized Alternative to "Personality"

KAREN L. SUYEMOTO

Brown and Ballou's *Personality and Psychopathology: Feminist Reappraisals* (1992) identified many problems with traditional personality theories from a feminist viewpoint (Espin & Gawalek, 1992; Kantrowitz & Ballou, 1992; Lerman, 1992; Okun, 1992; Romaniello, 1992). These criticisms included:

1. They use male norms, goals, and ideas of health.
2. They examine and evaluate the individual in relative isolation from the social context.
3. They fail to adequately recognize social influences and socialization, focusing instead on "human nature" which is historically gendered.
4. They fail to recognize the influence of external systemic and structural forces and the effects of power, privilege, and oppression.
5. They frequently fail to attend to the sociohistorically situated aspect of theory development (e.g., the basic acceptance of the inferiority of women) and address changes in time and context.
6. They fail to address cultural influences and relativity, assuming an ethnocentric stance of universal applicability.

A feminist postmodern constructivistic (rather than rationalistic, realistic, essentialistic, or positivistic) approach would add critiques of the imposition of external power that is implied in the definition, categorization, and measurement of personality and potentially misused in the application of personality theory to evaluations of health and pathology, and point to a need for greater emphasis on process rather than content and a nonnormative-based developmental theory (Gergen, 1999; Rigazio-DiGilio, 1997). New theory is needed to address these critiques and step away from foundations inherently fused with sexist ideology. This chapter explores an alternative theory proposing identity/self as actively self-constructed and reconstructed by an individual situated in a sociohistorical and cultural context. This construction is not internal but is inherently interdependent with others' co-constructions of both individual identity/self and the group referents that contribute to that construction.

As it is beyond the scope of this chapter to review constructivism and constructionism, I refer the reader to articles and books that attempt this daunting task (e.g., Sexton & Griffin, 1997). In this volume, Maracek's chapter presents a thorough critique of central points of personality theory from a constructivist and postmodernist viewpoint, freeing me from that task as well. Thus, this chapter begins with only a brief review of integrated constructivistic and constructionistic ideas that were used as the foundation for the current identity theory development.

AN INTRODUCTION TO THE
CONSTRUCTIVISTIC FOUNDATION

There are a great variety of constructivistic and constructionistic stances, which vary in their emphases: cognition (e.g., Lyddon, 1995; Neimeyer, 1993), developmental processes (e.g., Guidano, 1995a, 1995b, 1995c; Rigazio-DiGilio, 1997), narrative (e.g., Gonçalves, 1994; White & Epston, 1990), personal constructs (e.g., Kelly, 1955), social construction (e.g., Gergen, 1985; Wentworth & Wentworth, 1997), and so on. The variety in emphases and viewpoints perhaps should be expected, given the foundation that unifies constructivistic views: *people actively create their own realities*.[1] One creates a worldview in order to organize experience, maintaining consistency over time and situation, guiding attention, and contributing to interpretive processes. The foundation of multiple realities implies other important and relevant points such as (1) there are *multiple subjective realities*, each of which seems valid and true to the person constructing it, therefore there is *no absolute or universal truth*; (2) the creation of one's worldview or reality is ongoing, so the *process is continual*, such that subjective reality is reconstructed again and again; and (3) whether an external, "objective" reality exists is contested, with radical or strong constructivists suggesting it does not and more moderate constructivists conceding that a reality exists, but either way, as we cannot know reality directly (only through our constructions), *the existence of an "objective" reality is irrelevant*.

Constructivism, as utilized here, focuses more on process than on content. *How* people know what they know and how the meaning is created is more important than what they know specifically and, even more so, than how their knowledge or meaning parallels (or does not) an "objective" reality. But we do not construct our worldviews in a vacuum; rather, we construct our view within a sociohistorical context (Gergen, 1985, 1999; Wentworth & Wentworth, 1997). The social context has multiple levels of relationships (e.g., individual or dyadic relationships, family and group relationships, organizational and community relationships, cultural and national relationships, etc.). And the sociohistorical context is actively co-constructed within the relationships at and between these multiple levels (Gergen, 1985; Wentworth & Wentworth, 1997). The inclusion of the historical context acknowledges the changes that take place in individual and social worldviews and "truths" over time. The recognition that our constructive process is situated within and interdependent upon the social context enables a recognition that not all individual worldviews have the same influences on the social construction and the social construction does not affect all individuals in the same way (Doan, 1997; Gergen, 1985, 1999)—that is, not all realities are equally valued or validated. Thus, the existence and effect of power and privilege within and between individuals and groups is acknowledged. And this acknowledgment, combined with the basic foundation of multiple realities and its accompanying challenge to any single or universal Truth, means that taking such a constructivistic stance questions the dominant paradigm, the accepted truth, and the process through which that truth has been created, accepted, reaffirmed, and (frequently) imposed.

This kind of constructivistic foundation embraces many feminist goals and ideologies: an emphasis on multiple voices and truths; attention to the relational context and what is between people as well as what is within individuals; the validity of multiple ways of knowing and discovering; and the recognition of power differentials and their detrimental effects on individuals, groups, and societies. Using this foundation to theorize alternatives to traditional personality theories thus has the potential to address many of the feminist criticisms of these theories.

FEMINIST CONSTRUCTIVISTIC QUESTIONS OF SELF AND PERSONALITY

Given the foundation of multiple views, process rather than content, the sociohistorical context, and the consideration of structural power, many questions are raised in specific relation to personality theory. What really is personality? What is considered personality and what is considered something else (e.g., roles, situational determinants, identity, personas, socially imposed acceptable behavior, etc.)? Why are certain things considered "personality" and others not? Traditional theories of personality have within them assumptions about what is attended to and what is not, what is important and what is not, and what is considered to contribute to pathology and what to health. These assumptions are, of course, culturally and historically constructed (which means, as reviewed above, that they are usually andro- and Eurocentric).

Multiple subjective truths and worldviews call into question the idea that there can be a theoretical approach to, or understanding of, personality that is relatively universal—for example, that the personality "categories" suggested by the DSM-IV (2000) are applicable to all peoples in all cultures, or even to all peoples in one culture, with the same meanings for health and pathology. This categorizing approaches the terrain of essentialism (and a single Truth) where "personality" is constant, unchangeable, and possibly deterministic. Even developmentally focused traditional personality theories (rather than content-focused theory, e.g., Freudian or object relations developmental paths of personality) frequently assume a single or normative developmental path. This contradicts the view that we continually construct (and co-construct within social contexts) and reconstruct our own realities, which includes constructing our own "identities" or "selves" or "personality" (Rigazio-DiGilio, 1997). We also construct the *meaning* of "personality" to us and in our presentation of ourselves to others.

One of the most important questions that can be asked of traditional personality theorists is, Who gets to decide? Who determines what my (or your) personality is or is not; what is or is not generally called personality; and, perhaps most importantly, what is or is not healthy or pathological in personality? Historically, it has been psychiatrists and psychologists (traditionally male and European/white) who have the personal and social power to decide what is/is not important to attend to, based on their personally constructed experiences and views. And the personally constructed experiences and views that inform these decisions are particularly privileged ones that are strongly affected by mainstream social co-constructions, because historically these are the people who have had the privilege to become experts, to train in the established and accepted institutions as researchers, doctors, and therapists. Personality has been viewed as an objective thing that can (and should) be assessed from outside the individual (the development of "objective" personality tests is a prime example). Certainly, psychodynamic, neo-Freudian, object relations, and some rationalistic cognitive-behavioral theories have rested on assumptions that an external expert best evaluates personality tendencies, health/rationality, and pathology/ irrationality. Even humanistic personality theories that focus on the phenomenological experience (e.g., Rogers or Perl; see Lerman, 1992, for a feminist critique) have this external component, as it is rarely the individuals themselves who evaluate what is actualized, authentic, or fully "in contact."

From a feminist constructivist viewpoint, with a firm belief in egalitarian relationships and deconstructing power hierarchies that confer unearned privilege and dominance, we must question the impact of our theoretical beliefs: Does personality theory function to maintain some social constructions and not others? Does it privilege certain voices, views, and cultures? Does it pathologize socially oppressed groups such as women and racial/ethnic minorities? Does it fail to address and incorporate the social constructions of oppression and power inequities? The following view of personality as identity/self construction, co-construction, and reconstruction attempts the creation of a theory that answers "No" more than "Yes" to these questions.

Of course, any theory—even a feminist constructivistic theory—has some of the limitations discussed above because theories inevitably draw boundaries and focus attention on one thing rather than another, implying that the first thing is more important. It is not that I (as a constructivist) am proposing that we stop trying to understand the development of people, how people present to others, how people view themselves, and/or how people create relationships at multiple levels. But it is important that we fully recognize that our theories *are* constructions (Efran & Heffner, 1998), that these *are* open questions with multiple answers that are all culturally situated, and that the answers may be different for each person. Without this recognition, we will inevitably contribute to reifying some person's or group's truth over others. It is the process of constructing and continually reconstructing a worldview—always understanding this process as socially contextualized and interdependent with co-constructions—that shows more of the answer to the primary question (What is personality?), not the imposition of an outside, socially accepted construction (e.g., an accepted personality theory, label, or category). This leads to an emphasis on the developmental (but not normative) process of "personality" and an in-depth consideration of the individual in personal, social, historical, and cultural context.

IDENTITY/SELF AS PERSONALITY

Constructivism and constructionism (Dickerson & Zimmerman, 1995; Gergen, 1985) emphasize how the language we use actively contributes to (or even directly and primarily causes) the social constructions that create (and constrain) our realities. The language of "personality" is, I believe, a language that contributes to a positivistic, expert-based, power-hierarchied view. It suggests something that is separate from the person and yet has the power to define or determine the person. Both identity and personality focus on the organization of internal aspects of the person. Both contribute to coherence, helping us to define for ourselves the "kind of person we are." But the language of identity and self places the power of self-definition and organization more clearly within the subjective realm, maintaining the emphasis on the possibility of multiple views.

Historically, identity has been seen in psychology as a process (e.g., Erikson, 1968; Marcia, 1980) that entails consideration and active choice and commitment to views; this history emphasizes personal power and claiming. Identity is also a very broad area of inquiry and theorizing, which has explored both metalevels of personal identity (e.g., Blasi, 1988; Erikson, 1968) and more contextualized, specific, and group-referenced levels such as feminist identity and racial/ethnic identity (e.g., Fischer et al., 2000; Wehrley's [1995] review). This multileveled characteristic of identity allows simultaneous consideration of internal metaorganization and more contextualized, socially constructed, and referenced ideas of self; this enables incorporating a greater possibility of exploring the influence of social context in general, culture more specifically, and power and privilege associated with group membership and co-constructed identities.

What is identity? Identity is the process of trying to make sense of ourselves in the world.[2] It is one way in which we attempt to create some internal connection and continuity, so our experience of ourselves (vs. our experience of others or of the world around us, which are other constructions) is not fragmented into discrete moments of reflexive awareness and experience. While our ability to be in the moment and experience is important, it is our reflection on and explanation of that experience (James's [1890/ 1990] self as knower vs. the self as known; Guidano, 1995c) that creates the construction/map/schema that connects the moments into a seemingly coherent and consistent whole that we call our "identity" or "self" (Guidano, 1995b, 1995c; McAdams, 1997). Identity encompasses behaviors, roles, characteristics, and traits. However, because identity is an organizing *process*, it goes beyond any one behavior or characteristic to try to integrate and organize these into a sum that is greater than its parts (as in McAdams's [1997] ideas of "selfing"). So while I may teach, or have the role of a teacher, or a characteristic of openness to ideas (e.g., on the NEO-PI's scales), it is the integration of these along with other aspects and the meaning and importance that I give to them as they interact in their contributions to the identity as a whole that make me claim as one of my multiple identities an *identity* as a teacher and integrate this subidentity into my core personal identity.

Baumeister (1997) proposes that identity creation requires three processes: reflexive awareness (self-awareness, reflection), executive function (the ability to choose and the willingness to do so), and social context. The nature of the reflexive awareness changes developmentally and the awareness need not be conscious. The ability to choose is central to a feminist constructivist theory, and actively protects the theory from falling into an imposition of ideologies onto less privileged people. The social context is central, as we do not construct alone or in a social vacuum, so our choices and commitments are inevitably influenced by our relationships: individual dyadic relationships, larger group relationships, and even larger structural/ societal relationships. All of our constructions are co-constructed within our social contexts and we actively contribute to the creation of these co-constructions as well. The influence of the social context can limit available choices, either practically in terms of blocked opportunities, or psychologically, in terms of influencing the process of construction and what is available to reflexive awareness. But the individual is not helpless, for she or he can also influence and challenge the co-constructions of the social contexts. Finally, while we can talk about these three separate experiences, in the actual process of identity development they cannot be so easily separated.

Our self-understandings include both an overarching core personal identity and multiple contextual and group-referenced identities. The core personal identity is an integration of all the multiple group-referenced identities as well as other behaviors, roles, characteristics, or traits that may not have been elaborated or incorporated into one of the multiple group-referenced identities but that are seen as particularly important and self-defining. The core personal identity is the same as the central identity, core self, or basic "personality." This is, to use myself as an example, my "Karenness" (or me-ness). What distinguishes the core personal identity from the multiple group-referenced identities is that (1) it is a metalevel of organization in that it attempts to construct an identity that encompasses and integrates other identities and (2) it does not *explicitly* reference a group or external social construction. This latter point means that it emphasizes uniqueness and autonomy—no one else can claim "Karenness" (well, other folks named Karen, but this is an issue of language and the fact that names are inadequate identifiers of our unique me-ness). In addition, no one else can define or construct my "Karenness" or tell me what it ought to be or what it ought not to be. My identity is self-defined; it cannot be imposed or denied from outside (see below in "Social Context").

While my core personal identity *is* unique, this does not mean that it is essentially individualistic, in the commonly discussed meaning. It is certainly possible to have a core personal self that is collectively oriented, in that the choices made in the creation of that self are choices that reflect collective ideologies and values (e.g., the group before the individual, hierarchical relations, high-context communication, etc.). These choices are still individual choices, so the idea of a purely collective self without the coexistence of a private self is inherently disputed here.[3]

What we commonly refer to as *identities* are also parts of our core self that we emphasize at different times and in different contexts. We see them as identities because they are organized attempts at coherence and continuity that we cluster together and use to create connections (both internal and external) through the group references, just as we do with the core personal identity. We may see these as more or less stable, although one has to envision some stability and a relatively major relation to the core personal identity (salience to self, importance, etc.) in order to construct it and call it an identity and not a role: this is one manifestation of commitment and choice within our self constructions. The question of one versus multiple identities is largely one of language and attention. We seem to have multiple identities because we are emphasizing different *aspects* of our core selves, but these identities are inevitably interrelated and each affects the construction of the other, combining to contribute to the core personal identity, so they cannot really be separate. Thus, while I can talk (and think) about my identity as a multiracial person as seemingly separate from my identity as a woman/feminist that is separate from my identity as a teacher that is separate from my identity as a psychologist, actually this is a false separation. My lived experience does not have these lines drawn in it. The identities flow into one another, and largely influence the construction and lived experience of each other. Thus, I am a multiracial woman feminist teacher psychologist. My multiracial identity has been formed and reformed within my understanding of gender oppression, for example, and because I also claim these identities, my construction of my teacher identity within psychology includes a meaning that teaching psychology includes addressing oppression, fighting the silencing, and including multiple experiences. One could argue that identities that are formed first are the foundation and that others are lain upon that, suggesting a possible division. However, this is refuted by all identities being constantly reconstructed; each identity that we currently hold affects and permeates all others in our continuous reconstruction.

The separation of identities is an artifact partly related to language and our need to categorize and draw boundaries in order to describe, and partly related to social context. In order to talk/think about and/or define identities, we need to create these boundaries in our language. In order to share our *knowledge* (not experience) of them, we need to have words with referents, which means words that mean some thing(s) and not others. As we try to think and communicate about how these identities are constructed and the social construction influence, we create a tension, because we must maintain the constructions in order to use language in the process of trying to destroy them—for example, by talking about deconstructing race while using the language of racial groups and divisions or discussing gender-bending while using gendered language. When you draw boundaries, you reify what you are putting the boundaries around. When you try to deconstruct the boundaries using the language that establishes the boundaries, you reify them as well[4] (Kitzinger, 1995).

The Development of Identity

The core personal identity is that part of ourselves that we *construct* as central to the "I," that part or those identities and/or characteristics that we *see* as continuous, stable, and centrally defining and that we organize into a whole. However, it should not be forgotten that the central identity is created and re-created over time (McAdams, 1997); it too is *continually* constructed. While we may *think* that the central identity is unchanging, this is not really the case (Gonçalves, 1994; McAdams, 1997), which is part of how and why psychotherapy works (Guidano, 1995c). Certainly, our central identity changes developmentally from birth and basic self-awareness through childhood, adolescence, adulthood, and old age, as our social contexts, cognitive capabilities, physical abilities, spirituality, goals, and so on, change (Guidano, 1995a).

One criticism of traditional developmental and personality theories is that they focus almost exclusively on the individual (and sometimes the family), not attending enough to the context and social situation in a larger sense (Rigazio-DiGilio, 1997). Initially, as infants, our sense of identity is developed primarily familially because we are physically and emotionally family-based and also because cognitive capabilities such as categorization and abstraction do not develop until later (Guidano, 1995a, 1995b). As we expand our social contexts and develop the ability to categorize, we further organize our own self-constructions, developing reference groups (and nonreference groups) through noting similarities and differences. Our developing reflexive awareness thus begins to incorporate an examination of ourselves in active relation not only to individuals (e.g., within the family) but also to socially constructed group identities (Thoits & Virshup, 1997). We begin to construct our multiple group-referenced identities to help order and label these different organizations of parts of our core personal identity. But even before this time the larger social structure has a large influence as the meanings that are created within our families are inevitably affected, contextualized, and co-constructed by the larger social context, including social structures and systems of oppression (Rigazio-DiGilio, 1997). Our own and our parents' ideas of family are, like all else, socially contextualized.

Because abstraction and full reflexive awareness are not cognitive capabilities of young children, one might say that in children, the identity/ies are not yet formed, much as some traditional personality theory sees personality as in development in children and not fully formed until adolescence or adulthood. Meaning making—including the making meaning of our self-views that is called here the development of the core personal identity—is an ongoing developmental process. Development occurs through continual transformations in meaning (Carlsen, 1995; Rigazio-DiGilio, 1997), including changes in meaning or reevaluations due to increased cognitive capacity (e.g., the development of abstraction; see Guidano, 1995a). But the development of identity even in children does not follow a particular path or progress through specific stages. Because of the emphasis on awareness and choice, a constructivistically based view of identity and de-velopment explicitly steps away from the linear and hierarchical nature of developmental stages and the ways in which these stages and traditional de-velopmental theory prescribe a "normal" ideal (Rigazio-DiGilio, 1997). Even young children have some self-awareness and create their own devel-opmentally situated understanding of who they are (I am a sister, I like chocolate, I am in first grade, etc.; see Blasi & Milton, 1991; Guidano, 1995a). While some aspects of this *process* (e.g., object constancy or con-crete operations) may be common across children at particular ages, the meaning that each child gives to that process in her or his context inevita-bly varies considerably.

In spite of (or perhaps also because of) this continual reconstruction, we perceive continuity within ourselves, as we reconstruct our past stories and memories *to accord with* our current construction of our core personal identity (e.g., selective memories of the past, slightly changing stories or versions of events; see Gonçalves, 1994). We may subtly change our mean-ings over time in order to create this consistency, even as we may also rec-ognize major changes or differences that we see as less central. In extreme cases, we may see our core identity as changing so significantly that we view our past self constructions as false or externally imposed. The idea of a "false self" or an "inauthentic personality" is therefore understood as rooted in the experience of the self being reconstructed through current reflexive awareness and executive function in a way that seems so different than what was seen as core before that the prior construction is rejected as false. If one is aware of having a false self at the time one has it, it is not seen as "self" or "identity" even at that time, but rather as something foreign, a mask one dons or a role one plays. If one sees a false self only in retrospect, then it is a reconstruction; it is likely that most people who had a "false self" once thought at the time that it was their true self.

But what of those particular traits or characteristics that are seemingly part of who we are in that others (and perhaps even ourselves) see how they influence our behaviors, thinking, and feeling, and yet we do not see them as necessarily positive and may actively *not* claim them when we con-sider them consciously in isolation? Are these part of our core personal identity? If so, doesn't that refute the idea that we actively create our core personal construct through processes of consideration and choice within a social context? These questions stem from the assumptions that consider-ation and choice must take place on a conscious level and that it is possible to consider particular traits or characteristics in isolation for acceptance or rejection. Part of this assumption is related to the language of identity being used in this theory; traditional identity theory (e.g., Erikson, 1968; Marcia, 1980) has seemed to focus primarily on *conscious* consideration in a moratorium stage, and referenced identity theories have traditionally seemed to examine particular kinds of identity in relative isolation (e.g., ethnic/racial identity in isolation; see Root, 1997). But this current theory that uses the idea of identity as an overarching self-organizing construct that is self-created encompasses a more comprehensive and less focused approach and, with a constructivistic foundation, does not need to assume that consideration and choice take place consciously.

Mahoney and Gabriel (1987) describe how a cognitive constructivistic view embraces a greater incorporation of unconscious processes and possibilities. Guidano (1995c), Neimeyer (1993), and Arnkoff (1980) emphasize the interconnectedness and interdependence of the beliefs, stories, and views that we use to construct our worldview and, in this case, our core personal identity. Arnkoff (1980) and Gonçalves and Craine (1990) go on to discuss how much of the knowledge we have about ourselves and the world is tacit knowledge; they focus on how we use this knowledge to create "deep structures," similar to core constructs, which are frequently unconscious. The core personal identity construct is not, of course, a singular simple entity. It is instead a complex process and pattern of interconnections. Parts of this pattern and process likely begin their construction before we have full reflexive awareness and the cognitive capacity for fully conscious or explicit executive function and informed choice. And parts of the construct that may be seen as undesirable will also be tacitly connected so strongly to other parts that are valued that they cannot be easily changed without first changing the belief that the parts are inevitably connected.

Take, for example, a person who is bothered by an inability to take risks and try new relationships, resulting in a relatively lonely existence. This person might be seen on a personality scale as being introverted or having low openness; this approach looks at this "trait" in relative isolation. If one were to ask this person if she or he wanted to be that way (i.e., if she or he has chosen that trait), she or he will likely deny this and may even expound at length about the ways in which she or he has tried to change this. At the conscious level she or he experiences this "trait" as dystonic, dysfunctional, and possibly imposed. And yet it may eventually become clear that she or he also has a belief that to try to make new relationships is to be emotionally unsafe, accompanied by a high value on the feeling of safety, and/or a belief that she or he has little to give and trying to make new relationships will inevitably lead to disappointment and the confirmation of how interpersonally undesirable she or he really is. The person may therefore make an unconscious evaluation (or have made this evaluation much earlier and never fully reevaluated it) that it is better to be uncomfortably introverted than to be interpersonally rejected. And each of these beliefs and evaluations is connected and entwined with others because no belief or choice stands on its own but all are contextualized and informed by the overall worldview or story (see Contratto, Chapter 2, this volume). Furthermore, we can easily imagine several developmental and interpersonal scenarios that might have contributed to this small pattern, many of which may have taken place in early childhood. This example is a gross oversimplification of the complexity of the pattern and does not even touch on the way the content (the pattern) interacts with the process choices. But it does serve to illustrate how a seemingly not chosen and denied aspect of self may indeed be chosen and considered at some level.

The vast interconnectedness, the importance of context, and the likelihood of unconscious processing make it difficult to ever truly comprehend the full core identity construct. One never sees this fullness in another, as it is only the surface manifestation that is displayed, and inevitably only that part that is most salient to the current time, situation, and social context (Arnkoff, 1980). Similarly, one never fully comprehends the fullness of oneself either, as attention is a focusing process that inevitably creates boundaries within. Thus, to measure a particular "trait" or "type" is problematic without stressing the situational nature of that measurement and recognizing the context of other meanings for the individual (personal internal meanings, as well as interpersonal and broader social contexts that are co-constructed). An example of how multiple levels of context might interact in understanding constructed meaning is that of relational orientation in a given woman. Perhaps she is highly relational because she has actively chosen to be this way and would have done so in any context; or perhaps she is relational because she was expected to care for her siblings and developed these skills and feelings; or perhaps she is relational because she is expected to be so by society and wants to succeed socially, so she acquiesces by choice; or perhaps she is relational because she is oppressed by the social system of sexism and patriarchy and a relational orientation is part of her unconscious survival strategy. Or perhaps these are all correct at different times, in different situations, or all at once.

Social Context at Multiple Levels: Relationships, Power, and Privilege

Identity is the process of trying to make sense of ourselves *in the world*. As such, it is a process not only of trying to understand ourselves, but also of trying to understand ourselves *in social contexts*. This means understanding ourselves in relationship not only to other particular people such as our family in developmental processes (although this is very important) but also (1) in relation to groups and ideas (e.g., the idea of "feminist," which seems to unify the group) and (2) in relation to social structures and co-constructed meanings at multiple levels.[5]

I have been discussing the development of the core personal identity as something that the individual does through reflexive awareness and choice; the language necessary for this discussion implies that this may be an individual process. But it is impossible to have a truly individual process or to make a totally individual choice. Everything we do and think is socially contextualized: "knowledge is not something people process somewhere in their heads, but rather, something people do together" (Gergen, 1985, p. 270). Our worldviews from birth are constructed in relation to other people. Our meanings are shaped by other people's meanings. And by "other people's meanings" we must mean more than what particular individuals in our lives think or believe. We must also look at group co-constructed meanings as well as structures and systems that are a given society's constructed meanings. And we must realize that these co-constructed meanings not only *influence* our individual, internal constructions (in this case, our core personal identity), but also actively *create* and constrain these constructions. Co-constructed meanings are created between people, in the language, space, and process of their interactions (Dickerson & Zimmerman, 1995; Gergen, 1985, 1999; Rigazio-DiGilio, 1997; Wentworth & Wentworth, 1997). So, while we speak of the construction of a core personal identity as something the individual does, it is actually an interdependent process between all individuals, all "individual" meanings, and the shared meanings created by groups in the space between.

Thus far, I have been focusing primarily on the core personal identity construct and have mentioned only briefly the existence of multiple identities that are group-referenced. The interactions between the individual and the social context may be easier to see with these multiple, explicitly group-referenced identities, as the shared meanings are relatively bounded and placed in the foreground. Multiple identities, like the core personal identity, both create and are created by the social meaning construct that is co-constructed in a reciprocal manner with others—in the case of multiple identities, particularly others who claim the same or similar identities. Reference groups have their own group identities co-constructed by the group members and, like the individual identities we have been discussing, constantly being reconstructed. An individual's group-referenced identity will likely include some aspects of the group identity, or at least some aspects of another group's view of that identity (see discussion of defining in opposition, below).

In terms of creating an individual group-referenced identity, as we categorize and organize our world and our self-view, we use our reflexive awareness to consider what characteristics create affinities between some people (the ingroup) and not others (the outgroup). We then consider these characteristics within ourselves, in terms of their fit with other identities and characteristics and the way we organize these within a core personal identity. If I consider my core personal identity to reflect or embrace the affinity characteristics as a particular organized unit, I may then claim and construct a specific group-referenced identity and integrate this subunit into my core personal identity; if not, I may actively *not* construct that identity.

If I construct the group-referenced identity through a process of seeing similarities and acceptance by the group, then I am defining myself *in relation* to others and actively integrating the group's co-constructed meaning of group membership into my self-view—my core personal identity—through the construction of the group-referenced identity. One may also define oneself *in opposition* to others, as when we use reflexive awareness to consider, at the individual as well as at the group level, what we are not as well as what we are. External categorizations without active group acceptance (either due to group rejection or to the absence of the reference group) frequently lead to defining in opposition. In these cases, the meaning of what we are is linked to the social co-constructions of exclusionary meanings, as opposed to social co-constructions of shared meanings—for example, "I am not white" is the experience/reflection that may then lead to "I am a person of color."

Most identities are created through both processes—that of relation as well as that of opposition—in the inevitable process of drawing boundaries in the organizing attempt. However, when we define ourselves primarily in relation or primarily in opposition, it can have implications for the personal and social effects of the identities we create. Identities created primarily in relation contribute to social connection; the process inherently includes other people that help one understand and construct parts of the core personal identity through the offered explicit co-constructions of the meanings of the shared identity. But these identities may be less individually considered and integrated, and more strongly influenced by group co-constructions and agreed upon social meanings. And an ingroup may accept a person and expect her or him to develop or already have developed a particular identity (e.g., people of color who have a strong identity as such may expect other people of color to have a similar viewpoint and will be taken aback or even be judgmental when a given person only accepts the label but has not developed the identity) or to have particular shared meanings to that identity. Alternatively, identities created primarily in opposition are frequently isolating in that they are created in the context of social exclusion and the individual will need to construct her or his own meaning of the identity without the support of the ingroups' social constructions of meaning. While this can possibly be liberating, it can also be more difficult, as the individual will continue to be subject to the outgroups' social constructions about the ingroup, which can be quite negative.

To make this more concrete: I can define *in relation* as a multiracial person. If I grew up in San Francisco, I would probably have had an ingroup: I would have likely been exposed to many more multiracial folks, seen media, shared experiences, belonged to groups, and so on. I might have been exposed to group constructions of the meaning of a multiracial identity—for example, a bridge between two cultures, the wave of the future, the best of both worlds. I may also have had a particular view of being multiracial; I may have said "Hapa" instead of multiracial and drawn my boundary around Asian multiracials only, not considering as consciously the larger connections. Currently I do define in relation, but this came only after many years of self-definition mostly in the social context of exclusion—that is, defining *in opposition*. Defining *in opposition* as a multiracial person means not having the ingroup available (growing up in Boston in the 1970s), and negotiating the identity partly in response to the outgroup's demands (in this case the dominant white group first and then the minority Asian group). I can be told in a variety of ways that I'm not white, I'm not Asian, and that people don't know how to categorize me in the traditional race boxes. Because I don't have an ingroup referent (a group of other multiracial folks), I have to figure out for myself what this means. I have to find my own label and language (How to answer "What are you?"). While doing this, I am continually subjected to the more dominant (the outgroup in relation to me, in this case both the white and Asian groups) group's view of being multiracial. Thus, I have to define the identity for myself while negotiating outgroup messages that being multiracial means being confused, being different, being exotic, being strange, being too assimilated, being impure, and the like. It may be harder to define in opposition, although the ingroups' social constructions may be limiting and oppressive to the individual as well.

An identity cannot be imposed or denied from outside. If the ingroup, members of the ingroup, or anyone else asserts that I have the affinity characteristics or "belong" to a particular group, this does not necessarily mean that I will claim the identity and integrate this meaning into my understanding of who I am. And if a person or group excludes me from their group, that does not inevitably mean that I will not claim that identity. I may need to continually validate my claim to the group or I may be completely ostracized and rejected, but I may nonetheless maintain a group-referenced identity to this rejecting group that I see as central to my self-understanding. For instance, I may claim a Japanese American identity even if the group excludes me. If confronted with some other person's construction of us that is different, new, or dissonant with our own, we use reflexivity to consider it and either reject the other's construction or change our own (unifying all three of Baumeister's root experiences in one act of change). This is one of the major differences between this theory and traditional personality theory where one can have traits or types that are not chosen or considered.

While it is true that an identity cannot be imposed or denied from outside, this does not mean that the acceptance or rejection of the reference group, or the categorization by another group, does not matter. Within social contexts, there are multiple levels of interactions and co-constructions. To simplify, there is the individual (e.g., a multiracial African European American woman), a particular reference group (e.g., the African American group), other groups that are possibly larger or more powerful and that may or may not also be reference groups (e.g., the white/European dominant group), and a larger social/cultural/systemic structure within which these groups exist (e.g., U.S. society and "American" culture).[6] Each of these affects the meanings that are created by the others and each of these also can resist the effects of the others. Those individuals, groups, or systems with more power have more influence and more ability to resist change from others; those with less have less. Frequently, we attend more to how the group affects the individual or the society affects the group (downward influence), but the individual may also affect the group and the group may also affect larger societal meanings (upward influence).

When a group actively identifies an individual as "one of us," this affects the way the individual understands her- or himself in relation to the world, encouraging the consideration of possible affinity characteristics in an attempt to understand the meaning of the social interactions. Similarly, when a person is continuously categorized as "not one of us" (e.g., by a larger or more powerful group), she or he will find it socially necessary to apply *some* reflexive awareness to the categorization. The meanings that the individual makes about the group-referenced characteristics (e.g., race) may then be shifted by their exposure to others' meanings, particularly because all of these meanings are connected to other shared and co-constructed meanings and webs of meanings developed in a shared general context (e.g., the U.S. context and its overarching ideologies about race).

In both defining in relation and defining in opposition, the multiple levels of social context and the individual choice process of identity construction have been in relative accord. The ingroup has accepted the relational identity definition process or the outgroup has agreed upon the exclusion leading to the oppositional identity definition process. But one can claim and develop a contested group-referenced identity in *opposition to the ingroup's acceptance* and/or in *relation to the outgroup's exclusion.*[7] Whether and why one may choose to do so is likely related to other aspects of the core personal identity, as well as to the power and privilege of the individual and/or groups. It is also related to the social contexts' resistance to that claim, for while the social context (at any level—social system, group level, familial or dyadic interaction) cannot explicitly deny an identity (which is self-constructed and chosen), it can attempt to limit choice or influence the individual construction. It can also impose severe penalties for the public claiming or enactment of a contested identity (although nothing can be done about *internal* claiming, which is why identity cannot truly be denied). Claiming an identity that grossly contradicts agreed-upon social constructions will likely lead to social exclusion from *both* the ingroup and the outgroup, so it tends to be a lonely and isolated kind of choice unless the chosen affinity group comes to accept the identification and possibly change its own self-definition.

An example of a contested identity is a multiracial African European American woman who identifies as white while being externally categorized by both the European American white group and the African American group as black. She may be choosing a white identity in order to access structural power and privilege accorded to white people above people of color in a given society and historical time. Or she may be choosing a white identity because she feels a greater affinity with white people. Or she may be choosing a white identity to make a political statement about race categories and change. Her reason(s) may affect both how she displays this chosen identity and how susceptible it is to change under the influence of various social contexts. The way that these social contexts perceive her reason may also be important, as this may affect their response and whether her choice is seen as healthy or pathological within a particular social and historical context. In earlier eras, this identification may have been contested practically by the dominant white European American group by punishing

this woman's attempt at "passing" (claiming a white identity) by ostraciz-
ing, enslaving, or jailing her. Her family may have received similar treatment from the white society. In current days, she may still be ostracized,
questioned, or challenged. She may also be ostracized by the African American community for "selling out" (although note that the minority community has never had the structural power to impose the more severe legal/
physical penalties). Confronted with the repeated negative consequences of
her identification, her feelings of affinity may begin to change, affecting her
self-view and the construction of her identity. While the connection to
"personality" may seem vague, there are certainly many personality attributes historically associated with race and racialized gender that would accompany these social constructions and identities (e.g., conscientiousness,
personal drive and ambition, amiability, nurturance, etc.).

Choices can also be limited in a more intrapsychic manner. An example here is childhood trauma or neglect, where the development of reflexive
awareness itself is discouraged and derailed by the coping mechanisms necessary to survive (e.g., dissociation). A related example is the insidious
trauma of racism where the individual may internalize so much of the negative message that the traumatic effect is similar (Comas-Díaz, 2000; Root,
1992), closing off reflexive awareness and critical thinking, as well as the
possibility of alternative views. While the multiracial African European
American woman in the previous example *could* choose to identify as multiracial or as European American, centuries of oppression, and social and
legal institutionalization of the one-drop rule, may have such a strong effect
on the social co-constructions around and within her that she may not even
be aware of these possibilities.

These examples of influence and constraint clearly affect the identity
formation of the individual, but they also illustrate how group identity constructs can be influenced and constrained by larger or more powerful
groups, and the larger holding social structure and historical context. More
powerful groups can attempt to punish less powerful groups for certain
kinds of ingroup definitions through physical, social, and legal means (e.g.,
feminists were/are attacked, ostracized, vilified in the media, etc., for their
ingroup definitions of women as powerful, worthy, etc.). And sociohistorical co-constructions embedded in our society can be used to privilege some voices over others. In the example above, the dominant white
group's definition of African Americans as anyone with "one drop" and the
dominant groups' oppression of the group may have influenced the minority African American group's definition of itself and its potential members.
The power and privilege constructed and maintained by the dominant

group's definitions affects the co-constructed meanings of claiming particular identities within the minority group. This may lead the African American minority group to disallow a simultaneous multiracial or European American identity, which in turn influences the identity construction of the particular African American woman. At the group level of interactions, reflexive awareness may also be constrained through the deflection of attention, as when media and historical attention is focused on interminority conflict to divert attention from the dominant–minority oppression and the privilege and power of the dominant group (e.g., recent Korean American–African American conflict; encouraging conflict between working-class whites and African Americans; dividing race and gender issues). It is important to remember that just as our identity construction choices are not necessarily conscious, the ways in which we contribute to co-constructions influencing others and constraining others' choices may not be conscious either.

Thus far we have been focusing primarily on social influence from larger and more powerful social systems to smaller ones. But it is important to consider not only the downward influence, but also the upward influence, as herein lies the potential for the less powerful to effect change. Claiming a group-contested identity can be a primary way of challenging the boundaries and oppressive definitions of ingroups. As mentioned above, I can claim an identity as a Japanese American. Especially in the past, many Japanese American ingroups would not have accepted my identification because part of the co-constructed affinity characteristics used by the group to define itself was being monoracial. It is partly through continuing identity claims by multiracial Japanese Americans that the ingroup's definition is beginning to change (King & DaCosta, 1996). The socially co-constructed meaning of the group identity is influenced by the individual.

Claiming interacting identities or focusing on another identity in a given context can also challenge the boundaries and possibly contest the socially co-constructed ingroup meanings—for example, focusing on being a person of color in a feminist group can challenge the historically implicit meaning of "feminist" as white. In addition, the *interaction* of two (or more) specific group-referenced claimed identities is both a personal meaning-making process (internal—reflexive awareness and executive function) and also a social contextual issue, as, for example, where the socially constructed meaning of being a feminist is different for different racial/ethnic groups and therefore affects the personal meaning-making and identity process of those who claim that identity and also affects the co-constructed meaning of the groups themselves.

At all the multiple levels of interaction and change, power and privilege affect the constructions. Groups and individuals with more power have a greater likelihood of being able to self-define with little constraint from other groups or individuals. Groups that consist primarily of individuals who have more power and privilege in other referent groups will be influenced by that interaction as well. Individuals who have more power in one referent group may also have an undue influence on defining the meanings in another referent group (e.g., middle-class white women who have class/race power may have undue influence in defining feminism). Groups or individuals with less power will have to struggle more with imposed definitions and constrained choices that may interact within the individual and the groups with which she or he identifies (e.g., an Asian American lesbian working-class feminist; see Allison [1996], Kadi [1996], and Lee [1996] for further discourse about interactions and constrained meanings within groups). The desire to maintain power and privilege may lead more powerful or dominant individuals and groups to continue co-constructing social ideologies (e.g., meritocracy) that deflect attention from the process of oppression or decrease their own (as well as others') reflexive awareness. The same desire may lead groups and individuals within groups to resist attempts at upward change coming from within-group individuals.

Because power and privilege are relative, oppressed groups with relatively more power than some other groups, subgroups, or individuals may use similar strategies to maintain the amount of power and privilege they do have. A primary strategy to do this is to continually reconstruct the meaning of the group identity in a way that draws strict boundaries and excludes others. This, inevitably, leads to the tension of needing to maintain group boundaries to retain or establish political power while recognizing that the creation of these boundaries is part of what causes the oppression in the first place and therefore what needs to be deconstructed to truly change the political climate (Kitzinger, 1995). A possible solution would be to advance multiple definitions that include while also attempting to maintain the ingroup privilege—for example, maintaining the "strict" definition of GLB while creating a new referent of gender and "sexually oppressed peoples" to include transgendered people. This might be a way to begin to share power without "outraging" the most dominant group so that the power the GLB community has created is maintained rather than threatened. It is important to remember here that all of these maneuvers are necessary because those who truly have power and privilege (heterosexual middle-/upper-class white men) don't want to share it.

The social context clearly directly affects the construction of multiple group-referenced identities. These identities are integrated and constructed within the web of meanings associated with the core personal identity. In addition, all characteristics (even if not explicitly linked to an identity) that are integrated into the core personal identity are developed within the social context, if not in relation to a specific socially defined reference group, then in relation to the family, other dyadic or group relationships, or the meanings co-constructed at the societal level. In contrast to traditional views of personality, identity is actively constructed and chosen, but—also in contrast—there is an immense influence at all levels of the social contexts and their attending issues of power and privilege.

CONCLUSION AND IMPLICATIONS FOR THERAPY

Identity is the continual *process* of constructing and integrating the meanings considered and chosen within a constantly changing social, cultural, political, and historical context. Identity is always created in social context, and is therefore inherently affected by ingroup and outgroup meanings, references, comparisons, exclusions, and boundaries. Because social contexts are multilayered, identity at all levels is also affected by larger sociohistorical systemic meanings and the power and privilege that are afforded or restricted based on these meanings. Finally, because the meanings of social contexts themselves are co-constructed by individuals, these meanings can be challenged and changed and the influence of these meanings on individuals' identity development can therefore also be shifted.

Theorizing identity rather than personality challenges the ideas of self-organization (personality or identity) as deterministic and individualistic, the imposition of outside judgments and constructions, and the myth that all individuals have the same options for personal development and organization structures. Traditional personality theories have often been criticized as ethno- and androcentric, creating ideas of healthy personality from traits and characteristics seen as desirable for European (American) white males. Individuals who are neither white nor male were then judged against these theories, with no attention paid to the social contexts (both oppressed and dominant contexts) that considerably changed the meanings accorded to the traits and characteristics of "health." Theorizing identity instead allows the meanings of the traits and characteristics to be contextualized in the developmental and social realities of each individual. Developmentally, theorizing identity as the primary means of self-organization emphasizes the continual reconstruction and the interconnectedness of characteristics and choices. For therapy, this approach holds a promise of hope, for if we are continually reconstructing ourselves and our stories, then nothing is deterministic and unchangeable. It also suggests an openness to developmental focus and information, an awareness of deep structures as well as surface enactments, and a questioning of "resistance" as possibly a healthy reaction to an overly isolating approach that fails to attend to the connected meanings of targeted change. Finally, the developmental aspects of theorizing identity for self-organization suggest that we approach traditional "objective" personality testing with considerable care, as this process inherently isolates characteristics that may not be able to be fully understood out of developmental and social context.

Socially, theorizing identity as the primary means of self-organization emphasizes that all constructs are co-constructs, including the continual reconstructing of the core personal identity and multiple group-referenced identities. For therapists, this points to the need to attend to their own identities. The power therapists hold in their role affects the co-construction of therapy and identities affected by therapy; awareness of this power as well as the effects of prior social co-constructions for both the therapist and the client are imperative for nonoppressive therapy; "the personal is political" and the first step to cultural competence is self-awareness (Wehrley, 1995). The social contextualizing aspect of theorizing identity also affects the way therapists view the health and behavior of their clients, as it emphasizes the co-constructed meanings that affect choices and reflexive consciousness, including the group and societal pathologies (e.g., sexism, racism, homophobia, economic oppression) with which each particular individual contends. Therapists need to judge health within this social contextualizing, thereby recognizing that healthy "personality" or identity construction will inevitably look different for each person. Furthermore, because it is recognized that the individual's choices may be constrained and that the contexts may be oppressive, health and pathology can also be considered at multiple levels. A "personality trait" that may be unhealthy for a more privileged person may be quite adaptive for someone who is considerably more oppressed (e.g., "cultural paranoia" in African Americans [Sue & Sue, 1999] or less emotional expression in Asian Americans [Uba, 1994]). And perhaps it is not the individual that is unhealthy, but rather the group or the society. Theorizing identity points to the social contexts' responsibility for growth and health, making it clear that social change, not just individual change, is needed.

ACKNOWLEDGMENTS

This chapter owes much to ideas co-constructed with the students in my first Constructing Identities class: Claudia Fox Tree-McGrath, Xóchitl Kountz, Tammy Leary, Atsushi Matsumoto, Robert Su Prescott, and Steven Saranga. I thank them for the opportunity to teach and learn with them. I also want to thank Pata Suyemoto and Claudia Fox-Tree McGrath for their suggestions and edits, and Mary Ballou for her continual encouragement to think beyond.

NOTES

1. See Mahoney (1991), Mahoney and Lyddon (1988), Sexton (1997), and Shreiner and Lyddon (1998) for discussions of the historical and philosophical context and development of the basic constructivistic ideologies, including those presented here.

2. While this chapter focuses primarily on the self and socially constructed identity, I need to introduce a brief tangent here. In order to consider what identity is, one must also consider what it is not. Identity is not essential, but the possibility of the existence of an essential aspect that affects identity must be considered. In traditional personality theory, this essential aspect may be discussed as "human nature," separated from any discussion of spirituality and theorized as displayed as those parts of the personality that are inherent and unchangeable. This is different than those parts that are unconsciously created or accepted. But the idea of "human nature" comes mighty close to the idea of the "soul" when historically situated (see Danziger, 1997). While I do not believe in a deterministic (and gendered) human nature, I do believe it is important to recognize the possibility of a spiritual aspect, particularly given the strong influence of religion and spirituality on the majority of people now and throughout history and also in order to break down the traditional (constructed) boundaries between mind and body and soul, between psychology and spirituality, that contribute to the idea of objectivity and science as the major (or only) vehicle toward knowing "reality" or "Truth." Identity (or personality) is not something separated from the spiritual self.

3. As an aside, I must note that generally the whole identity construct is culturebound and, of course, I can only construct my ideas and models from my own personal/cultural/historically situated stance.

4. Special thanks to Peter Parker for pointing me in this direction.

5. We must also recognize the context of time and historical situating, not only within the individual (i.e., developmentally), but also historically, as this influences the meaning of co-constructions and creates the social context. For example, in Brown and Ballou's edited volume, Okun (1992) discussed the need to evaluate object relations personality theory from both the zeitgeist of the original time it was developed and from the current zeitgeist with its very different views of gender, human nature, and relationships. Specific to identity theory, Danziger (1997) has a fascinating chapter on the historical view of identity and

self, reflecting upon how the current construct with its definition including re-flexivity, choice, and executive function is a relatively new one that is in signifi-cant contrast to earlier ideas of self as soul or self-reflection as self-centeredness. While the importance of the historical context is noted here, it is beyond the scope of this chapter to explore it in depth.

6. Of course, there are other groups as well, including many other reference groups, some of which will be more or less privileged, in relation to the refer-ence group we are discussing here (the African American group), in relation to each other, and in relation to other groups that are not reference groups. These groups may contribute (or not) to other multiple identities.

7. This, of course, is another example of the social construction of reality. The lan-guage of ingroup and outgroup suggests that only certain people have access and others do not. It is less discussed who has the power to determine which groups are ingroups and which outgroups for a given person or group of people. If one identifies with what others consider an outgroup, then is it an ingroup (personal perspective) or an outgroup (social perspective)?

REFERENCES

Allison, D. (1996). A question of class. In I. E. Rosenblum & T. C. Travis (Eds.), *The meaning of difference: American constructions of race, sex and gender, social class, and sexual orientation* (pp. 188–193). New York: McGraw-Hill.

American Psychiatric Association. (2000). *Diagnostic and statistical manual of mental disorders* (4th ed.). Washington, DC: Author.

Arnkoff, D. B. (1980). Psychotherapy from the perspective of cognitive theory. In M. J. Mahoney (Ed.), *Psychotherapy process: Current issues and future directions* (pp. 339–361). New York: Plenum Press.

Baumeister, R. F. (1997). The self and society: Changes, problems, and opportunities. In R. D. Ashmore & L. J. Jussim (Eds.), *Self and identity: Fundamental issues* (pp. 191–217). New York: Oxford University Press.

Blasi, A. (1988). Identity and the development of the self. In D. K. Lapsley & F. C. Power (Eds.), *Self, ego, and identity: Integrative approaches* (pp. 226–242). New York: Springer-Verlag.

Blasi, A., & Milton, K. (1991). The development of the sense of self in adolescence. *Journal of Personality, 59*, 217–242.

Carlsen, M. B. (1995). Meaning-making and creative aging. In R. A. Neimeyer & M. J. Mahoney (Eds.), *Constructivism in psychotherapy* (pp. 127–153). Washington, DC: American Psychological Association.

Comas-Díaz, L. (2000). An ethnopolitical approach to working with people of color. *American Psychologist, 55*, 1319–1325.

Danziger, K. (1997). The historical formation of selves. In R. D. Ashmore & L. J. Jussim (Eds.), *Self and identity: Fundamental issues* (pp. 137–159). New York: Oxford University Press.

Dickerson, V. C., & Zimmerman, J. L. (1995). A constructionist exercise in anti-pathologizing. *Journal of Systemic Therapies, 14*, 33–45.

Doan, R. E. (1997). Narrative therapy, postmodernism, social constructionism, and constructivism: Discussion and distinctions. *Transactional Analysis Journal, 27,* 128–133.

Efran, J. S., & Heffner, K. P. (1998). Is constructivist psychotherapy epistemologically flawed? *Journal of Constructivist Psychology, 11,* 89–103.

Erikson, E. (1968). *Identity: Youth and crisis.* New York: Norton.

Espin, O. M., & Gawalek, M. A. (1992). Women's diversity: Ethnicity, race, class, and gender in theories of feminist psychology. In L. S. Brown & M. Ballou (Eds.), *Personality and psychopathology: Feminist reappraisals* (pp. 88–108). New York: Guilford Press.

Fischer, A. R., Tokar, D. M., Mergl, M. M., Good, G. E., Hill, M. S., & Blum, S. A. (2000). Assessing women's feminist identity development: Studies of convergent, discriminant, and structural validity. *Psychology of Women Quarterly, 24,* 15–29.

Gergen, K. J. (1985). The social constructionist movement in modern psychology. *American Psychologist, 40,* 266–275.

Gergen, K. J. (1999). *The place of the psyche in a constructed world* [Online]. Available: *http://www.swarthmore.edu/SocSci/kgergen1/manu.html* [2001, January 2].

Gonçalves, O. F. (1994). From epistemological truth to existential meaning in cognitive narrative psychotherapy. *Journal of Constructivist Psychology, 7,* 107–118.

Gonçalves, O. F., & Craine, M. H. (1990). The use of metaphors in cognitive therapy. *Journal of Cognitive Psychotherapy, 4,* 135–149.

Guidano, V. F. (1995a). A constructivist outline of human knowing processes. In M. J. Mahoney (Ed.), *Cognitive and constructive psychotherapies: Theory, research and practice* (pp. 89–101). New York: Springer/American Psychological Association.

Guidano, V. F. (1995b). Constructivist psychotherapy: A theoretical framework. In R. A. Neimeyer & M. J. Mahoney (Eds.), *Constructivism in psychotherapy* (pp. 93–108). Washington, DC: American Psychological Association.

Guidano, V. F. (1995c). Self-observation in constructivist psychotherapy. In R. A. Neimeyer & M. J. Mahoney (Eds.), *Constructivism in psychotherapy* (pp. 155–168). Washington, DC: American Psychological Association.

James, W. (1890/1990). *Principles of psychology.* New York: Holt.

Kadi, J. (1996). *Thinking class: Sketches from a cultural worker.* Boston: South End Press.

Kantrowitz, R. E., & Ballou, M. (1992). A feminist critique of cognitive-behavioral therapy. In L. S. Brown & M. Ballou (Eds.), *Personality and psychopathology: Feminist reappraisals* (pp. 70–87). New York: Guilford Press.

Kelly, G. A. (1955). *The psychology of personal constructs.* New York: Norton.

King, R. C., & DaCosta, K. M. (1996). Changing face, changing race: The remaking of race in the Japanese American and African American communities. In M. P. P. Root (Ed.), *The multiracial experience: Racial borders as the new frontier* (pp. 227–245). Thousand Oaks, CA: Sage.

Kitzinger, C. (1995). Social constructionism: Implications for lesbian and gay psychology. In A. R. D'Augelli & C. J. Patterson (Eds.), *Lesbian, gay, and bisexual identities over the lifespan: Psychological perspectives* (pp. 137–161). New York: Oxford University Press.

Lee, J. (1996). Why Suzie Wong is not a lesbian: Asian and Asian American lesbian and bisexual women and femme/butch/gender identities. In B. Beemyn & M. Eliason (Eds.), *Queer studies: A lesbian, gay, bisexual, and transgender anthology* (pp. 115–131). New York: New York University Press.

Lerman, H. (1992). The limits of phenomenology: A feminist critique of the humanistic personality theories. In L. S. Brown & M. Ballou (Eds.), *Personality and psychopathology: Feminist reappraisals* (pp. 8–19). New York: Guilford Press.

Lyddon, W. J. (1995). Cognitive therapy and theories of knowing: A social constructionist view. *Journal of Counseling and Development, 73*, 579–585.

Mahoney, M. J. (1991). *Human change processes: The scientific foundations of psychotherapy.* New York: Basic Books.

Mahoney, M. J., & Gabriel, T. J. (1987). Psychotherapy and the cognitive sciences: An evolving alliance. *Journal of Cognitive Psychotherapy, 1*, 39–59.

Mahoney, M. J., & Lyddon, W. J. (1988). Recent developments in cognitive approaches to counseling and psychotherapy. *Counseling Psychologist, 16*, 190–234.

Marcia, J. E. (1980). Identity in adolescence. In J. Adelson (Ed.), *Handbook of adolescent psychology* (pp. 159–187). New York: Wiley.

McAdams, D. P. (1997). The case for unity in the (post)modern self. In R. D. Ashmore & L. J. Jussim (Eds.), *Self and identity: Fundamental issues* (pp. 46–78). New York: Oxford University Press.

Neimeyer, R. A. (1993). Constructivism and the cognitive psychotherapies: Some conceptual and strategic contrasts. *Journal of Cognitive Psychotherapy, 7*, 159–171.

Okun, B. (1992). Object relations and self-psychology: Overview and feminist perspective. In L. S. Brown & M. Ballou (Eds.), *Personality and psychopathology: Feminist reappraisals* (pp. 20–45). New York: Guilford Press.

Rigazio-DiGilio, S. A. (1997). From microscopes to holographs: Client development within a constructivist paradigm. In T. L. Sexton & B. L. Griffin (Eds.), *Constructivist thinking in counseling practice, research, and training* (pp. 74–97). New York: Teachers College Press.

Romaniello, J. (1992). Beyond archetypes: A feminist perspective on Jungian theory. In L. S. Brown & M. Ballou (Eds.), *Personality and psychopathology: Feminist reappraisals* (pp. 46–69). New York: Guilford Press.

Root, M. P. P. (1992). Reconstructing the impact of trauma on personality. In L. S. Brown & M. Ballou (Eds.), *Personality and psychopathology: Feminist reappraisals* (pp. 229–265). New York: Guilford Press.

Root, M. P. P. (1997). Multiracial Asians: Models of ethnic identity. *Amerasia Journal, 23*(1), 29–41.

Shreiner, G., & Lyddon, W. (1998). Constructivist counseling: A primer. *Texas Counseling Association Journal, 26*(2), 79–90.

Sexton, T. L., & Griffin, B. L. (Eds.). (1997). *Constructivist thinking in counseling practice, research, and training.* New York: Teachers College Press.

Sexton, T. L. (1997). Constructivist thinking within the history of ideas: The challenge of a new paradigm. In T. L. Sexton & B. L. Griffin (Eds.), *Constructivist thinking in counseling practice, research, and training* (pp. 3–17). New York: Teachers College Press.

Sue, D. W., & Sue, D. (1999). *Counseling the culturally different: Theory and practice* (3rd ed.). New York: Wiley.

Thoits, P. A., & Virshup, L. K. (1997). Me's and we's: Forms and functions of social identities. In R. D. Ashmore & L. J. Jussim (Eds.), *Self and identity: Fundamental issues* (pp. 137–159). New York: Oxford University Press.

Uba, L. (1994). *Asian Americans: Personality patterns, identity, and mental health.* New York: Guilford Press.

Wehrley, B. (1995). *Pathways to multicultural competence: A developmental journey.* Pacific Grove, CA: Brooks/Cole.

Wentworth, W. M., & Wentworth, C. M. (1997). The social construction of culture and its implication for the therapeutic mind-self. In T. L. Sexton & B. L. Griffin (Eds.), *Constructivist thinking in counseling practice, research, and training* (pp. 41–57). New York: Teachers College Press.

White, M., & Epston, D. (1990). *Narrative means to therapeutic ends.* New York: Norton.

Chapter 5

Toward a Feminist Ecological Theory of Human Nature
Theory Building in Response to Real-World Dynamics

MARY BALLOU
ATSUSHI MATSUMOTO
MICHAEL WAGNER

Feminism, along with other critical theories, is critiquing the 19th- and 20th-century privileges of logical positivist, empirical, and rational forms of intellectual inquiry and their intersections with domination (of knowledge, resources, and institutional control). Many important questions are raised about the ways Western intellectual history has come to its underlying assumptions. For example, some of these assumptions are that universal laws underlie reality, that science can come to comprehend and control them, and that rationality is composed of a sort of dichotomous ordering of pre-defined constructs with a linear and causal relationship. Our attempt in this chapter is to move toward a description of human nature and experience that is not mired in the limitations of these traditional forms of inquiry. It is not our task to replace existing theoretical constructs with a grand theory of our own; rather, we attempt to move toward an understanding that is based more fully in the reality of people's lived experiences.

The process of writing this chapter has been a delightful one. We three authors came together to discuss our thoughts about what a feminist ecological model might look like and the literatures and contemporary thinking from which it might draw. We identified multicultural theory (particularly transformative positions), critical theory, systems theory (especially humanized systems theory), ecological thinking (from relational and systems earth-based views), and of course the myriad of feminist standpoints, especially feminist therapy theory.

At each of our meetings we spent time exploring thoughts about contemporary feminism, its coordination with other critical points of view, and their service in building points of view from the scaffolding of an ecological model. For instance, Bronfenbrenner's ideas were applauded as a language system and as an early example of interactivity and multiplicity, but were found wanting regarding a broader understanding of culture and structural factors. We talked too of the need for multicultural thinking to reflect on the meaning and implications of difference on mainstream thought. We decided to distinguish between inclusive and transformative multicultural theory and thinking. Additionally, we wanted to think broadly about feminism: academic and activist, women's studies and therapy, essentialist and constructivist, as well as postmodern, spiritual, and political. Finally, we wanted to consider the perspectives of critical theory, but not forget the connection back to the personal. That is, to remember that the lived experience of people ought not to be neglected, especially for particular nondominant groups/categories, or for the challenge to the mainstream that this approach presents. We formed a thinking and creating community as we struggled, and enjoyed bringing our own and others' ideas together in a somewhat coherent fashion. This chapter is the result of our thinking, somewhat proscribed by the requirement of the text.

THE THEORIES INFLUENCING
OUR FEMINIST ECOLOGICAL MODEL

In our developing feminist ecological model, we have been influenced by several critical theories. Critical theories offer rich potential for building a new theory of personhood, in part because they break with set-in personality theory, and they also challenge several of the underlying assumptions about 20th-century theory. Critical theories share similarities in taking issue with conventional assumptions and processes, yet they are too often silent about one another. Our attempt in this chapter is to build a model about human nature that includes contributions from several of the critical theories that have influenced our thinking.

Feminist Psychology

Feminist psychology is a large and exciting area. Though a few have already tried to explore it, its actual boundaries are still to be mapped, because it includes so much and is still expanding its territory. Two examples are *Shaping the Future of Feminist Psychology* (1997) by Worell and Johnson and Hope Landrine's edited *Bringing Cultural Diversity to Feminist Psychology Theory, Practice and Research* (1995). Several psychology of women's texts, written for academic courses in psychology and women's studies, are also widely acclaimed. These efforts, along with journals and professional organizations, have been and continue to be valuable and defining. Yet they do not contain all of the perspectives, activism, or indeed the international contributions to feminism that sometimes find their way into influencing the development of feminist psychology. Feminist psychology includes so much interdisciplinary and out-of-the-academy thinking, action, and history that it might just be more accurate to think in terms of *feminism's psychology* instead of implying that *feminism modifies psychology*. Instead, perhaps feminism is the subject—a subject influencing psychology by offering directions for its expansion, renovation, and reconstruction.

By now, there are several strands resting on different assumptions within feminism and feminist psychology. These various positions hold implications for and have had impact upon theory, practice, and modes of inquiry within psychology and many other disciplines. They have also had influence on ways of thinking and acting and making social policy. Feminism is, in the end, more of a worldview that has not only informed academic disciplines but has provided an assumptive value base for orientation and action in the lives of some women and men. It has served as the political position to ground political action, as the value base organizing interactions in women's collective activities, and as the principle from which new thinking, critical challenges, and new actions/inquiries have advanced.

Not only have these multiple activities been characteristic of feminism, but the several strands have attempted to maintain a pluralistic stance with one another. For example, in feminist psychology, liberal feminists who might wish to reform biased and noninclusive practices have tried to keep faith with their more radical sisters who want to excavate political, institutional, and disciplinary hegemonic linkages. Keeping faith is also attempted with sisters and brothers who wish to call into question the participation of the profession and the academy in power dynamics that maintain basic monocultural capitalist, racist, classist, sexist, and heterosexist assumptions and rewards. The insistence on women's lived experiences, pluralism, the influence of external forces, a questioning stance, and an interdisciplinary perspective has enabled feminism to be a powerful subject.

In our model, we draw from the principles of feminist therapy because they seek to maintain a broad and inclusive view of liberal and more radical feminist psychology, and because they inform us of theory, inquiry, practice, and actions in psychology and beyond.

Feminist Therapy Theory

Feminist therapy theory is a pluralistic and multifaceted perspective that informs theory, research, and practice. It encompasses a diverse area of theoretical orientations, epistemologies, worldviews, professional roles, and change. Feminist therapy theory developed out of the women's liberation movement of the 1970s. The discussion in early years of the political dimension of therapy itself, and psychology as a discipline, was followed by the development of principles of feminist therapy theory. Active consideration of the complexities of power and privilege in recent years contributed to our efforts to identify ways to understand and appreciate differences while maintaining a common ground. Most recently, an attempt to expose and understand the experiences of women and to honor the voices of women and girls around the globe has begun.

The developments in feminist therapy theory are informed by and built upon feminist theory. There are several "schools" of thought within feminist theory. However, they all share a commonality in their understanding that gender oppression is a social fact that operates to produce inequalities against women in the social, cultural, political, and economic domains. Through consideration of the various ways in which these dimensions affect the lives of women, feminist theory aims to provide ways to work toward social change.

Feminist therapy theory is an enactment of feminist theory on an individual level in real-world contexts (Ballou & Gabalac, 1985; Brown, 1994; Kitzinger, 1991). The sociopolitical analysis based on feminist theory is an essential aspect in the practice of feminist psychologists. It offers a way to consider how inequalities shape and affect the lives of women. In addition to their grounding in feminist theory, feminist therapists develop skills to consider how the effects of the external world are played out to produce psychological suffering in the daily lives of women.

The principles of feminist therapy theory reflect the double perspectives of the psychological and sociopolitical (Hill & Ballou, 1998) that guide us as the foundations for theory, research, and practice. These principles are centered around five themes. The first is its emphasis on valuing women's experiences (Ballou & Gabalac, 1985; Brown, 1994; Hill & Ballou, 1998; Kaschak, 1981). Feminists seek to rewrite the reality of women's experiences by centering women's lived experiences as they are shared by women themselves. The second is its focus upon the psychological distress as deeply rooted in sociocultural factors (Ballou & Gabalac, 1985; Brown, 1994; Comas-Díaz, 1991; Hill & Ballou, 1998; Kaschak, 1981). Feminist therapy provides multiple levels of analysis in considering the intertwined nature of individual locations and the ecological system. The third principle is concerned with power in interpersonal relationships and also in a larger system (Ballou, 1990; Ballou & Gabalac, 1985; Brown, 1994; Enns, 1993; Hill & Ballou, 1998; Jordan, Kaplan, Miller, Stiver, & Surrey, 1991). Feminist therapy attempts to redistribute power in all relationships including those between clients and therapists, participants and researchers, and oppressed groups and dominant forces.

The fourth principle consists of an analysis of "intersectionality" (Crenshaw, 1994), and the ways in which oppression that is based on race, ethnicity, class, sexual orientation, age, religion, ableness, and geographical locations intersects with gender (Comas-Díaz, 1991; Hill & Ballou, 1998; Kaschak, 1992). This integrated analysis of oppression acknowledges that gender is intertwined with other forms of oppression, and that the experiences of women are shaped differently depending on power and privilege accorded to each of various intersecting oppressions. The fifth principle reflects the goal of feminist therapy theory to engage in social change (Ballou & Gabalac, 1985; Brown, 1994; Enns, 1992; Hill & Ballou, 1998). Feminist therapy and research guided by feminist therapy theory are creating social change by increasing awareness of inequalities and providing different ways in which individuals cope with their distress (Hill & Ballou, 1998). At the same time, feminist therapy's principles encourage direct social action as an essential part of the responsibility of feminist psychology. These principles are widely accepted at the bases of feminist therapy and its continued development. They have also been used as a principled structure in analysis and development in several areas.

These feminist principles, for example, have also informed feminist epistemology, which in turn influences theory and research. For instance, a questioning stance toward mainstream assumptions has led feminist scholars across the disciplines to engage in a critique of the scientific method and its underlying logical positivism epistemology. Beyond critiquing logical positivism assumptions—that knowledge is located "out there" in the world and is accessible through applications of neutral, objective, and systematic scientific methods of investigation—feminists have provided alternative approaches to knowledge. These alternatives can be labeled as *feminist empiricism, feminist standpoint epistemologies,* and *feminist postmodernism* (Harding, 1993; Riger, 1992).

Feminist empiricists maintain some of the epistemological assumptions and scientific methods of logical positivism. They believe that truth can be accessed through rigorous scientific methods accompanied by truly neutral and bias-free experimental conditions. Feminist empiricists attempt to eliminate androcentric bias in their search for truth. Feminist standpoint epistemologies, in contrast, locate truth as residing in the experiences of women (and men) as reported by women (and men) themselves. Their focus on the experiential methodology reflects the assumption that participants or clients, not researchers or therapists, are the experts concerning their own experiences. Listening to voices of women and girls is thought to be the best way to understand how they make sense of their worlds. Feminist postmodernism, better known as social constructionism in psychology, attempts to interrogate the underlying oppressive values and assumptions of the dominant knowledges by utilizing reasoning methodology. It aims at breaking down essentialist claims, and exposes how modern science (or psychology) maintains the interests and values of certain segments of populations at the expense of others. In doing so, feminist postmodernism focuses upon language or discourses to articulate its belief in multiple realities and knowledges.

Currently, feminist postmodern positions have excited the enthusiasm of many across the disciplines. At the same time, however, some have engaged in a productive criticism of feminist postmodernism (such as Linda Nicholson, Susan Friedman and Nancy Fraser, to mention a few). Some feminist scholars warn us that, although the emphasis placed on language and discourses by feminist postmodernism do have certain explanatory powers, these factors alone may not bring transformative change in society. By taking what is useful from feminist postmodernism, renewed interests in social action appear to be in order. In our own development of the feminist ecological model, we hope to integrate multicultural, critical, and liberation psychologies to further strengthen the areas of the ecological model while utilizing a feminist perspective as a guiding force in producing transformative change.

Critical Psychology

Our feminist ecological model builds with several theories, including feminist therapy theory, liberation psychology, and transformative multicultur-

alism. Although these theoretical stances differ in their emphasis on theoretical concerns and the intellectual contributions they provide, they do
share common theoretical underpinnings and hence are broadly considered
critical theory. Critical theory holds that the unquestioned authority of assumptions, values, and normative standards in mainstream psychology
contributes to injustices to people it seeks to serve rather than promotes
better human welfare. With a commitment to identifying ways to articulate
reality more fully and accurately from the perspectives of the nondominant,
critical psychology has paid greater attention to exposing ways in which the
status quo is maintained in psychology. As Prilleltensky and Fox (1997) indicate, critical theory attempts to transform the discipline of psychology by
encouraging psychologists to serve as "agents for social change rather than
agents of social control" (p. 5).

Critical theory is explicit in its critique of the underlying assumptions
in mainstream psychology. For example, feminist therapy theory and
transformative multiculturalism provide sharp views on traditional personality theory by taking a critical questioning stance as to who gets to establish the normative standards of health. Critical psychology also holds explicit assumptions in areas of knowledge, issues on power, questioning
stance, professional ethics, impacts of sociopolitical dimension upon individuals, and notions about the "good society." For example, in contrast to
mainstream psychology, which tends to see problems as residing within individuals, critical theory holds that much of psychological suffering experienced by individuals is grounded in external factors that surround them.
With this difference in understanding the cause of psychological suffering,
the approach to intervention also differs. While critical theory focuses on
both personal and social factors, mainstream psychology remains focused
on inducing or altering behaviors of individuals so as to help them adjust
or fit in to existing external conditions. The failure to see the impact of external factors upon individuals, however, leads to blaming the victim.

Foregrounded Themes and Values in Critical Theory

The book *Critical Psychology: An Introduction*, edited by Fox and Prilleltensky (1997) provides much insight into the underlying themes and values shared by critical theory. The opening chapter by Prilleltensky and Fox
introduced three themes in critical theory. These are individualism and
meaning, oppression and inequality, and intentions, consequences, and
dilemmas. They see mainstream psychology as supporting the values of
economic and social institutions that encourage people to achieve meanings in their lives through consumption of greater material goods. The

pursuit of individual satisfaction became a norm in current society to a degree where individual satisfaction is desired even if it means increasing the sufferings of others. This capitalist ideal has contributed to separating individuals from engaging in the community and maintaining a sense of connection with others.

Negative consequences of the values and norms of capitalist systems work to produce suffering among those who are powerless. Indeed, inequalities and oppression are pervasive. This exploitation of the oppressed by the dominant and the powerful is naturalized and normalized as if it was the "fact" about societies. Psychologists may be reinforcing oppressive systems, despite their good intentions, because their theory, practices, and professional customs are colored by the traditions and values of mainstream psychology, which in turn are shaped by a particular group of individuals. Coupled with a narrow focus on the individual level of intervention, it often results in forcing individuals to fit into normative standards defined by particular groups with power and interlocking interests.

The themes mentioned above are built upon the values critical theory promotes. While traditional thinking in psychology understands that values are the source for bias, which interrupts objectivity and neutrality, critical theory rests on values that have potential in enhancing human welfare. These values central to critical theory include social justice, self-determination and participation, caring and compassion, and health and diversity. The authors suggest that, when applying these values in psychology, first, each of these values needs to be considered by maintaining the balance among other competing values. Also, the need for advancing values toward better human welfare is dependent upon the social climate and the needs of particular groups and individuals and their histories. Lastly, although all values do have potential in transforming psychology and social institutions, some values may have more potential to do so compared to others. It is important that critical psychologists establish a capacity to identify which values or combination of values works best to enhance the needs of individuals and the communities that they wish to serve.

Social Justice in Psychology

Prilleltensky and Nelson (1997) discuss reconstruction of community psychology from a critical theory perspective that is also useful to the development of a feminist ecological model. They recognize that all values are interrelated, and argue that balance among them must be carefully considered. When values are separated from one another, a collaborative and joining process among people to work toward creating a better society is at risk. Current social, political, and historical forces, unfortunately, reflect the tendency to promote one value over another—for example, promoting capitalist and patriarchal values (profit and control for those on top of the hierarchy) and dismissing the value of social justice. The lack of implementing the value of social justice is likely to reinforce unjust and unethical actions.

Social justice is defined as a value consisting of "the full and equitable allocation of bargaining power, resources, and burdens in society" (Prilleltensky & Nelson, 1997, p. 177). Some nonmainstream psychologies have begun to incorporate the value of social justice by advocating equal distribution of resources and equal access to care. Such an approach is a crucial ingredient that needs to be emphasized in theory building, yet it also needs to be extended further to understand the deep-rooted causes of the problem at the systemic level. Indeed, the amelioration or first-order change within the discipline of psychology is important, but it also needs to be supplemented by efforts to bring a transformative change in the system itself.

The contributions made by critical theory offer us a value structure to support building theory, while at the same time encouraging the discipline of psychology to be more responsive to implementing the value of social justice. As feminism's "personal is political" and liberation psychology's "critical consciousness" reflect, psychology needs to actively engage in sociopolitical analysis by bringing awareness of inequality and oppression in the daily lives of individuals and communities. At the same time, such a process must be accompanied by efforts to develop a sense of connection among all individuals who are involved in a promotion of better society. As highlighted in the principles of feminist therapy theory, the focus on establishing the egalitarian interpersonal relationship that promotes social change is a crucial ingredient in transforming the discipline of psychology. Lastly, the relation between the powerless and those who stand in positions of power must be considered as well. Psychologists hold potential in assisting those with power to redefine their goals and positions, and to create an environment where both ends can engage in negotiation for redistributing power.

Critical theory and its self-reflexive stance may contribute to a reconstruction of assumptions, values, and normative standards in mainstream psychology. Also, such a process may contribute to advancing critical theory itself in identifying ways to transform both psychology and society. While critical theory remains within psychology, liberation psychology—which also highlights values and social actions—draws from interdisciplinary perspectives. Indeed, changing the discipline of psychology itself is important, but a shift in focus beyond psychology in also needed. Rather than simply "add" values in theory building, research, and practice, psychology needs to go outside of its terrain to consider political and moral theories if our focus is to bring social justice in action.

Liberation Psychology

Liberation psychology was developed from and rests upon liberation theology. Liberation theology was developed by a group of bishops who focused on the defense of human rights and the defeat of colonialization in Latin America. These bishops, holding a socialist stance, recognized that capitalism pervaded Latin America. They viewed the colonialization of Latin America in all its dimensions—economic, material, and political—by the industrialized world as unethical (Hollander, 1997). They also extended their critique of colonialization to the spiritual and psychological dimensions of people, finding it equally unjust in these realms.

Later, liberation psychology was developed by the social psychologist Ignacio Martin-Baro. His works have enriched our understanding of the intertwined nature of structural inequalities and psychological sufferings. For Martin-Baro, psychology was both a theoretical and a practical endeavor that held the potential to facilitate people's participation in social activism to work collectively towards social change. Liberation psychology is, however, informed by peoples' commitments to social justice and activism. The focus is on making a change in the lives of individuals through actions that attempt to alter the existing social structure. It shares ground with feminism in that both are concerned greatly with making a change in the everyday lives of individuals through direct intervention in external influencing factors. Just as feminism modifies feminist psychology, social change at a structural level modifies liberation psychology.

Martin-Baro (1994) proposed three essential factors in making psychology more responsive to the needs of individuals in real-world contexts. First, he called for a radical transformation of society that would not only emancipate all oppressed groups, but would liberate each individual. Second, he argued that psychology needs to generate knowledge from listening to the experiences of people whose lives are shaped by the inequalities enforced upon them by those with power, necessitated in part because the oppressors render powerless the socially invisible. Third, he called on psychologists to work and collaborate with the dominated rather than with the powerful.

The image of psychology that emerges from the points made above differs dramatically from that of mainstream psychology as it remains behind the door of the academy. In contrast to the supposedly neutral and objective stance of modern psychology, liberation psychology provides us with roles as active agents who assist people in their process of personal, spiritual, and collective empowerment. The ultimate goal of liberation psychology is to ground action as a means of social change. Such a psychological perspective helps highlight the blind spots in mainstream psychology, in particular those concerning a lack of structural analysis in theory building that accounts for social change and political analysis. In the following discussion, we provide some tenets of liberation psychology that may serve to expand our theory building.

The psychology of liberation highlights particular themes necessary to gain understanding about individuals and their problems in living. One of the themes shared by those whose works represent the framework of liberation psychology is their effort in situating the lives of individuals in a larger context of history and geopolitics (Comas-Díaz, Lykes, & Alarcon, 1998; Enriquez, 1992; Martin-Baro, 1994). The daily experiences of individuals are shaped by and inseparable from the effects of history and politics. By placing an emphasis on sociohistorical events, liberation psychology not only attempts to see and analyze the dynamic forces of past historical events shaping the experiences and reality of individuals at present, but it also attempts to link past, present, and the future by recognizing the agency of individuals and their collective efforts in creating the future. This understanding of individuals and groups reflects the notion that people are not mere passive recipients of sociopolitical events, but instead are capable of effecting them based on their reflections about past events.

Liberation psychology explicitly argues that much of the psychological suffering experienced by people is tied to social inequalities at a structural systemic level. Therefore, sociopolitical analysis becomes a crucial ingredient in understanding how those who sit on top of the hierarchical system utilize their power to promote their own interests at the expense of others. Establishing and utilizing critical ways of seeing the world is thought to uncover the root of the problems experienced by the oppressed. In the United States, the effects of external factors, including distribution of resources, politics, the economy, and social policy, are recognized to effect individuals differently depending on their social status. Indeed, inequalities produced at a structural level are played out in the daily lives of individuals as psychological suffering. Yet mainstream psychology fails to acknowledge this profound social control facilitated by the system, and resorts to focusing only on making individuals adapt to this condition. Just as the principles of feminist therapy indicate, liberation psychology encourages us to utilize the double perspectives of the personal and the political.

In addition to understanding the operation of inequalities in the systemic base, the psychology of liberation encourages psychologists to join the people that they serve and to consider how oppression is played out in their daily lives. With the development of such awareness, psychologists work with them to further help them establish critical analytical skills in considering a variety of forces that surround them as well as others.

One of the themes that is highlighted in liberation psychology is the development of critical consciousness. Psychologists need to join with people and consider how oppression is played out in their daily lives. In this process, liberation psychology prescribes a role for psychologists to facilitate peoples' critical analytical skills in considering a variety of forces around them. With the development of critical consciousness, liberation psychology brings forward the notion that such analytical skills must be tied into action at all levels of our daily lives. Psychologists together with the people they serve can identify ways in which they can take an active part in social activism to alter the existing structural condition.

Another important point liberation psychology brings forward is the stance that critical perspectives must be tied into action in every aspect of our daily living at varying levels, including interpersonal and intrapersonal, group/collective, and sociopolitical. Identifying specific ways in which people can take an active part in social activism to alter the existing structural condition is an essential principle of liberation psychology. As Prilleltensky and Fox (1997) indicated in their discussion on critical psychology, liberation psychology shares a value of critical psychology in its focus on social justice where all individuals are given "the full and equitable allocation of bargaining power, resources, and burdens in society" (p. 177). Both liberation and critical psychology progressively attempt to reduce the gap between rhetoric and action.

Social justice requires that psychologists go beyond psychological theories to consider other tightly connected areas of concern. These may be, for example, ethics, human rights, social movements, community organizing, and social policy. An interactive collaboration with people that we seek to serve may be particularly sound in empowering individuals and their communities. In addition, as agents for social change, psychologists need to monitor developments in the sociopolitical sphere to make sure that no particular group or individual is targeted as a scapegoat, or that the interests of certain groups are not promoted without inclusive consideration.

Liberation psychology expands the territory of theory building. In order to implement action and social change in theory, psychology needs to go beyond traditional constructs of personality in its theory to explore how structural forces affect human nature and the ways in which action can be actualized. To this end, an interdisciplinary approach is necessary to understand the factors influencing human nature. For example, thinking about geopolitics, social movements, human rights, social policy, and community organizing may provide us with other ways to think about human nature and to realize how it is indeed shaped by structural forces. At the same time, it is important to remind ourselves that theory building must be grounded in the lived experiences of people and ways to bring about social change.

Transformative Multiculturalism

It is clear that there is a need for theories of human nature that are adequate enough to address the complex needs of an increasingly diverse yet interconnected global population. This need has been well-documented in the multicultural literature by such authors as Sue, Ivey, and Pederson (1996) and others. Multiculturalism in psychology and related disciplines developed largely as a response to the recognition that most dominant theories of human nature have been products of a Eurocentric perspective based on assumptions, for example, that personal autonomy, achievement, and responsibility are the driving forces for all humans. These orientations, including the psychodynamic, cognitive-behavioral, and existential-humanistic, have been examined in terms of their failure to adequately acknowledge the impact of culture on an individual's existence, particularly regarding non-Western, nonmale, and noncapitalist viewpoints.

According to the multicultural literature, non-Western values and worldviews have not been adequately considered in psychological theory building, research, and practice (Sue, Ivey, & Pederson, 1996). In fact, the issue of the culture-boundedness of mainstream theory has been well-documented in multicultural discourse and analysis. In response to these limitations, theories of human nature based on cultural variables have emerged prominently. Such theories, while more comprehensive and inclusive than theory in the mainstream, have not acknowledged the extent to which they have profited from feminism.

Multicultural theory, in its most basic form, examines the relationship between the individual and his or her social and cultural environments, with an emphasis on a broad definition of culture. Fowers and Richardson (1996) suggest that culture can be regarded as "the set of shared meanings that make social life possible. . . . These meanings and assumptions orient members of a culture and structure their lives through exemplars, norms, and standards of behavior" (p. 610). A multicultural perspective examines these meanings and assumptions across cultural groups in order to make sense of the differences among those groups and to work toward acceptance and appreciation of those differences.

Traditional forms of multiculturalism in psychology and related fields have focused on the building of awareness about and the acceptance of the differences between the practitioner and the client based on variables such as race and nationality or one's identification with those variables. These forms of multiculturalism have immense value in creating an atmosphere in which practitioners can be maximally effective in working with people who are culturally different from themselves.

With its emphasis on a close examination of the influence of cultural differences within the client–counselor relationship, however, multiculturalism has given relatively little attention to the structural forces and power dynamics that impact on an individual's experience in the world and her or his functioning outside of the therapeutic dyad. It is important to note that multiculturalism in psychology is a product of Western cultural beliefs and norms, and is modified by traditions and social practices within Western thought (Fowers & Richardson, 1996). Given this heritage, multiculturalism is predisposed toward an emphasis on the levels of the individual and his or her culture/community, with less focus on questioning the economic, political, and other larger structural forces that impact individuals and groups. For that matter, psychology itself is embedded in Western philosophy and moral discourse, a discourse that tends to deemphasize the impact of political, economic, and gender-based power differentials.

Our challenge, then, is to foster an openness to truths as they are defined in other cultural traditions, to analyze normative structures that cross cultural boundaries, and to attempt to move multiculturalism in a direction that emphasizes egalitarian relationships, equalized access to resources, and social action. Inherent in this process is the need to recognize and alleviate the impact of oppression and marginalization based on particular cultural attributes (which multiculturalism has begun to do on some levels). Furthermore, we must force ourselves to look critically at our own beliefs and assumptions, just as we look critically upon those of others.

Fowers and Richardson (1996) have captured the thrust of the movement by stating that "multiculturalism is a moral movement that is intended to enhance the dignity, rights, and recognized worth of marginalized groups" (p. 609). This statement suggests that, in taking a multicultural perspective, we have a moral obligation to work actively to make changes in the lives of marginalized groups, which is to work to transform the lives of the oppressed.

The practice of transformative multiculturalism is an act of deconstructing our mainstream, logical positivist, empiricist viewpoints, and moving toward an integrative and practical approach to facilitating social change regarding cultural issues. Particularly important is our obligation to address the needs of individuals and groups that have been marginalized, oppressed, and singled out for unequal and differential treatment based on such identifying characteristics as gender, sexual preference, age, physical disability, language, ethnicity, and race (Ballou, 1996; Nuttall, Sanchez, & Webber, 1996). It is a move away from individualism toward socially focused understanding and action.

Liberation psychology informs transformative multiculturalism. Through the lens of liberation theory, psychology can be seen as a theoretical and practical endeavor (Martin-Baro, 1994), which is affected by historical events, power struggles, oppression, sociopolitical issues (such as racial policies, white dominance, access to the media, etc.). Transformative multiculturalism assumes that there are diverse ways of knowing, all of which have validity and importance. This idea can be supported by feminist principles, as outlined previously. As in the psychology of liberation, transformative multiculturalism prescribes developing a critical consciousness in a Friereian sense, which demands action and participation on the part of the oppressed. It involves increasing people's understanding of their own realities through a reflection on their own social experiences, rather than what the media or those in power (government, military, etc.) would suggest.

Multiculturalism and the Concept of Difference

Historically, there has been a bias toward studying white, European American heterosexual males as a basis for comparison in research and creating a standard for understanding "difference." As practitioners and theoreticians, we have a moral obligation (based on the ethical codes and principles of the American Psychological Association, the Feminist Therapy Institute, the National Institute of Mental Health, and other organizations) to promote human welfare, which means that we must not be blind to differences between groups and within groups. Ignoring the fundamental aspects of a person's identity and his or her experiences undermines our attempts to understand and to offer adequate assistance. It is not correct to see difference as variation from the mean.

In her discussion of difference in terms of the development of racism, sexism, ageism, elitism, classism, and other forms of dominance, Audrey Lorde (1992) recognized that the differences among people based on age, race, sex, and other characteristics are very real. It is not the differences themselves, however, that separate people. Rather, it is people's "refusal to recognize those differences, and to examine the distortions which result from our misnaming them and their effects upon human behavior and expectation" (p. 402). The failure to recognize differences leads to the active ignoring of oppression when it occurs. There are socioeconomic and structural reasons why this happens: those in power hierarchically don't want to recognize differences because they take away from the assumptive position of dominance that they hold.

Essential to our perspective is the recognition that there is a hierarchical valuing of particular ways of being and behaving; difference, then, is defined in terms of hierarchically valued categories that are determined by people and structures that have the dominant voice. Such hierarchically determined values include individual achievement, competence, performing versus emoting, and doing rather than valuing. Those in oppressed, marginalized, or nondominant groups are told, "Who and what you are is not valued." Part of the purpose of our model is to respond to the middle-class white male "ideal" by pointing out the ways in which this "ideal" is politically and structurally supported and reinforced.

Hope Landrine (1995) suggested that understanding culture and gender as contexts that impact women's experiences is a necessary step toward understanding those experiences. This process involves integrating cultural diversity into feminist psychology, and putting beliefs (or worldview) in the context of women's knowledge of gender, of themselves, of culture, and of difference. This idea implies that we must seek to integrate gender and culture generally, and that we must decode gender-based beliefs and culturally based beliefs. In seeking this integration regarding ways of knowing, however, we must be careful not to assume that the term "culture" necessarily refers to anyone who is a non-white, non-European female. As Landrine suggests, "to persist in the belief that knowledge that is based almost solely on studies of middle-class, European American women and men is knowledge of gender, while readily admitting that women of color are cultural products, is to render culture exotic, superfluous, and relevant to people of color alone" (p. 15).

While examining difference across groups, it is also important to recognize the diversity that exists within groups. Rhoda Unger (1995) proposes that race and gender are not essentialist conceptions that can be used to describe all people who fit into these categories. There are vast differences within gender and racial groups: these differences are due in part to sociocultural and political structures, and in part to the individual variability that one can observe in everyday life. It is clear, then, that the self is not completely socially constructed. Rather, as our feminist ecological model suggests, there is a *reciprocal interactivity* between characteristics of the person (personality, temperament, developmental issues, genetics, etc.) and elements in the person's cultural/social/political environment. It is this interactivity that generates difference.

Basing Our Work on Lived Experience

Transformative multiculturalism tells us that there is much to learn from the ways that other cultures live in the world. In taking such a perspective, perhaps other cultures' ways of knowing and doing can transform our own ways of knowing and doing. We can expand our understanding of ourselves and of our connectedness with the community, with the earth, and with our spiritual selves. We are driven to ask about our relationship with the earth and how we understand this relationship.

Writing about the generation of knowledge and its relationship to lived experience, Ballou (1995) suggested that "basing knowledge claims in actual lived experience is an effective way of generating knowledge because it requires careful attention to the actual experience, rather than imposing structure on that experience. It is especially useful in it attempts to gain cross cultural and other contextual understandings" (p. 12). This perspective, based in feminist spirituality, guides a focus on understanding reality through lived experience. Being spiritual and experiential involves connecting with and reflecting upon our experiences, and using that process to move toward multiple ways of knowing and being.

In applying these ideas to the individual, we might be able to conceptualize human nature in a broader perspective (away from pathology) such as describing the person in terms of his or her connectedness with the earth, and seeing through the multiple lenses through which diverse people interpret the world and make meaning of it. This openness to other ways of knowing must be grounded in an appreciation of the lived experience of those whose voices have been suppressed by the dominant forces (Ballou, 1996).

An appreciation for and understanding of the lived experience of others is especially important for the way in which it recognizes the commonalities and linkages among diverse groups of people, especially those who have experienced oppression by the hierarchy and whose shared experiences of oppression binds them together. Those who have experienced oppression have the potential to use their common experiences to learn from each other, to teach others, to share strategies for coping with marginalization and oppression, and to work together with the common goal of acting against oppression in the future. By looking through a transformative multicultural lens, we as practitioners and theory builders open ourselves to broader conceptualizations of human lives based on an examination of lived experiences—including experiences of wellness and pathology, and of dominance, marginalization, and oppression.

Ecopsychology

Ecopsychology is a relatively new and developing field, but has received an increasingly important emphasis in psychology. It contributes to our thinking and to the development of our feminist ecological model. A defining text edited by Roszak, Gomes, and Kanner entitled *Ecopsychology: Restoring the Earth, Healing the Mind* (Brown, 1995), offers a view of the range and diverse points within ecopsychology.

The relationship of our awareness and behavior with the condition of the earth is one of the themes within the text. Sarah Conn calls attention to the problems that we fail to understand in ourselves and in our earth because we have disconnected from the earth. Alan During points out that the future of the earth depends on whether consumers in first-world nations can learn to turn to nonmaterial sources of fulfillment. Sounding a slightly different theme, Anita Barrows uses ecopsychology to look at child development, and questions what would happen if states of communion were valued as highly as rational consciousness. Mary Gomes and Allen Kanner take a gender/feminist psychology view to explore opening up to a world of increasing richness, complexity, and beauty when we move beyond defensive attitudes of separation and domination. Other themes explored include cultural diversity, symbolic representations, and political engagement. In general, ecopsychology is exploring what ecology means to psychology and mental health.

Lester Brown (1995) perhaps captures it best when he writes that "ecopsychologists are drawing upon ecological science to re-examine the human psyche as an integral part of the web of nature" (p. xiii). Theodore

Roszak, writing in "Where Psyche Meets Gaia," the first chapter in the ecopsychology section of the book, brings ecological science to psychology by presenting both the personal and the planetary links between environmentalism and psychotherapy. He explores both levels as cultural activities with much in common. While politics and economics are so vastly important to our understanding of the influences on human development, environmentalism brings an invitation to set these forces in a more diverse, multiapplied, and variously apprehended territory. The mutually interactive systems, the inclusion of the symbolic, the multiple points of origin, the numerous epistemologies and the relevance of political and economic factors, cultural perspectives, feminist sensitivities, and notions of healing from numerous traditions make the potential of this area very broad indeed. Ecopsychology has also offered perspectives that have enhanced our views in building more adequate models to describe personality and the influences on it.

Capra (1996) brings a breathtaking advanced theoretical physics perspective to systems thinking. The interconnections between spheres and their relationships that he posits is extremely informative and promises to transform our understanding of process, relationships, and reality. Essential to the ecological perspective is an understanding of the interconnectivity of all living systems (Capra, 1996). In recognizing that humans and the earth are interconnected and mutually influential, we understand that working with people within their various contexts demands that we develop reasonable and earth-preserving solutions to problems. That is, human behavior impacts the environment as much as the environment impacts humans; therefore, we must work toward solutions that sustain and renew the earth. Capra describes this process as part of *deep ecology*; he states that "deep ecological awareness recognizes the fundamental interdependence of all phenomena and the fact that, as individuals and societies, we are all embedded in (and ultimately dependent on) the cyclical processes of nature" (p. 6). Capra goes on to describe the importance of developing an *ecological literacy* in order to be able to develop effective practices that are responsive to the demands of the interconnected systems in the world.

THE FEMINIST ECOLOGICAL MODEL

Feminist theory building in general, and the feminist theory discussed in this chapter, is quite different from more usual theory. Theorems, postulates, and corollaries are the thinking structures for those who believe in the old constructs of individualist Western male images, who believe that universal truths both exist and function in human nature. These sorts of notions are the stuff of intellectual systems in the West and elsewhere. They have contributed greatly to our specific understanding in physical reality. They have also been used in theory building and formalized description in many other realms of reality.

Our task in this chapter, however, is to begin to build feminist theory that does not hold with easy assumptions of universal laws and other mechanisms of intellectual historical discipline. Instead, we present a model that holds ideas in relationship that are common or complementary, drawn from several lines of contemporary critical thought. We offer a model that rests in feminist principles, and attempt to call attention to the multiple and pluralistic influences on human beings. We do not set out logically or otherwise our beliefs about partial, linear, and value-based qualities of human nature. Nor do we write personal and interpersonal history over time, which is more often termed "development." Moreover, we do not imply which favored aspect to engage to hasten a certain direction for development or to change a trait, state, attribution, or behavior.

We do, however, set forth a representation of multiple dimensions of human existence, of real-world complexity, of multiple modes of living and ways of knowing, of multidirectional interactions between the person and her or his contexts, and of direct, contiguous, and distal influences. Moreover, we invite others to join in the process of building a better, more just, more inclusive, and more accurate likeness of women and men.

The theoretical models that we will be drawing from in this chapter address human diversity in an inclusive and practical manner. They are responsive to the needs of an increasingly diverse and yet interconnected world. These models each take a multidimensional approach to conceptualizing human experience on the levels of the individual and the group, and also prescribe actions that promote and sustain growth, and that address the multiple levels of environmental forces with which people interact, including the physical environment.

The feminist ecological theory we describe draws from the principles of ecological theory, feminist therapy theory, multicultural psychology, liberation psychology, and critical psychology. Feminist ecological theory outlines a comprehensive and several-dimensioned approach for conceptualizing human nature and influencing professional practice. Our task is to examine the connectedness of these various theories and to explore ways in which their combination might more adequately address the complex nature of human existence than other single existing theoretical models.

The model is presented in Figure 5.1. Its lineage is identified at the bottom of the figure. Several years of discussions within a doctoral seminar course that one of us teaches, presentations at American Psychological Association and at Feminist Therapy Institute meetings, and our present thinking also facilitated its continued development and certainly its use in this chapter. Other influences are the political and economic dynamics globally, in North America, and in the professional disciplines.

The model is designed to represent the multiple spheres of influence in people's lives. Ideally, this figure might be presented in three (or more) dimensions. Since holographic images remain beyond texts, we present Figure 5.1 in two dimensions, as a set of concentric rings that give a structure to our thoughts.

The individual, with multiple aspects, lies within the center ring. Each ring that encircles those within represents influences and interactive factors that are more distal in relation to the individual. The factors in the outer rings do not necessarily have less influence on or interactivity with the life experience of the individual, and may indeed have more influence and interactivity with the person. The factors within each ring constantly and dynamically interact with the person and with each other, as will become clear in the descriptions that follow.

The Inner Circle (the Individual)

The inner circle of the feminist ecological model is the level of the individual. This level is the focus of much of traditional personality theory. The first three forces—psychodynamic, cognitive-behavioral, and humanistic—are largely chronicles of the individual-self-personality, though more recently some theories have shown growing attention to interactions with others and immediate environments: family systems, feminist, multicultural, and biopsychosocial models.

Much of conventional psychology focused nearly exclusively on the individual level, and remained silent about institutional and structural forces. Indeed, Western intellectual history is filled with a preoccupation with the individual. Our disciplines, our folk culture, and our laws and customs all feature the individual, and indeed hold separation, autonomy, independence of self, and productivity as quintessential values. This position is so strong that it often serves to blind us to the interactions with and support of others that inevitably surround an individual's accomplishments. This position also serves to impair our vision of the value of the group or community.

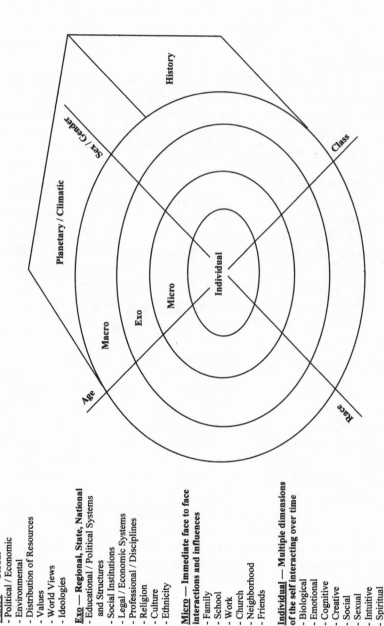

Macro — Global
- Political / Economic
- Environmental
- Distribution of Resources
- Values
- World Views
- Ideologies

Exo — Regional, State, National
- Educational / Political Systems and Structures
- Social Institutions
- Legal / Economic Systems
- Professional / Disciplines
- Religion
- Culture
- Ethnicity

Micro — Immediate face to face interactions and influences
- Family
- School
- Work
- Church
- Neighborhood
- Friends

Individual — Multiple dimensions of the self interacting over time
- Biological
- Emotional
- Cognitive
- Creative
- Social
- Sexual
- Intuitive
- Spiritual

FIGURE 5.1. The ecological model.

In a similar reductionistic manner, conventional psychology holds certain aspects of individuals central. Just as the intellectual and physical (biological) aspects hold priority for many conventional psychological theories, so too do the rational and material aspects demonstrate the hegemonic linkage with economic, government, mainstream disciplines, and conventional professions. Some current work (e.g., Gardner, 1993; Goldman, 1995) on multiple intelligence, for example, carries multiplicities further than the conventional theories. But this work still emphasizes intelligence as the productive use of rationality, while underplaying the contextual and structural influence in Western cultures.

Not only are certain dimensions of individuals privileged, but also the very modes of understanding they use to direct understanding in certain ways. That is, in the academic and scientific West, our preoccupation with rationality and empiricism has directed and defined our conceptualization in ways both powerful and blinding. It is undeniable that the advances of Western science and reason in material realms are breathtaking. We have begun to unlock and redesign material nature, as well as the primary assumptions that direct human organization and rules. While the organizational, scientific, and technological advances in our era are tremendous, the very reasoning processes that have contributed to these accomplishments have distanced, dimmed, and muted other modes of knowing and the related quality of things known. For example, in our model, we have represented the intellect as one of many dimensions of the individual. We point toward some of the expanding work that moves conceptualization of this dimension more broadly. Yet, unless we also move beyond mere empiricism and rationality, we are unlikely to understand higher consciousness, or to honor empathic knowledge and intuitive knowing. To come to apprehend the connections among compassion, insight, enlightenment, creativity, and intuition, or the felt patterns in living in harmony with nature, with others, and with the earth, is a different sort of knowing. These experiences and the sorts of cognition/knowing to which they relate are unlikely to be available through the conventional mind-structuring rules of rationality and empiricism.

In contrast, the feminist ecological model represents many aspects of individuals and their interaction with other influences as well. Our model recognizes intellectual, emotional, physical, and spiritual dimensions of the person, and it indicates that the coordinates of race-ethnicity, class, sex-gender, and age all interact profoundly with these dimensions of the individual. Moreover, the other levels of the model are more inclusive of environmental, social, and political factors. They are ever-present in their

interactive influence, and are set within a historical period and within dynamic planetary and physical conditions. These are factors that themselves
interact with and influence individuals and groups. Feminist theory, multicultural perspectives, and ecological thinking all have inherent influence
upon these ideas. Further, feminist and other critical theories direct our attention to the gendered and structural factors along with their hegemonic
linking as they contribute to the multidimensional interactivity of human
existence.

The figure presents the multiple aspects of an individual. We have represented emotional, spiritual, physical, and intellectual aspects, though
these may not be inclusive. Indeed, some would argue that aesthetic, moral,
interpersonal, and psychic factors should also be represented. Some would
also argue the discrimination is not fine enough, for example, to lump huge
and separate areas of biology and behavior under the physical self. We
would not disagree. The particular number or even the labeling is not our
concern at this time. Rather, we wish to show the multiplicity, interactivity,
and mutually influencing nature of multiple aspects of the individual. We
also wish to illustrate through this figure the mutual influence among the
various aspects of the individual and between levels of the model. Finally,
the figure points out that certain coordinates—age, sex-gender, race-ethnicity, and class—have consistent influence across levels, and all are set in history time and in planetary conditions. We wish to further demonstrate that
merely focusing on one aspect within the individual level or at the individual level itself is inadequate and perhaps incompetent for theory.

Another consideration of the model is reflected within the words car-
rying the ambiguity of the ontological status of the specific dimensions. Is
human nature really captured with words of intellect, emotion, the physical
and spiritual, or even the psychic or aesthetic, for that matter? Or are these
words, which are artifacts of language and culture, used to offer the illusion
of mastery and control, as postmodern linguists would have us consider?
Our purpose here in not to engage that postmodern debate, but to acknowledge that words, and the constructs they create, often mediate between our
comprehension and our experience.

The Microsystem

As discussed above, taking the ecological perspective demands an examination of the connections between multiple aspects of the individual and the
larger structural forces that exist in the environment. The first ring of the

model outside of the individual is the microsystem, which includes elements in the person's environment offering immediate, face-to-face interactions and influences. At this level of the model, we consider those factors in the individual's immediate environment with which he or she interacts daily. The reciprocal interactivity between the person and the immediate environment is more readily observable than the interaction with more distal political, economic, and structural forces. In fact, the factors at this level are perhaps less important in and of themselves than the nature of the person's interaction with those factors. Seen in this way, the feminist ecological model represents the experiential nature of living, rather than representing static elements in fixed positions.

This level of the model includes such factors as the neighborhood or community in which a person lives, the township or city, local government, the school system (including quality of educational resources and access), and resources for employment.

The microsystem also includes intimate relationships and the immediate and extended family. It is important to mention that, in our model, the definition of family is not limited to biologically based conceptions of family relationships, but rather is based on all the affectional commitments that bind people together. In taking this approach, we want to include the variety and breadth of ways in which people interrelate. Relationships with friends, peers, and participation in community activities are also considered at this level, such as church/religious/spiritual organizations and leisure activities.

The influences at this level particularly impact on individual growth and development in terms of the belief systems and expectations of a person's parents, teachers, mentors, spouses, partners, close friends, and other associates, and how those beliefs and expectations shape that person's cognitive and emotional development, expectations, and worldview. These social and familial factors present the person with a set of normative values and roles that he or she is expected to accept without question. The hegemonic influence of such values and roles often goes unrecognized. It is important to recognize that any set of values comes from a certain social and political point of view. In order to allow for differences among people, these values and roles must be recognized and questioned.

The microsystem level of analysis regarding the more immediate interactions and influences draws from multicultural and gender theories, as well as from social psychological perspectives. A person's gender or cultural heritage plays an important role in how he or she interacts with his or her family and immediate community, informs the belief system that person develops, and impacts the expectations that he or she has for daily life in his or her community, school, and work.

The environments or norms at work and school, for example, share an interaction with groups and individuals, which is mediated by culture and gender. The workplace has a culture or set of norms with a particular set of expectations for work behavior in terms of how long and how often one works, how one's progress is measured, and to what extent this progress is expected in order to maintain job security or earn advancement. The person enters work with a set of expectations about working—whether that might be in terms of expected pay, achievement, regard from others, or material gain.

An example of the interactivity between the person and the norms of work may be seen in the experience of traditionally oriented Native Americans. Imagine a Native American from a small southwestern town who has had an upbringing based strongly on traditional cultural values. Imagine that this person moves to a big city far from home that does not value traditional cultural belief systems. This person finds a job, and is expected to arrive at work on time and be there 8 hours a day 5 days a week, often without a specific set of expectations for productivity or outcome. Imagine the experience of that person in this new environment. How does culture play a role in shaping that experience, and how does that experience interact with the various aspects of that person, as described in the description of the individual level?

In this example, the norms of work in the dominant society often leads to working for the sake of working, rather than working for the attainment of specific goals or resources. These work expectations may be at odds with the cultural ethos of some Native American groups regarding working as a form of trade—that is, one works not for goods in and of themselves or for individual gain, but rather to trade labor for the benefit of the community. Another aspect of this ethos embraces the idea of having as little impact on the environment as possible, and maintaining a balance with the physical and spiritual realms; this is an ethos that does not mesh well with the consumer-driven, product-oriented economy of mainstream America. In addition to having a different view of labor and the purpose of work, some Native Americans have a different concept of time. Time is not in itself something that can be traded, so working an 8-hour work day may not necessarily be meaningful, unless in that span of time some specific task was achieved that benefited the person's community. This example could be carried further, but let us move to another example.

The school system is another aspect of this first ring; an individual's or group's interactions with this system are driven by factors at the individual level, factors within the community in which the school exists, and factors about the school itself. One must examine the educational expectations of the community, of the school system, and of the particular school. Prayer in the schools is an example: What is the belief or practice about prayer? Is that belief or practice based on whether the school is parochial or public, and what does that say about the norms in that school? How do those norms affect the individual? At a more distant level, what are the policies of that school system, what is the perspective of the state educational system, and what is the tenor of the discussion at a national level?

Curriculum development in the school is another issue that exists at multiple levels in the ecological model, and must be examined in terms of the beliefs and assumptions of the individual, the community, the local school system, and so forth. The example of curriculum development is particularly relevant when we examine how knowledge and ways of knowing are privileged based on what persons or groups in the school system have the dominant voice. It is usually the case that the type of knowledge that is valued is based on mainstream viewpoints, in which empiricism and rationalism are given the dominant voice. What, then, happens to intuitive knowledge and the other ways of knowing that students from nondominant groups might value?

The Exosystem

The next circle of the feminist ecological model is the exosystem, which consists of various institutions at the regional, state, and national levels. Some of these include, for example, the legal system, governments, educational systems, religious institutions, professional groups, and academic disciplines. The aim of these institutions is to oversee the interests of the public and identify ways to respond to them through establishing sets of guidelines, rules, and programs. While institutions hold potential to serve as a source for social change by responding to the needs of people, they are not currently structured to do so and remain at a marginal level in accommodating the diverse needs of individuals. Those who are located in positions of power within institutional settings too often make an assumption that they are capable of setting effective goals and determining the means to achieve them without listening to the daily experiences of individuals whose lives are affected by their decisions. For instance, the development of a welfare policy that continuously fails to become inclusive of the voices of the poor, or of laws defining "domestic" violence that are primarily concerned with physical evidence while discounting the psychological sufferings and terror experienced by victims of violence, are just a few examples that illustrate how exclusions of lived experiences contribute to further marginalizing individuals that social institutions are meant to serve. It is crucial to understand that negative consequences enforced upon individuals through the workings of the exosystem are in material and economic resources, and also on the psychological and spiritual aspects of individuals. Bridging the gap between the exosystem and individuals is clearly needed.

A close look at health care systems, in particular insurance policies and mental health care, offers an example of how private insurance corporations attempt to maximize their profits at the expense of others. The policy imposed by insurance companies regulates the number of visits an individual can make, as well as requiring that service providers diagnose their clients with "mental disorders." This contributes to the further marginalization of those individuals who are most in need of the services. While affluent individuals are likely to be able to afford services, poor individuals may not have any options in continuing to receive services. In addition to the impact on individuals by health care systems, these policies implicitly effect other arenas of institutions simultaneously. For example, the "efficiency" and profit-maximization approach taken by insurance corporations leads to reductionistic medical models and external judgments of medically necessary treatments. It further leads to guidelines authorizing only empirically supported most effective treatments. It is no surprise that the behavioral and biological approaches are most readily measured. Those psychotherapies and treatments measured as most effective are more likely to receive grants for further empirical research. Moreover, they also receive the most attention in professional journals and impact the education and training students receive.

As the impact of social institutions discussed above indicates, the lives of individuals are embedded in the exosystem. This brings challenges for psychologists. Although mainstream psychology has begun to acknowledge the effects of the larger systemic base upon individuals, actions are yet to be incorporated in many psychological theories. In order to work toward social change, psychologists need to work with people in identifying ways to intervene with social institutions. The emphasis of liberation psychology on the development of the critical consciousness, feminism's "personal is political" or its inverse "political is personal," and formation of a coalition based on shared differences foregrounded by transformative multiculturalism may serve as a first step to organize collective actions. Additionally, it is crucial that disciplinary boundaries be negotiated among researchers, practitioners, and students to take on multiple perspectives in understanding ways to actualize social change. In particular, collaboration among diverse disciplines may serve to identify ways to better transform societies without losing sight of the empowerment of individuals within them.

Traditional mainstream psychology has dismissed the link between individuals and the larger structural base, and has often attributed psychological distress within individuals. However, as the impact of social institutions discussed above clearly indicate, individuals and the microsystem are embedded with inequalities produced within the exosystem. The challenges for psychologists are thus situating the lives of individuals within a larger systemic base and working with others to identify ways to intervene with the social institutions.

The Macrosystem

The next and the last ring of our feminist ecological model is the macrosystem. It consists of a variety of structural and environmental forces, including values, worldviews, human rights, global distribution of resources, politics, and the economy. Not only do these factors directly interact with the immediate circle of the exosystem, but they further extend their influences in shaping the experiences of groups and communities, as well as the daily lives of individuals. The consideration of issues from the macrolevel is crucial in that it makes us realize social change requires us to use the frame of double perspectives, to connect the personal and the political, theory and actions. For example, understanding and helping individuals who are experiencing psychological distress requires us to consider their current concerns and immediate surroundings (meaning first-order change). In addition, it requires us to consider ways to promote changes in structural forces that would support and advocate their empowerment (meaning second-order change). Our efforts to help individuals with their immediate concerns by intervening with their current surroundings are important, but they may be limited in terms of success unless they are also accompanied by efforts to challenge inequalities produced in the macrosystem and to identify ways to contribute to altering structural forces and alleviating their impact.

One example is the distribution of resources and its impact upon children in the United States and globally. Children who live in poverty are affected by multiple consequences that may contribute to limiting their psychological and physical development and growth. Despite rhetoric in the United States that children are the future of our society and that education is central to our nation's future, opportunities available for children to maximize their development are far from equal. Opportunity is accorded by class distinction, which often determines, for example, the type of education and care a child receives. One must understand the economic structure and related political systems within national and global policies and practices to comprehend or account for the paradox that underlies valuing yet underresourcing children. Valuing children is empty or misleading rhetoric if social policies and institutional interventions and resources are not followed up with actual implementations.

In a similar manner, distribution of resources in a global context highlights its consequences upon children in poor nations. Third-world nations that do not have structures to sustain their economy rely on international transactions and the exchange of their cheap labor for material goods from the "industrialized" nations. Under this international economy, children are forced into a labor market to work in slave-like conditions, and some are traded as objects with a price in a global sex-slave economy. Despite reports of these incidents taking place around the globe, human rights are not extended to children, and there remains little effort in identifying ways to help poor nations in a nonoppressive manner. Nor are linkages between these human rights abuses and the hegemonic imposition of an advanced capitalist economy being widely discussed.

The example discussed above is a highly complex issue, and it is not easy to provide an ultimate solution. There may be multiple opinions, each colored by the values and worldviews of nations and individuals. Having indicated so, we believe that consideration of values in relation to ethics may serve as a key to start building a foundation in forming a coalition. Although complex in nature and challenging to action, it is very clear that large structural forces impact strongly on the lived experience of individuals, and understanding human nature and experience requires the broadest of views.

Planetary/Climatic Conditions

The level of planetary/climatic conditions is one dimension of our model that is often attended to by U.S. environmentalists, the Green Party in Europe, and by those with more intuitive and spiritual connections with the earth. Ecopsychology, Capra's systems thinking, feminist spirituality, some cultures' nature orientations, and environmentalists have already developed theories, beliefs, and analyses about the need to consider human interactions with the planet. Evidence of a profound lack of awareness about the planet, and the harmful effects of human behavior on planetary conditions, can be seen in many contemporary circumstances. One such area is the general disregard of the earth in corporate materialism, which is implicated in pollution, global warming, distribution of food to countries by economy rather than by population, overuse of natural resources, and demands for energy to fuel the increasing pace of technobusiness. Another general area is failure to attain relationships with the global community, as evidenced by interpersonal violence and violence against nature, civil and national wars, ethnic conflicts, and the loss of relationships with one another and with other life forms.

These and other conditions illustrate ever-present concerns that must hold prominence in our model. Climate and planetary conditions are occasionally dramatic, as is the case with natural disasters; however, these conditions are more often subtle and too easily ignored. Climate and planetary conditions affect our lives and our health in many ways. For example, one of the largest building booms near Disney World in Orlando, Florida, in recent memory has accompanied a serious 3-year drought in Florida. The six new golf courses in the area threaten not only the wildlife in the rivers and swamps, but also the fertility of the few remaining agricultural fields. This example pales in the face of floods, drought-induced starvation, and the destruction of once-fertile lands due to overuse without replenishment of the earth. These examples are the more dramatic—but are all considered in the planetary and climate conditions. We examine our effects on the earth and its effects on us—the interaction is easy to see, particularly if we take a long view over time and events.

The climate and the planet need to be a part of the feminist ecological model. The model makes them visible by reminding us that we are linked to other living systems in mutually interdependent ways. This linkage has systematic effects on our personality, social structures, and physical lives. We see these effects over time as well. Adults living in this era now seek work in the service industry instead of in agriculture and horticulture, pointing to a growing disconnection with the earth. Children now growing up have entirely different images from those of previous generations of what work is and might be. Change, transience, people pleasing for profit—these are qualities fast replacing the ethic of caring for and working with the land for productivity, commitment, and authenticity. A quite different and more hopeful area is the symbolic understanding of the mutual interactions among living systems, which is seen in earth-based spiritual practices, and in the balance and harmony of Buddhism, Taoism, and the practices of several indigenous peoples.

The physical aspects of the planet and climate span the levels of the feminist ecological model, and require that we think both out-of-the-box and across disciplines. We must consider the beliefs and practices of cultural groups and earth-based mystics, as well as of sciences, social studies, and humanities. The climate and planetary support structure, as with its twin of history, invite consideration outside of hegemonic constraints. Including both of them in our model brings a reality to the mutual influence of multiple systems and conditions.

Time/History

In the ecological perspective, the concepts of time and history are very important. Time and history affect the individual at all levels of the model, and interact with structural, political, economic, and geophysical forces to inform the life experiences of individuals and groups. Time involves environmental events, processes of transition that take place in the life course of individuals and groups, and the flow of sociohistorical events and conditions.

Not only does time affect people, but people affect time as well. There are a myriad of ways in which people measure and experience the flow of time. They define time in ways such as linear, circular, and static moments that are marked more by events than by date or period in history. Time has relatively more or less impact in the experiences of individuals and groups depending on how it is defined.

In the ecological model, time is defined according to particular categories. Personal or biographical time refers to the individual's personal experience of time, including events and experiences in that person's lifetime, such as significant life events, the changing meaning of membership in dominant or nondominant groups, and relationships with other people and institutions. Historical time refers to the era or period in history in which a person lives, with its particular mix of social and geopolitical forces. Historical time defines how and when social and political normative standards are structured and codified. Historical time also describes which groups, institutions, and ideas become the dominant forces, and which become marginalized or oppressed. A third aspect of time is cross-generational time. This aspect of time encompasses the ways in which normative standards and sociocultural mores are passed along through generations (of family, social and cultural groups, institutions, etc.).

For personality theory, an interactive example of time in relation to the individual might consider that the stability of personality over the lifetime is affected by the structural opportunities that are presented to individuals at particular points in history, mediated by present and cross-generational social effects.

Ideas from liberation psychology mesh well with an ecological perspective on time. Liberation psychology focuses prominently on sociohistorical events that shape the lives of individuals and the collective experiences of groups. Not only does liberation psychology attempt to see the dynamic forces of past historical events shaping the present, but it also attempts to link past, present, and the future by recognizing the agency of individuals and collective efforts in creating the future. Individuals are thought of not only as passive recipients of historical events, but as capable of effecting the future based on reflections of the past. For example, understanding historical events consisting of the exclusionary practices of "others" requires multilevel analysis of power and privilege, while at the same time listening to how individuals and groups make sense of the impact of historical events that shape their present conditions and their hopes for the future.

Coordinates of the Feminist Ecological Model

Certain demographic categories within human experience at particular points in history seem to function as signifiers across the levels of the ecological model. Sex-gender, race-ethnicity, age, and class are shown as such categories in our feminist ecological model. These categories—called *coordinates* in our model—are represented as lines that cut across the multiple levels of the model. The coordinates, unlike the phenomena, structures, and process within levels of the models are signifiers at all levels. Their interactivity with all levels of the model is constant, particularly in terms of their impact on the individual's experiences with and interpretation of daily life.

The literature within feminist psychology, and more generally women's studies, is quite compelling regarding the influence of gender on personality and its development. The various influences of race-ethnicity are also becoming clarified. While neither sex-gender nor race-ethnicity holds a central position in mainstream psychology, there are studies, chapters, and communities of people that are helpful in increasing awareness about these issues. Class and age are enormously consequential but have received less attention in the psychological literature.

Class, for instance, is a significant factor at the individual level. Class is certainly a strong influence on one's sense of self or identity, and is complex and very potent in one's experiences in life. Not only are social and economic resources affected, but so are the expectations for and perceptions of the self. For instance, a child of poverty might typically go to a neighborhood school without an adequate building, books, teachers, or support services. This child may walk to school through violent and dispirited communities and participate at school after a relatively poor level of home attention to dress and homework. This child will speak in the language patterns and share the interests of her family, friends, and neighborhood. Further, the level of need and security within the child's life space will affect the child's motivation toward school as well as the reinforcement that child can expect to receive for school performance. All are factors influencing self perceptions, attributions, and the expectations of others.

Class determines school-related behavior at both ends of the economic spectrum. The school experiences of both poor kids and rich kids might, for example, deemphasize the importance and authority of the public schools, but for very different reasons. The rich child might have the opportunity for basic socialization at the primary-public-school level, but certainly will continue her or his education in private schools aimed at fostering the elite. So for some rich children, public schools may not hold much importance. The poor child, on the other hand, may have an ambivalent experience with the public school, but it does not necessarily lead to the middle-class expectation of opportunity opened up through meritorious performance. Given the trend of housing displacement that poverty often fosters, the poor child may change schools so frequently that a sense of place and belonging does not develop. The physical needs and dangers of living in a poor community take precedence over academic achievement, and therefore may require most of the child's attention for which the school also competes. The home environment may be marked by so many demands and strains that regular parental attention to and support for schoolwork is unavailable. Further, given the threats to security and economic viability, school performance and excitement about the progressive gaining of skills may be overwhelmed by the demands for money to pay rent and buy food, both today and tomorrow. The experience of the middle-class child is perhaps the only one that may approach the safe, nurturing learning community where parents, teachers, and community leaders alike attend to and support the child's school experience. This single example, restricted to individual and microsystem levels, though stereotypical, does give some sense of how very important it is for us to pay close attention to differences and similarities by class. Class—not just the economic resources, but the differential experiences and needs, attributions, and self-perceptions of individuals—is necessary to consider deeply in the feminist ecological model.

Class also holds second- and third-order influence in the outer levels of the ecological model. Typically, the regional, state, and national exosystems, as well as governmental law and policy, are neither inclusive of nor structured toward the needs and experiences of the poor. Similarly, economic resources and influence through professional organizations, disciplines, religion, and other social institutions are not often oriented toward the poor. Few honors are given to high school kids who work as much as possible to contribute to the family income, or to children who manage to pass their grade levels from the homeless shelter. Nor are voices of the poor solicited when welfare policies change to allow budget surpluses and tax cuts.

At the macrosystem level, distribution of resources, political and economic factors, consideration of the environment, and worldviews and values are not influenced by nor responsive to the poor nations. Third-world nations typically have huge national debts and very little educational and economic infrastructure through which to win a place at the competitive global table. Instead, whatever resources may exist are drained to support other more powerful nations: timber from old-growth trees, meritorious students and scholars, inexpensive labor for manufacturing, and so on. Poorer nations are often more populous, and have high needs for nutritional, economic, educational, housing, employment, and environmental resources. These demands, however, are often critically underresourced in the poor nations.

Sex-gender, race-ethnicity, and age each hold similar patterns structurally. At every level of the model, each of them is responded to differentially—directly or indirectly. For example, human rights are often not extended to kids. The elderly are frequently underserviced in legal and educational areas. Black men are not typically presidents of banks or of governments in the Western worlds. Women continue in some situations to be owned and abused by fathers, brothers, and husbands.

These coordinates of class, sex-gender, race-ethnicity, and age are critically important influences across all levels of our model. These coordinates are very important to consider because they are the design of our global and immediate social and structural environments. They unequally distribute power, authority, and credit to some while silencing and oppressing others. Our model is not intended to be a disconnected, abstract drawing of multiple influencing factors and structural forces, but is instead a statement about relationships and impacts on people. These and other coordinates exert substantial influence on the development, experiences, and status of people. Without some awareness of these influences in theories of personality, health, and development, efforts to describe human nature are inevitably misdirected.

CONCLUSION

Within mainstream psychology theories of personality are too limited. Our feminist ecological model seeks to define some of the many influencing factors, structures, and interactions well beyond these familiar but limited and defining constructs. Though gender roles are more permeable within the family, and although families have taken on many forms in the last few decades, personality theories have not kept pace with these dramatic changes. Conventional personality theory describes the needs and effects of the unfolding or developing human nature conceptualized as a self, within the context of institutions such as the family, the school, or the workplace. Each institution defines personality and sets the standards for health. Traditional notions of family, for example, suggest that a family consists of mother and father engaging in a gendered division of labor in which the mother is serving as the caretaker within the private sphere while the father is serving as a worker in the public sphere to obtain the income necessary to provide material resources for his family. The gendered division of parenting assumes that the attentiveness and the caring provided by a mother to a child are critical factors in the unfolding nature of a child. Gendered parenting and roles also describe the nuclear family as the only legitimate form of the family, and it dismisses multiple forms of families and meanings of what "family" is. It is essential to note that the familial environment is important, but is only one of many factors that impact personality or human nature. Maintaining an assumption that personality is only effected by what appears to be immediate, such as the familial context, is quite limited, and works to perpetuate our focus only on individuals as they interact with a single point of influence. Human nature does not depend only on the family environment or the microsystem alone, but it is also affected by time, additional levels of influence within our model, and by certain coordinates (such as gender, ethnicity, and class—to name three among others), as well as by history.

While we attempted to provide directions for thinking about the multiple and interacting factors on human nature over time, our model does not give specific content regarding the nature of human beings. In this way, we acknowledge that we have violated the usual expectations of personality theory. Yet our feminist ecological model is liberating in that it may serve as a first step in thinking about "personality" beyond the grand theories that have contributed to unilateral thinking about human nature. Indeed, ego-development, trait-factor, sense-of-self, meaning-making, varieties of learning (including classical, operant, cognitive, and social learning), or even socially and culturally constructed identities, all have a substantive impact on personality. Yet we think that these very *familiarities* within personality theory are what actually constrain our thinking. Our model tries to capture integrated thinking and move beyond conventional theories of personality. Our hope is that we offer readers a sense of liberation to free themselves from the constraints imposed by familiar personality theories.

A multiplicity of interacting factors have begun to be recognized in psychology. Yet the use of dominant methodologies, structured or reinforced by multivariate analysis, for example, fails to articulate the connectedness of external factors by reducing them to separate parts. However, if we are to think differently, we need to come to a renewed consciousness through grounding ourselves in interdisciplinary collaboration, the interactivity of multiple levels of analysis, and the intersubjectivity among people as well as between individuals and the social world. Indeed, this challenging task requires us to reflect, rethink, and rewrite the whole process of theorizing in order to make it more attuned to the actual experiences of diverse people. To this end, we brought together theories of critical theory, liberation psychology, multiculturalism, and human systems. What brings this combination to yet another level is that it is informed by principles of feminist therapy theory. We believe that it not only allows for the advancement of our understanding of human nature in a nonoppressive, egalitarian, and ethical manner, but it also holds potential to impel us to work toward a transformation of society by linking the personal, the political, and action.

The proposed combination of feminism, ecological thinking, critical theories, transformative multiculturalism, and human systems thinking that we present in this chapter, may be a sign that a fourth force is emerging in psychology. Despite claims by some that multiculturalism is the fourth force, the ideas fastened together in this chapter may offer a broader and more profound scaffolding for creating a new force. We hope that the ideas presented here secure and draw together the overlapping, similar (or sometimes competing) claims within many of the progressive thoughts of our time within psychology, other disciplines, and activist communities. In addition to the contents of multiple theoretical stances, our model also offers a grounding in the values of the sociopolitical realm and feminist modes of inquiry.

As briefly discussed earlier, the principles of feminist therapy theory rely upon women's experiences—that is, upon recognizing, valuing, and learning from differences; egalitarian prescriptions of power differences in interpersonal and at multiple levels; and external influences upon people including multiple oppressions according to categories of nondominance. At the same time, these principles highlight the need to take a critical questioning stance toward how ideologies and social control at systemic levels are played out in our daily lives. The same principles apply to disciplinary theory and practices. Multiple epistemologies, methodologies, methods, advocacy, and commitment to social and structural change are essential components of the stance we take as feminists. The principles noted above overlap with an orientation to the themes within our chapter. It is these themes that we would like to address in the following paragraphs—that is, to discuss new codes for building theory in feminist psychology.

We have emphasized the multiple factors of influence by extending dimensions of the external world and of the individual. The consideration of micro-, exo-, and macrolevels of influence are also unique in that each level is colored by sociopolitical dimensions. To take such a perspective is not yet seen in North American mainstream psychology. For example, we extended interacting dimensions by introducing time and history. Including time and history are essential in understanding how individuals as well as groups make sense of their experiences in the present and in the past. Geopolitics in the past and historical events are intertwined with the present, particularly in terms of how they influence the ways individuals or groups view the world. At the same time, considering time/history may provide us with ways to engage in creating the future in a nonoppressive manner.

At a content level, another factor that distinguishes our feminist ecological model from various social-psychological models may be our emphasis on the dialectical process between the psychological and the sociopolitical, and interactions between individuals and multiple levels of ecological factors. Here, we would like to emphasize that we do not assume that individuals are shaped only by external factors. In traditional and mainstream psychology, it is assumed that individuals are passive recipients of external influences, and thus the focus is typically placed upon helping individuals to become responsive to and fit into the existing demands of a social world. In a similar manner, mainstream sociological thinking is heavily one-sided in that it places so much focus on external factors, while failing to recognize the psychological suffering or problems in the lived experience of individuals.

In contrast, our model focuses on reciprocal interactions between individuals and interacting external factors by recognizing double (or multiple) perspectives on the psychological and the sociopolitical. Our model is driven by our core principle to recognize the agency of individuals—to influence and take a part in transforming external conditions. All of the theories that we drew from value the agency of individuals. Liberation psychology and feminism in particular provide ways to connect personal and collective emancipation through direct social interventions.

Indeed, the importance of our personal and collective actions as well as social movements is beginning to be recognized in psychology, yet it rarely appears to be articulated in detail. For example, mainstream multi-cultural theory tends to highlight the particularities of different groups and the ways to work toward actualizing the interests of each group. Differing needs and political struggles of multiple groups are legitimate; yet in this process of validating differences, it appears that all groups become quite fragmented from each other without any sense of coalition among themselves. It is perhaps crucial that we identify ways to form a coalition and a shared sense of affinity based on common differences among groups, to collectively work toward social change. It may be a time in which we move beyond theories in psychology to consider ways to actualize actions and social change.

In addition, we also would like to note that considering interests or problems experienced by groups is important in shaping the actions they choose to take. It is equally important, however, to acknowledge that personal problems in living and psychological suffering are just as important to consider. As feminism, liberation, and critical theories suggest, the empowerment of individuals is necessary to attain social change, just as the transformation of our social world can be called social change only when it brings personal empowerment to people.

In order to understand human nature, just as feminism based its knowledge claims in women's experiences, we also privilege experiences of individuals as they describe themselves and their experiences. One of the points shown by our model is that the inequalities produced at such levels as the micro-, the exo-, and the macrosystem shape the daily lives of individuals. The effects upon individuals are highly dependent upon coordinates and the locations of individuals within the hierarchical system. Listening to and validating the experiences and realities of those who are placed in a subordinated position may provide a less distorted picture of reality. As Comas-Díaz and colleagues (1998) suggest, standing alongside people whose knowledge claims are subjugated is a crucial starting point in building a theory that actually "works" in a real-world context. Such an approach assumes a dialectical process of individuals, environments, researchers, and the people with whom they work. These points anticipate the paradigm shift in the social sciences.

A paradigm is a set of assumptions, definitions, accepted methods, and rules that are established to organize and process understanding of individuals in a social world. Working within the context of a paradigm applies not only in doing academic research, but also to practices, activism, and the web of relationships and contacts we make in our daily lives. In this chapter, we discussed feminist epistemologies as examples of paradigms. In mainstream psychology, the experiences of individuals are evaluated through empiricist epistemology. In contrast, the fourth force that we use as our paradigm insists upon emphasizing the lived experiences of individuals as described by their own words, and to consider it as a rich source of information to understand how people make sense of their worlds. In our chapter, principles of feminist therapy theory bring us to phenomenological epistemology. In addition to valuing lived experiences, we highlight the equal distribution of power, the importance of valuing pluralism, the interlocking nature of oppression produced by external forces, and a commitment to social justice and change. All these values serve to create a structure or a direction in which theory building needs to move.

In addition to the principles of feminist therapy theory, critical theory encourages us to reflect values embedded in each theory. Critical theory gives us a direction in which ethical principles are brought forward. It teaches us the importance of reflecting upon the values that each theory brings forward and others that are placed in the background. This chapter is not an exception. In building this model, the authors have come to sense a shared vision, and thus this model is embedded with our values and worldviews.

In closing, we invite readers to join with us in reconsidering ways to think about human nature. We also would like others to consider and reappropriate values in psychology and the professions, while at the same time thinking critically about the values promoted in society as well as globally. Our hope is that this chapter served to open up the process of theory building to all of us concerned with human nature. Our model is filled with the complexities of interactions that are based on multiple levels and coordinates; additional dimensions, in turn, influence these levels and coordinates. Yet we chose to create our model on the grounds that theory building needs to be situated in real-world contexts. It is also our hope to provide a framework that may reflect organizations of structures that are less distorted and more accurate from the multiple standpoints of individuals. Radway (1998) indicated the necessity to "insist on the importance of remembering that feminist intellectual work on gender emerged within the context of a social and political movement devoted to changing the everyday lives of women as well as the social policies and social forms underwriting that [customary] existence" (p. 40). We stand with her spirit. With this in mind, we also encourage others to co-construct our model of human nature.

REFERENCES

Ballou, M. (1990). Approaching a feminist-principled paradigm in the construction of personality theory. In L. S. Brown & M. P. Root (Eds.), *Diversity and complexity in feminist therapy* (pp. 23–40). New York: Haworth Press.

Ballou, M. (1995). Women and spirit: Two nonprofits in psychology. In J. Ochshorn & E. Cole (Eds.), *Women's spirituality, women's lives* (pp. 9–20). New York: Haworth Press.

Ballou, M. (1996). Multicultural theory and women. In D. W. Sue, A. Ivey, & P. Pederson (Eds.), *A theory of multicultural counseling and therapy* (pp. 236–246). Pacific Grove, CA: Brooks/Cole.

Ballou, M., & Gabalac, N. (1985). *A feminist position on mental health*. Springfield, IL: Charles C Thomas.

Brown, L. R. (1994). *Subversive dialogues: Theory in feminist therapy*. New York: Basic Books.

Brown, L. R. (1995). *Ecopsychology: Restoring the earth, healing the mind* (T. Roszak, M. E. Gomes, & A. D. Kanner, Eds.). San Francisco: Sierra Club Books.

Capra, F. (1996). *The web of life: A new scientific understanding of living systems*. New York: Anchor Doubleday.

Comas-Díaz, L. (1991). Feminism and diversity in psychology: The case of women of color. *Psychology of Women Quarterly, 15,* 597–609.

Comas-Díaz, L., Lykes, M. B., & Alarcon, R. D. (1998). Ethnic conflict and the psychology of liberation in Guatemala, Peru, and Puerto Rico. *American Psychologist, 52*(7), 778–792.

Crenshaw, K. W. (1994). Mapping the margins: Intersectionality, identity politics, and violence against women of color. In M. A. Fineman & R. Mykitiuk (Eds.), *The*

140 DEVELOPING FEMINIST THEORIES

public nature of private violence: The discovery of domestic abuse (pp. 94–117). New
York: Routledge.

Enns, C. (1992). Toward integrating feminist psychotherapy and feminist philosophy.
Professional Psychology: Research and Practice, 23, 453–466.

Enns, C. (1993). Twenty years of feminist counseling and therapy: From naming biases to implementing multifaceted practice. *Counseling Psychologist, 21*(1), 3–87.

Enriquez, V. G. (1992). *From colonial to liberation psychology: The Philippine experience.* Quezon: University of Philippines Press.

Fowers, B. J., & Richardson, F. C. (1996). Why is multiculturalism good? *American Psychologist, 51,* 609–621.

Fox, D., & Prilleltensky, I. (1997). *Critical psychology: An introduction.* Thousand Oaks, CA: Sage.

Gardner, H. (1993). *Multiple intelligences: The theory in practice.* New York: Basic Books.

Goldman, D. (1995). *Emotional intelligence.* New York: Bantam Books.

Harding, S. (1993). *The racial economy of science: Toward a democratic future.* Bloomington: Indiana University Press.

Hill, M., & Ballou, M. (1998). Making therapy feminist: A practice survey. *Journal of Women and Therapy, 16,* 1–16.

Hollander, N. C. (1997). *Love in a time of hate: Liberation psychology in Latin America.* New Brunswick, NJ: Rutgers University Press.

Jordan, J. V., Kaplan, A. G., Miller, J. B., Stiver, I. P., & Surrey, J. L. (1991). *Women's growth in connection: Writings from the Stone Center.* New York: Guilford Press.

Kaschak, E. (1981). Feminist psychotherapy: The first decade. In S. Cox (Ed.), *Female psychology: The emerging self* (pp. 387–401). New York: St. Martin's Press.

Kaschak, E. (1992). *Engendered lives: A new psychology of women's experience.* New York: Basic Books.

Kitzinger, C. (1991). Politicizing psychology. *Feminism and Psychology, 1*(1), 49–54.

Landrine, H. (Ed.). (1995). *Bringing cultural diversity to feminist psychology theory, practice and research.* Washington, DC: American Psychological Association Press.

Lorde, A. (1992). Age, race, class, and sex: Women defining difference. In P. Rothenberg (Ed.), *Race, class, and gender in the United States: An integrated study* (pp. 402–414). New York: St. Martin's Press.

Martin-Baro, I. (1994). *Writing for a liberation psychology* (A. Aron & S. Corne, Eds.). Cambridge, MA: Harvard University Press.

Nuttall, E., Sanchez, W., & Webber, J. (1996). MCT theory and implications for training. In D. W. Sue, A. Ivey, & P. Pederson (Eds.), *A theory of multicultural counseling and therapy* (pp. 125–136). Pacific Grove, CA: Brooks/Cole.

Prilleltensky, I., & Nelson, G. (1997). Community psychology: Reclaiming social justice. In D. Fox & I. Prilleltensky (Eds.), *Critical psychology: An introduction* (pp. 166–184). Thousand Oaks, CA: Sage.

Prilleltensky, I., & Fox, D. (1997). Introducing critical psychology: Values, assumptions, and the status quo. In D. Fox & I. Prilleltensky (Eds.), *Critical psychology: An introduction* (pp. 3–20). Thousand Oaks, CA: Sage.

Radway, J. (1998). Gender in the field of ideological production: Feminist cultural studies, the problem of the political subject, and the aims of knowledge production. In S. V. Rosser, J. Radway, & N. Fobre (Eds.), *New perspectives in gender studies: Research in the fields of economics, culture, and life sciences* (pp. 37–59) Linkoping, The Netherlands: Linkoping University, Department of Gender Studies.

Riger, S. (1992). Epistemological debates, feminist voices: Science, social values, and the study of women. *American Psychologist, 47,* 730–740.

Sue, D. W., Ivey, A., & Pederson, P. (1996). *A theory of multicultural counseling and therapy.* Pacific Grove, CA.: Brooks/Cole.

Unger, R. (1995). Cultural diversity and the future of feminist psychology. In H. Landrine (Ed.), *Bringing cultural diversity to feminist psychology* (pp. 413–432). Washington, DC: American Psychological Association Press.

Worell, J., & Johnson, N. G. (1997). *Shaping the future of feminist psychology: Education, research, and practice.* Washington, DC: American Psychological Association.

Part II

Psychopathology

Chapter 6

Somatoform and Pain Disorders

DENISE WEBSTER

WHAT IS THE CURRENT SITUATION?

In the early 1960s there was great excitement on the psychiatric service of a prestigious teaching hospital. A "true conversion reaction" had been admitted to the unit. These were seen relatively rarely these days, we were told, and most educated people were obviously reticent to seek psychiatric treatment. But the pretty young woman exhibiting these blatant symptoms was from a remote area of Kentucky, which would explain her ignorance about the condition. For weeks, she had displayed convincing fainting spells and claimed not to know at first where she was when she "awoke." As no underlying physical cause had been determined, it seemed apparent that we were witnessing a loss of voluntary motor function, the manifestation of a primitive defense mechanism motivated by unconscious psychological conflicts. The goal of treatment would be to unearth the primary conflict and identify the secondary gains she obtained from others' concerns about her mysterious malady. Unfortunately, from an educational standpoint, the nurses noted a definite pattern to the spells: they all occurred about 30 minutes after she took her anticonvulsant medication and were accompanied by a precipitous drop in her blood pressure. A change in medication stopped the fainting.

Many aspects of medicine, psychology, and psychiatry have changed in the intervening decades. However, the psychiatric diagnoses included in the categories of somatoform and pain disorders remain among the most difficult to accurately diagnose and effectively treat. These diagnoses include somatization disorder or Briquet's syndrome (a long history of complaints of multiple unexplained symptoms), conversion disorder (neurological symptoms inconsistent with pathophysiological knowledge), hypochondriasis (preoccupation with/fear of disease), body dysmorphic disorders (excessive concern about imagined body defects), and pain disorders (pain complaints disproportionate to physical evidence) (American Psychiatric Association, 1994). In medical practice, physical symptoms that cannot be medically explained are often called *functional somatic disorders* (Wessely, Nimnuan, & Sharpe, 1999). Lying in the sizable gap created by conceptualizations of the mind and the body as separate, these conditions defy dominant contemporary medical explanations for disease. Positivist and determinist philosophies predominate in the medical model—that is, objective signs of pathology must support subjective reports of symptoms and treatments should provide consistent responses in different people having the same condition. If patients reporting these conditions are suspected of feigning symptoms or of manufacturing evidence to support a medical diagnosis, the more likely diagnosis would be either factitious disorder or malingering. In factitious disorder (called Munchhausen's by proxy if an adult is responsible for inducing injury or illness in a child), the apparent intent is to take the role of a patient and/or to be hospitalized. Malingering is suspected if false or exaggerated symptoms appear intended to permit the complainant to avoid responsibility (often legal), gain financial reward, or obtain drugs (Rogers, 1988). References detailing assessment, differential diagnosis, and treatment issues related to the range of somatoform conditions are available in several sources (American Psychiatric Association, 1994; Cassam, Stern, Rosenbaum, & Jellinek, 1997; Kaplan & Sadock, 1998; Kroenke, Spitzer, deGruy, & Swindle, 1998; Maxman & Ward, 1995; Rogers, 1988; Williams & Silk, 1997). This chapter focuses primarily on somatization and pain disorders.

Medically unexplained symptoms are highly prevalent in primary care (Katon & Walker, 1998). Some estimate that 40% of all primary care visits are for 14 common physical symptoms, with only 10–15% of these determined 1 year later to represent an organic diagnosis (Kroenke & Mandelsdorff, 1989). Among the symptoms that often have unexplained causes are chest pain, fatigue, dizziness, headaches, edema, back pain, shortness of breath, insomnia, abdominal pain, and numbness. Medically unexplained symptoms are described as a major problem in health care because they lead to unnecessary specialty referrals, drive up the costs of health care, and threaten the quality of the doctor–patient relationship. The relationships between psychological distress and physical symptoms are variably described. Prior illness, underlying personality, and family environmental factors are often cited as predisposing to unexplained physical complaints. Major mental disorders and personality disorders are also described as common among those with unexplained physical complaints (Katon & Walker, 1998). Lifetime prevalence of somatization disorder is estimated at less than 0.2% for men and from 0.2 to 2% in women. Conversion disorder rates vary widely, but are estimated to occur in women 2–10 times more frequently than in men. Pain disorders are very common (10–15% of adults are work-disabled for some period each year due to back pain) and women are reported to have more headaches and musculoskeletal pain (American Psychiatric Association, 1994).

Explanatory Models

Issues of ontology and epistemology are unavoidable in the politics of naming any phenomenon. Nowhere is this more apparent than in the naming of conditions that reside on the boundaries of powerful fields. Border skirmishes and outright battles can emerge from differing explanatory frameworks regarding what is real, how reality is recognized, how it is named, who gets to do the naming, and how to deal with those who use different concepts and names to describe the same phenomenon. Ideas about health and illness are powerfully, deeply, and often invisibly embedded in social and cultural views of what it means to be a person, how and why we and the universe came to be, and what the consequences are for defying whatever gods a society honors at a particular point in time. The following models refer primarily to the more prevalent current Western models of health and illness. These models seldom address issues of culture, race, social class, or gender directly, although through examples or omissions there may be serious implications for those with limited power to name their own experience and/or have it heard (Kleinman & Becker, 1998).

Psychiatric and psychological explanations and treatments for somatoform disorders tend to fall into three major categories: psychoanalytic/ psychodynamic, cognitive-behavioral, and biological. Classical psychoanalytic views of somatoform disorders were first described by Freud and continue to prevail in some "New Age" as well as in classical explanations for illness. In this view, psychological trauma, having been repressed, nevertheless has a life of its own, through unconsciously motivated symptoms. The underlying personality of the person (usually a woman) with these tendencies betrays characteristics of dependency and ambivalence. Freud's description of his work with Dora is considered one of the first descriptions of psychological conflict manifesting as physical problems. (Dora has since been discussed as sexually abused by feminist therapists

[Kreig & Goodwin, 1993] and the case as reflecting anti-Semitism by others [Blum 1994; Gilman, 1997]). In such conditions, "greed for love" was seen to be at the root of learning to use illness to get love and attention, as a weapon for maintaining position, or to manipulate a distant husband to be more solicitous (Freud, 1990). Erik Erikson (1994) implicated conflict during the developmental stage of initiative versus guilt as associated with paralysis or impotence, on the one hand, or overcompensation, on the other. Pathological regression related to conflict at this stage was often demonstrated psychosomatically (Kaplan & Sadock, 1998, p. 237). Similarly, conversion disorder is linked with oedipal conflict, while psychosomatic children tend to fear they are not living up to others' expectations. Personality patterns are sometimes associated with specific psychosomatic diseases—for example, oral needs manifest in asthma, and peptic ulcers are linked to ongoing frustration of intense dependence needs (Kaplan & Sadock, 1998, pp. 797–805). Psychodynamic treatment utilizes interpretation of conflict and insight, based on interpretations of transferences in the therapeutic relationship (Taerk, 1998; Wilson, 1989). Several contemporary writers seeking to create a field of psychoanalytic health psychology acknowledge that one major barrier to the task will be convincing therapists to develop and value research on psychodynamic concepts in health and illness that extend beyond therapist-reported studies of individual cases (Duberstein & Masling, 2000).

Cognitive-behavioral approaches have been successful in treating many conditions of chronic illness, including some that are considered to have strong psychosomatic components. Often combined with stress-based biological theories of illness described below, cognitive-behavioral treatments focus on modifying thoughts and behaviors that precede or accompany symptoms such as pain, anxiety, and depression. Negative thoughts and behaviors are hypothesized to amplify reports of physical symptoms directly and/or indirectly through interpretations that increase feelings of helplessness and hopelessness. Maladaptive pain behaviors (such as physical "guarding" and physical inactivity) and ineffective coping (such as catastrophizing or self-blame) are often targeted in cognitive-behaviorally based self-management programs presented individually or in patient groups (Sanders, 1996). Education about the medical understanding and treatment of specific medical conditions is often provided (Keefe, Beaupré, & Gil, 1996). If family therapy is provided, the focus may be on reducing behaviors seen to "reinforce"/reward illness or pain behaviors in the identified patient (Kerns & Payne, 1996). In contrast to psychodynamically based approaches, cognitive-behavioral approaches are less concerned with historical or developmental explanations about how a condition developed than with how current behavioral goals can be identified and positively reinforced.

Stress models have become increasingly popular in the fields of health psychology and behavioral medicine to provide explanations for the use and effectiveness of a range of stress-reduction approaches. These models are based on early physiological studies by Cannon and Selye, who hypothesized, using animal models, the limitations of the human body to withstand unremitting stress without the development of physical symptoms and eventual death (Lovallo, 1997). Lazarus and Folkman's (1984) work on stress and coping emphasizes the role of cognition in the interpretation of events and symptoms as mediators that could facilitate or interfere with adaptation to stress. In contrast to psychodynamic models, stress models usually emphasize generality rather than specificity in the stress response and suggest a range of stress-reduction and coping approaches seen as having wide application across a range of conditions. Programs for stress reduction are often combined with cognitive-behavioral self-management programs (Eimer & Freeman, 1998; Lehrer & Woolfolk, 1993; Lorig, 1996).

Stress–diathesis models hypothesize that a person with a specific vulnerability (diathesis), in the presence of a stressful influence, may develop symptoms. Integrating biological, psychosocial, and environmental factors, this model presents stress and diathesis as potentially environmental, biological, or both. Environmental stressors can psychological (e.g., family problems or the death of a loved one) or biological (e.g., infections or allergens). Other epigenetic factors may further shape the biological basis of a diathesis (e.g., psychosocial stress and trauma or substance abuse; Gatchel & Weisberg, 2000; Paris, 1999).

Biologically based theories of somatic phenomena, including the above stress-based theories, reflect the rapidly changing fields of neurology, immunology, endocrinology, genetics, and pharmacology. The National Institutes of Health-declared "Decade of the Brain" and the Human Genome Project have raised many questions about human behavior in the process of answering others. The emphasis on funding biologically based studies (including twin and adoption studies) has resulted in growing evidence that much of human behavior is genetically based, although the ratio of hereditary to environmental influences varies depending on the characteristic under study (Cloninger, 1999; Paris, 1999). Most major mental illnesses are now strongly attributed to genetic predisposition. In the case of somatoform disorders, the major genetic links identified thus far are related to personality disorders in patients or their families of origin, as well as to somatization tendencies in female relatives (Morrison, 1990). For example, several adoption studies link somatization disorder in women to first-degree relatives with antisocial personality and alcoholic biological fathers (Bohman, Cloninger, von Knorring, & Sigvardsson, 1984; Cloninger, Sigvardsson, von Knorring, & Bohman, 1984; Sigvardsson, von Knorring, Bohman, & Cloninger, 1984)

Other biologically oriented models describe differences in genetic temperament that may reflect differing levels of neurotransmitters, such as dopamine, norepinephrine, and serotonin, associated with personality traits of reward dependence, harm avoidance, and novelty seeking (Stallings, Hewitt, Cloninger, Heath, & Eaves, 1996). Similarly, there is some evidence that introversion is an inherited tendency that reflects a high level of internal stimulation and arousal (Ornstein, 1993). In the presence of stressors, it might be expected that physiological and neurological responses would be different for those with different temperaments. Several studies support differences in pain threshold and tolerance, based on extraversion–introversion (Phillips & Gatchel, 2000).

The concepts of neurological sensitization and kindling have been used to explain increasing behavioral and physiological response to repeated stimuli. Phenomena explaining the intensification and spread of seizure activity have been implicated now in several psychiatric conditions, including posttraumatic stress disorder, depression, and bipolar disorder (Kendler, Thornton, & Gardner, 2000; Wolpert, Berman, & Bornstein, 1999). Proposed models suggest that "acute or repeated stressors may not only leave permanent memory traces, but also affect the biochemistry and microstructure of the brain, potentially by impacting immediate-early-gene and late-effector-gene expression" (Post, Weis, & Smith, 1995, p. 203). Other neurological models have been offered to explain why some people eventually experience even neutral or usually pleasurable touch as painful (a condition called *allodynia*) (Bennett, 1999).

Recent interest in the growing field of psychoneuroimmunology holds promise for improved understanding about the complexities of neurological processing, immune response, hormonal influences, and how much of human physiology might be amenable to conscious as well as unconscious influences (Rossi, 1993; Schwartz, 1990). Explorations of sex-, ethnic-, and age-related differences in health-related human response are still in their infancy (Watkins, 1997).

In the biological model, pharmacological interventions for biologically based diagnoses are the norm—but controversies about diagnoses, causal explanations, and treatment philosophies abound in relation to conditions assumed to be psychogenic in origin and somatic in presentation. Consequently, a wide range of different pharmacological protocols have been suggested by some to address specific symptoms, such as depression, anxiety, and insomnia, while others believe providing medications and treatment for the unsubstantiated physical symptoms inappropriately reinforces medical explanations for the complaints (Morrison, 1990; Williams & Silk, 1997).

In addition to psychiatric and psychological explanatory models, social analyses of somatization disorder have also been suggested (Barsky & Borus, 1999). Historical and contemporary perspectives on somatoform disorders represent a predictable range of controversies regarding the relative weight of personal and political factors. Feminists and nonfeminists have joined "nonbelievers" who see unexplained physical complaints as the result of media influences and self-diagnosis, mass hysteria, and gullible physicians. This group calls such conditions "iatrogenic," meaning that they are the result of medical intervention, that is, the "creation of " various "nondiseases" by the act of naming and treating them as if they were legitimate, either because they are overly anxious to help or fear legal reprisal (Barsky & Borus, 1999; Shorter, 1992; Showalter, 1997). Another group of historians and postmodern feminists have concluded that the condition represents a nonverbal protest against oppressive conditions, leaving open the question of whether this makes them "legitimate" because sickness as protest may be justified in the context of relative powerlessness (Ehrenreich & English, 1978; Hunter, 1983; Leavitt, 1984; Mitchell, 1974; Smith-Rosenberg, 1985). Still others imply that the conditions reflect the physical consequences of modern women's role strain, as they try to be all things to all people (Silverstein & Perlick, 1995).

Relatively little acknowledgment is given in the mainstream psychiatric and medical literature that cultural beliefs are central to all interpretations of symptoms, their causes, and their treatment. For example, a visitation from a dead relative providing advice for healing is seen as fortuitous in many cultures, whereas most psychiatrists would hear such a report as evidence of psychotic tendencies. Zborowski's classic (1952) study of cultural components in response to pain illustrates the wide variation even within dominant and acculturated groups about the meaning of pain and appropriate ways to express it. The need for awareness and respect for non-Western views of illness is becoming more evident as health care providers work with increasing numbers of immigrant and indigenous groups, as well as with other ethnic groups, who often have more holistic views about health and healing (Escobar, 1995; Friedman, 1997; Helman, 1994; Kramer, Ivey, & Ying, 1999; Lee, 1998; Spector, 1996).

Finally, at the intersection of the social, psychological, and biological models there is persuasive evidence that violence is a risk factor for many chronic health problems long after the acute effects of trauma have apparently resolved (Davidson & Foa, 1993; Dohrenwend, 1998; Friedman, Charney, & Deutsch, 1995; Miller, 1998; van der Kolk, McFarlane, & Weisaeth, 1996; Wilson & Keane,1997). A history of abuse, whether physical, sexual, or both, has been associated with somatoform disorders, eating disorders, and personality and dissociative disorders, as well as with many chronic pain conditions. Childhood sexual abuse has been particularly implicated as a factor predisposing to "chronic pelvic pain without organic cause" as well as other symptoms considered indicators of somatoform disorders (Farley & Keaney, 1997; Heim, Ehlert, Hanker, & Hellhammer, 1998; Reilly, Baker, Rhodes, & Salmon, 1999; Thakkar & McCanne, 2000). The relationships between a history of abuse and physical disease, unexplained physical symptoms, diagnoses of personality disorders, mood, anxiety, and other psychiatric disorders have been described and disputed from each of the above perspectives.

WHY IS THIS A PROBLEM FOR WOMEN?

The Eye of the Beholder

To understand the effect on women of theories of somatoform and pain disorders, it is essential to grasp the extent to which deeply held beliefs about women and health permeate the formal and informal education of those in the health care professions. A 1990 National Institute of Mental Health publication addressed in detail some of the differential diagnoses and challenges of treating "somatization disorder in the medical setting" (Smith, 1990). Prominently featured is a mnemonic aid for recalling the DSM-III-R criteria for somatization disorder: Somatization Disorder Besets Ladies And Vexes Physicians. The highlighted letters stand for shortness of breath when not exerting oneself, dysmenorrhea, burning in sex organs (not related to intercourse), lump in throat, amnesia, vomiting, and painful extremities. Having only two of these symptoms was considered highly suspicious for a diagnosis of somatization disorder (Othmer & Desouza, 1985). These guidelines were adopted for DSM-III-R. DSM-IV has reduced the number of symptoms used for screening for somatization disorder from the 35 in DSM-III-R to four symptom groups, each requiring a specific number of symptoms: pain (4), gastrointestinal (2), pseudoneurological (1), and sexual (1) (American Psychiatric Association, 1994). Somatization is considered rare in males, except in Veteran's Administration settings, where is it presumed to be reinforced by potential financial benefit. In a study of men with somatization disorder the point was made that many were homosexual (Morrison, 1990). The implication would seem to be that homosexual men are not "really" men and/or that they are more like women than like men.

Combined with this predisposition to see women as having somatization disorder is the subjective determination of appropriate levels of symptom complaint. One or more somatoform diagnoses can be given even in the presence of an identifiable medical condition if the complaints associated with the condition seem "excessive." Having a single symptom (e.g., fatigue, dizziness, gastrointestinal, or urinary) that persists for more than 6 months without identifiable and sufficient organic explanation makes one eligible for a diagnosis of "undifferentiated somatoform disorder" or a "pain disorder" (American Psychiatric Association, 1994). Another medical term often used to describe "functional somatic" symptoms is "psychosomatic," a term interpreted by laypeople and many professionals to mean a condition is "not real," that is, it is "in the head" rather than "in the body." The term originally was intended to acknowledge the inherent unity of mind and body—the reality that all conditions of health and illness are affected by psychological factors and vice versa. (Kaplan & Sadock, 1998, p 797). While some would prefer a return to the term "psychophysiological" to describe this unity, the current DSM-IV uses several different classifications in addition to somatoform disorders. "Psychological factors affecting medical conditions" refers to an extraordinarily inclusive diagnostic category requiring an Axis III diagnosis of a general medical condition and evidence that the psychological factors affect the course of the disease. The list of "psychological factors" can range from Axis I mental disorders to personality traits, stress-related physiological responses, "maladaptive" health behaviors or coping styles, as well as to religious, interpersonal, or cultural factors.

Drawing Battlelines and Naming the Enemy

Modern Western medicine is grounded in allopathic medicine, which seeks to treat disease with remedies producing an effect opposite to symptoms of the disease (Weil, 1995). Thus, many biologically based treatments have within their names the assumption of the battle being waged—for example, anti-biotics, anti-depressants, anti-hypertensives, anti-inflammatories, and so on. Consequently, the view that a condition is either physical *or* mental brings to the fore territorial battles between those who see a condition as lying within their purview or, more likely in the case of somatoform disorders, within someone else's. As medical care is increasingly rationed, it seems likely that the tendency to see difficult-to-treat conditions as someone else's problem will only increase. In the case of somatoform disorders, the absence of a clear and valid enemy creates frustration for the physician and the patient. In such instances the targets of frustrations often become interpersonal and degenerate into destructive name calling, for which a burgeoning list of psychiatric diagnoses is readily available.

Much of the difficulty in diagnosing somatoform conditions is the loss of the more convenient term historically used to describe a wide range of disruptive female complaints: *hysteria*. In its place, the World Health Organization's ICD-10 uses the term *dissociative (conversion) disorder* while DSM-IV has fragmented the term into different diagnoses in different categories, primarily the somatoform and personality disorders. Conversion is listed under somatoform disorders but is considered by many to be a dissociative disorder (Sims, 1995). Both ICD-10 and DSM-IV retain the "histrionic personality disorder" to describe personality characteristics associated with (but not exclusive to) hysteria. Nearly any presentation can be interpreted as hysterical (e.g., "la belle indifférence" indicates a lack of distress at the condition). However, other suspect presentations may include anxiety, depression, anger, or hostility. Symptoms presumed to be of possible hysterical origin include sensory, motor, and pain symptoms, as well as alterations in consciousness, including multiple personality (dissociative identity disorder). Diagnosis of borderline personality disorder shares many similarities to the criteria for somatoform disorder and high levels of comorbidity have been associated with the entire range of somatoform disorders. Body dysmorphism and hypochondria are seen as associated with narcissism, "especially associated with ageing [sic] and the fear of growing old" (Sims, 1995, p. 228). "Neurasthenia" (a condition of "nerve weakness" or "nervous exhaustion") is sometimes presented as the historical male equivalent of hysteria, seen more often during wars among nonofficers (Young, 1995). The condition was classified during the 19th century as a medical condition, and later fell out of favor and into a psychiatric classification (Gosling, 1987; Veith, 1993). Neurasthenia was retained in ICD-10 and is commonly diagnosed in European and Asian cultures as a chronic stress condition, rather than as evidence of unconscious conflicts (Kaplan & Sadock, 1998, pp. 646–653). DSM-IV lists symptoms of neurasthenia as "undifferentiated somatoform disorder" (American Psychiatric Association, 1994, p. 451). Conversion disorders are reported to occur twice as often among African Americans, while somatization disorders are described as more common among African Americans, those with less formal education, and in lower socioeconomic groups (Maxmen & Ward, 1995)—groups with less social power and those who may not have "learned" that the mind and body are separate (i.e., retain a holistic perspective).

The predominance of women among those with many poorly understood conditions puts women at considerable risk of being diagnosed with one or more somatoform disorders and/or personality disorders. Some conditions, such as osteoarthritis, osteoporosis, and breast cancer, have observable and measurable "markers" and there has been some progress in identifying possible biologically based explanations for the conditions, which makes them "legitimate" within the Western medical model. Some conditions occurring almost exclusively among women, such as pelvic pain, are seen by some as a somatoform disorder (Ehlert, Heim, & Hellhammer, 1999). Several other conditions having a greater female to male ratio have a strong autoimmune component—for example, autoimmune thyroid disease (15:1), systemic lupus erythematosus (9:1), scleroderma (4:1), rheumatoid arthritis (3:1), multiple sclerosis (1.5:1), and Sjogren's syndrome (National Institute of Allergy and Infectious Diseases, 1997–1998). Many of these conditions were considered primarily psychogenic until physiological markers (usually immune responses) were identified .

Several other poorly understood conditions that are diagnosed far more often for women are the source of considerable controversy within and between those in medicine and psychiatry. Katon and Walker (1998) list a number of medical specialties and their "problem patients." Among these are patients with complaints of pelvic pain, premenstrual syndrome, temporomandibular syndrome, fibromyalgia, chronic fatigue syndrome, irritable bowel, hypoglycemia, and multiple chemical sensitivity. Irritable bowel syndrome, chronic fatigue syndrome (CFS), and fibromyalgia syndrome (FMS), are seen relatively frequently in primary care settings, while the painful bladder condition interstitial cystitis is often treated as "nonbacterial" cystitis. Each of these conditions occurs more frequently among women than men. High rates of comorbidity of these conditions further complicate the assessment and treatment processes. All of these conditions are essentially diagnoses of exclusion, dependent on subjective reports of patients, with no clear or consistent physiologic "markers." As such, they are the source of ongoing debate regarding their classification, etiology, and treatment. In fact, some researchers claim the similarities between these conditions, their predictors, and their treatments support the need for a classification system that is less prone to the artifactual idiosyncracies and limited perspectives of medical specialization (Wessely et al., 1999). Not surprisingly, all have been and/or are currently considered by many health care professionals to be somatoform disorders (Greenberg, 1990; White, 1989). One textbook widely used in medical schools even has a chapter titled "Neurasthenia and Chronic Fatigue Syndrome" (Kaplan & Sadock, 1998), which presents the conditions as synonymous.

Lennane and Lennane (1973) questioned contemporary wisdom that three conditions experienced by women were primarily psychogenic, despite evidence to the contrary. Included were pain in childbirth, dysmenorrhea (painful menstruation), and infant rumination (babies who spit up frequently). Each of these conditions was then considered evidence of a woman's rejection of her femininity. The Lennanes attributed these explanations to a male bias in medicine and a tendency to "blame the victim." More recently, Morrison (1990) refuted a prominent psychiatrist's criticism that somatization disorder was a "product of male chauvinism" by pointing out that the concept "instilled a considerable degree of order" into the study of a misunderstood and mistreated population (p. 554). The same claim, of course, could be made for the historic diagnosis of "drapetomania," which provided a psychiatric explanation for the tendency of some slaves to try to run away from their masters (Tavris, 1992, pp. 176–177).

Despite a move in mainstream medicine to provide "evidence-based practice," there is also paltry evidence that treatment for somatoform disorders is either consistent or effective (Kellner, 1991). An Internet search for practice guidelines identified one set for chronic pain (American Society of Anesthesiologists Task Force on Pain Management, 1997) and others that were cross-listed as anxiety or depression. Several major textbooks providing guidelines for psychotherapy or most major psychiatric classifications omit information on treatment of somatoform disorders (Hersen & Bellack, 1999; Roth & Fonagy, 1996; Van Hasselt & Hersen, 1996). Some critics believe patients meeting the diagnostic criteria should be managed by psychiatrists, despite some estimates that only 1–10% of diagnosed patients seek mental health treatment (Jonckheere & Stockebrand, 1999). A frequent recommendation is that internists or general practitioners should have regular scheduled appointments with these patients to provide reassurance and limit inappropriate tests and treatments (Kaplan & Sadock, 1998; Smith, 1990; Williams & Silk, 1997). A built-in Catch-22 for patients is that the higher rate of visits could potentially be used as evidence supporting a diagnosis of somatoform disorder or as unwise reinforcement for illness behavior (Kouyanou, Pither, & Wessely, 1997). The viability of these options is questionable in the context of medical reimbursement systems that seek to control costs by limiting visits and supporting pharmacological treatments over psychologically based therapies.

Risks to Women

The diagnosis of somatoform disorder carries with it several risks for patients and providers. First and foremost is the risk of misdiagnosis. Klonoff and Landrine (1997) concluded that between 41 and 83% of people given psychiatric diagnoses, including schizophrenia, are later determined to have neurological or other physical disorders. Conversion disorders, which mimic neurological conditions, later have been found to have documented neurological bases in 25–50% of cases (Kaplan & Sadock, 1998, p. 636). Furthermore, even patients who have long and impressive histories consistent with somatization can get sick (Taylor, 1990), injured, or have serious medication-related complications. Much of the emphasis in psychiatric differential diagnosis is on which competing psychiatric diagnosis is most prominent or comorbid (see American Psychiatric Association, 1994; Kaplan & Sadock, 1998), despite changes in DSM-IV that caution about first ruling out physical conditions or substances that might explain a presentation. From a medical perspective, careful differential diagnosis must consider conditions that are themselves difficult to diagnose, have symptoms that vary over the course of the illness, and are much more common among women, especially systemic lupus erythematosus and multiple sclerosis, both of which would be likely to have neurological symptoms that can present intermittently as apparent conversion reactions (e.g., loss of movement, vision, balance, etc.). Lengthy lists of competing diagnoses and the tests necessary to rule out obscure conditions are both costly and time-consuming in busy practices that limit patient visits to less than 15 minutes (Katon, 2000).

On the other side of the equation, extensive explorations mean patients may also be exposed to expensive, invasive, and time-consuming tests and treatments that are not necessary if the presenting symptoms prove to be self-limiting. Iatrogenic problems can also include responses to treatments for presumed conditions. For example, one major source of fatigue is use of over-the-counter or prescribed medications that have depressant effects. Self-medication with herbal and over-the-counter medications can have serious interaction effects with prescribed medications, which often have their own sedating side effects (Pies, 2000). Alcohol and other substances provide additional and substantial risks to client safety and accurate diagnosis. The current tendency to prescribe multiple medications to treat resistant conditions often makes it difficult to know if lethargy is disease-related or the consequence of combined pain relievers, mood stabilizers, antidepressants, sleep medications, muscle relaxants, or any of the hundreds of prescription drugs that are now being marketed directly to the public (Critser, 1996).

Barriers to Learning about Poorly Understood Conditions

The fragmentation of medical specialization and research centers facilitates study of highly specialized phenomena while at the same time limiting the likelihood that findings in one area will be shared with and/or translated into the language of another. For example, basic science studies related to syndromes with similar symptoms or high comorbidity are housed in separates sections of the National Institutes of Health: chronic fatigue syndrome is studied under Allergy and Infectious Disorders, depression and sleep disorders are in different sections of the National Institute of Mental Health, irritable bowel disorders are relegated to Diabetes, Kidney and Digestive Diseases, and fibromyalgia is under Arthritis, Musculoskeletal and Skin Diseases. Immunologists, endocrinologists, and neurologists often use different terms to refer to identical phenomena. As one immunologist noted, "we would rather use each other's toothbrushes than each other's language" (Felton, 1993).

Funding for studying poorly understood conditions is often difficult to obtain. However, even when funds are available, they may be used to study tangentially related or more "interesting" topics. The 1996 book Osler's Web (Johnson, 1996) provided a detailed chronicle of the appearance and politics of chronic fatigue syndrome, described by some as inflammatory and part of the problem (Kouyanou et al., 1997; Showalter, 1997). Johnson, a reporter, documented a disturbing account of the deadends in researching conditions that are not considered "real." Four years later, it was reported that the Centers for Disease Control and Prevention (CDC) "admitted to misusing $12.9 million of $22 million allotted over the last four years by Congress for the study of chronic fatigue syndrome." An official audit found $8.8 million had been diverted to the study of polio and measles. There was insufficient documentation to determine how an additional $4.1 million were spent. The investigating committee was told that chronic fatigue syndrome (CFS) research funds were used to "balance the books at the end of each fiscal year." The committee eventually *recommended* that the CDC spend $12.9 million (the amount diverted) on research for studying CFS (*Fibromyalgia Health Letter,* October 1999, p. 3; emphasis added). No further sanctions were reported

Barriers to Reducing Diagnostic Predestination/Predetermination

Professionals and patients share the tendency to understand things in ways that are familiar (Langer, 1989). As a consequence, diagnoses may represent conclusions based on obsolete beliefs or incomplete understandings. When evidence contradictory to one's beliefs or inconsistent with one's explanatory paradigm is presented, such findings may be devalued and minimized or ignored altogether. For example, peptic ulcer was considered largely psychosomatic until the discovery of the gram-negative bacillus *Helicobacter pylori* and the development of effective pharmacological treatments. While acknowledging the role of infection, Kaplan and Sadock (1998) identify "chronic frustration of intense dependence needs" as a specific factor and stress and anxiety as nonspecific factors in the etiology of peptic ulcers. Duodenal ulcers are still considered to have a psychosomatic cause requiring relaxation therapy and psychotherapy addressing dependency conflicts (p. 805), as well as medication and dietary control. Because the dominant medical model is based on biological evidence, any hope for legitimizing poorly understood conditions will probably be dependent on biological findings that may also be consistent with psychological explanations for specific syndromes.

Similarly, the belief that somatic complaints often represent "masked depression" has been refuted by several studies indicating that, far from repressing emotional cues, people with many physical symptoms also report high levels of psychological distress (Simon & VonKorff, 1992). Some pain researchers take the position that the pain experience is inherently both affective and sensory because both processes occur in parallel and simultaneously (Chapman, 1998). For example, in the study of intestinal disturbances, there is growing evidence that the brain directly affects the gut and vice versa (Ringel & Drossman, 1999).

A few researchers have criticized the lack of biological research into somatization disorder during the "Decade of the Brain" (Bell, 1994). In contrast to the view that CFS is a psychiatric condition, a recent review of research by Kaplan and Sadock (1998) in the area concluded that CFS probably represents several different presentations and etiologies and should not be seen as a single diagnostic entity: "CFS may have an originally infectious origin; stress and psychosocial factors may disrupt the immune and neuroendocrine responses required to fight the infection; and chronicity ensues" (p. 266). The reviewers recommend studies combining stress physiology, psychological mechanisms, and immune measurements as well as those exploring the possibility of encephalopathy (Johnson, DeLuca, & Natelson, 1999). Noting that fibromyalgia syndrome and CFS are examples of "boundary conditions," Engleberg and Demitrack (1997) point out that while fibromyalgia is often secondary to other arthritic conditions, the overlap between fibromyalgia and CFS indicates both may be attributable to underlying neurological pathology. Further support for studying the complex relationships between neurologically based phenomena associated with depression, anxiety, sleep disorders, and pain comes from evidence that interruptions in Stage 4 sleep in study participants without sleep or pain disorders can result in complaints of muscle pain replicating symptoms of fibromyalgia (Lentz, Landis, Rothermel, & Shaver, 1999; Moldofksy, 1994, 1995; Moldofsky & Scarisbrick, 1976).

Beyond biological challenges to simple solutions/conclusions/diagnoses are a range of studies based in psychology, sociology, and anthropology that further complicate any rush to easy judgment. For example, Schwartz and colleagues have reported multiple studies documenting "response shift" in self-reported health-related quality of life in chronic illness. Measurements comparing baseline reports to later ones may be compromised by a variety of antecedent factors (such as sociodemographics, personality, expectations, and spiritual identity) and mediating factors (such as coping, social comparison, social support, reprioritization of goals, reframed expectations, and spiritual practices). These health adaptation factors have been shown to modify perceived quality of life through "response shifts" including changes in internal standards, values, and conceptualizations of the situation (Schwartz & Sprangers, 2000). The role of expectations is increasingly acknowledged as a common factor in meta-analyses of outcomes in psychotherapy (Hubble, Duncan, & Miller, 1999) and in treatment response in health care (Kirsch, 1999). Ongoing controversies about the role of expectations as placebos generally share the same tensions associated with the mind versus body, psychopathological versus "real" debates about somatization. Based on the medical model, placebo effects are nuisance factors that confuse "real" treatment response with the unfortunate effects of suggestibility. Others see the "placebo effect" as the capacity for healing that can be released in given situations, including expectation on the part of patients, their family and friends, and the clinician, as well as whatever "active" factors may be attributed to a particular medication or treatment (Harrington,

1997). Expectations are inextricably linked with theories of health and illness as well as with other socialization influences including the culture and gender of patients and providers (Devins, 1999; Escobar, 1995; Kramer et al., 1999). Incompatible or unrealistic expectations about the normalcy of fleeting aches and pains and the ability of medicine to eliminate all human suffering are an invisible source of mutual dissatisfaction, in which patients can feel cheated and clinicians defeated. The demand (or desire) to assume expert status may contribute to the tendency to seek absolute conclusions even when information is sparse or contradictory.

Psychopathologizing

The tendency to psychopathologize conditions that fall outside particular cultural norms has been critiqued from feminist, cultural, and other social perspectives (Alarcon, Foulks, & Vakkur, 1998; Ballou, 1995; Brown & Ballou, 1992; Fancher, 1995; Leavitt, 1984). A long history of seeing white, middle-class males as the norm for purposes of classification and research is being addressed through a variety of efforts intended to broaden knowledge and understanding about similarities and differences related to a wide range of variables.

The potential for stigmatizing women with unexplained physical symptoms includes not only any somatoform diagnosis, but a whole range of personality disorders putatively associated with these classifications—for example, histrionic, dependent, borderline, and antisocial. Perhaps the greatest danger associated with psychiatric diagnoses of physical symptoms is the denial of another's reality, an experience that can create the very sense of isolation so often attributed to people with chronic pain or other chronic health conditions (Biordi, 1998). A desire for any name/explanation for frightening symptoms may become replaced with a humiliated or trapped sense of having been labeled forever as unable to trust one's own experiences, and of not knowing exactly what is real or who is in the best position to determine what is real. When pain is interpreted to patients as "really" depression, anxiety, or some other experience that does not resonate with their experience or self-identity, the negative placebo effect (*nocebo*) is quite possible (Hahn, 1997), which may then lead to a continuing search for a better explanation, more consistent with personal experience (often negatively referred to as "doctor shopping"). The potential for such misunderstandings is amplified when cultural differences between the diagnosee and the diagnoser are great, as are described in the book *The Spirit Catches You and You Fall Down* (Fadiman, 1997).

The links shown in studies suggesting a history of abuse or current life stressors can become additional sources of misunderstanding if they are presumed to apply to an individual patient. While there is impressive evidence for the relationships between stress, including abuse, and many chronic conditions, such relationships are far from universal. When abuse has been part of a woman's history, there is no guarantee that "working through" the experience will reverse physical symptoms that may or may not be a consequence of the abuse. Furthermore, the therapist who seeks to normalize the symptoms that might be diagnosed as somatoform by giving a diagnosis of posttraumatic stress disorder may find the shift does not change the playing field for the patient, since many critics dismiss posttraumatic stress disorder as "real" or put it in the same category as neurasthenia and hysteria (Sparr, 1995; Young, 1995).

WHAT IS THE EXPERIENCE OF WOMEN?

Nearly 50 years ago Talcott Parsons described the sick role in capitalistic and Calvinistic (North) American society. First, the role must be conferred on a person by an expert in the health care profession. Only after this occurs may a sick person be exempted from performing expected social obligations, including caring for themselves, while ill. Accepting help from others is expected as part of the sick role. Legitimization of the sick role is often temporary, however, as being sick is seen as undesirable and one is expected to recover as rapidly as possible and return to one's duties (Parsons, 1966). When the limits of these criteria are exceeded, or when experts disagree, the legitimacy of the patient role is called into question.

Women with poorly understood conditions or unexplained physical symptoms may feel caught between several worlds, where they don't know the meaning of the language or where to seek safe shelter (Ruzek, Olesen, & Clarke, 1997). In addition to whatever health concerns they have about the meaning of their symptoms, they often find themselves in the midst of several double-binds. Controversies about the diagnosis and treatment of chronic pain, for example, means that while one pain consultant may recommend taking narcotics "as needed" to manage pain, other clinicians may interpret treatment compliance with addiction or evidence of inappropriate drug seeking (Maxmen & Ward, 1995). Complaints of pain exceeding the expectations of evaluators may raise questions about the patient's desire for questionable disability claims and make providers wary to treat someone they suspect has litigious tendencies. Using distraction or self-hypnosis to manage pain may be called "dissociative" tendencies by some professionals, while hesitancy to try these approaches may be seen as lack of motivation or "noncompliance" by others. Response to placebo may be seen as akin to failing a lie detector test. In essence, if there is a mismatch between client and professional views about who is responsible for a condition and who is responsible for its resolution, implicit questions about integrity and morality will be raised (Brickman et al., 1982; Webster, 2000). Once an "expert" has raised questions about the legitimacy of patient claims, families and friends may withdraw support from the complainant, increasing a woman's sense of alienation from her body and her social network. For clients who have a history of childhood abuse, the experience of "not being heard" or believed may be disturbingly similar to their earlier experiences (Morse, Suchman, & Frankel, 1997).

Name calling between those holding disparate professional views often deteriorates into name calling of patients who align themselves with these disparate views. "Crocks," "whiners," and "frequent fliers" are some of the common and less demeaning names applied to patients behind their backs. More than one author displays obvious disdain for patients who appear to "enjoy ill health" and gravitate to each new "fashionable diagnosis" popularized in the media (Ford, 1997), even accusing patients of "see[ing] themselves as victims worthy of a star appearance on the *Oprah Winfrey Show*" (Bohr, 1995, p. 380).

Even when women find a clinician willing to treat their symptoms as "legitimate" (i.e., physically based), they may find themselves frustrated when exaggerated claims for treatments (whether actually given or simply hoped for) are not met. Disappointment, anger, and guilt may contribute to a cycle of feeling "seduced and abandoned" as they seek health care providers who can tolerate their own frustration, disappointment, guilt, and anger with patients whose conditions may not respond adequately to proffered treatments. The process of seeking treatment may become a major source of stress and the roller-coaster experience of rising and dashed hopes leaves many unwilling to risk the hope that things will ever get better. Treatment regimes and unwanted side effects of treatments may become additional sources of physical, emotional, and financial stress.

What Are the Preferred Ways to Think (and Speak) about It?

Even when therapists hold holistic perspectives on health and illness, it is difficult to think and talk about somatoform and pain disorders without using language that reifies the diagnoses and ideas of a mind–body split. In practice, while many clients have holistic perspectives and can articulate the social and cultural beliefs that support these views, many share the belief in mind–body split and would find reinterpretation of their views dismissive. Further, because tensions surrounding ways of understanding these conditions represent ingrained philosophical differences in preferred ways of knowing, nearly any position taken can be used to support alternate viewpoints. Evidence for these ongoing tensions can be seen in the range of feminist critiques of hysteria and related conditions. These have included reanalyses of famous cases to expose sexist assumptions of theorist/clinicians (Lerman, 1986), deconstructing language and meanings (Micale, 1995), explaining and justifying hysterical behavior in oppressive social contexts (Smith-Rosenberg, 1985), offering alternative medical explanations for observed symptoms (Klonoff & Landrine, 1997), hypothesizing greater stress and stress-related conditions in women's lives due to sexism (Klonoff, Landrine, & Campbell, 2000), and dismissing unexplained physical conditions as evidence of the gullibility of overanxious doctors and media-driven public frenzy (Showalter, 1997).

Nor is it clear that a particular viewpoint can be effectively translated into positions and practices that will provide consistent therapeutic outcomes and that women with unexplained physical conditions will find supportive. The range of people with unexplained physical conditions will include those who have been misdiagnosed, misunderstood, and mistreated, as well as those who have had excellent, thorough, and caring treatment. When we see women in practice who have these conditions, we will find ourselves challenged with the range of their presentations, stories, and requests. A few have fixed, often bizarre, delusions (from Western perspectives) that may be unresponsive to any therapeutic intervention or might best be served by a spiritual healer whose beliefs and practices are culturally congruent with those of the clients. However, the vast majority of those whom we see in practice are simply suffering, often exhausted, and want to find some relief. Few patients who have a long history of unexplained physical symptoms seek psychotherapy as a way to treat their condition (Maxmen & Ward, 1995). However, many who have unexplained symptoms or who have been seen as resistant to treatment are willing to seek supportive therapies to help them improve their quality of life, make decisions about changing priorities, seek assistance with relationship problems, and develop more effective ways to manage pain and other distressing symptoms.

While some authors and physicians have found it beneficial to teach their patients about somatoform disorders to help them accept the label (Morrison, 1990), feminist therapists are hesitant to label clients with potentially stigmatizing diagnoses (Worell & Remer, 1992). In practice, the use of whatever terms the clients uses to describe the condition are most likely to support the development of the therapeutic relationship. The terms "poorly understood conditions" can also be used to emphasize the evolving nature of knowledge about many conditions—how they are seen differently in different cultures, during different eras, and from conflicting worldviews. It may be possible to encourage cautious hopefulness for those who are strongly committed to the need for medical understandings that research may eventually provide understanding that currently elude us. Some of this research may be in relation to specific conditions, while other research will help us understand variability within conditions. For example, the Office of Research on Women's Health is dedicated to learning more about how sex differences mediate differential responses to pain and pain medication (Berkley, 1997; Bodnar, 1998; Cook, 1997). Other studies are exploring how and why women's perceptions may differ in several ways from men's (Gijsbers van Wijk & Kolk, 1997). Greater understanding of the complexities of trauma experience and response may provide additional information that will improve treatments and help women make sense of their experience and feelings (Brady, 1997; Solomon & Davidson, 1997; Teicher, 2000). While reducing a sense of isolation by referring to the universality of their experience, it is crucial to acknowledge the existence of highly individual and unique experiences and responses. The need to seek and maintain validation for the legitimacy of their experiences is one of the major concerns that brings women to therapy. Maintaining realistic hopefulness can be challenging, as we help women make decisions about trying new treatments and encourage them to notice what situations and actions make them feel better or more hopeful. Some women will find condition-specific support groups extremely helpful, while others come away from them with more fears and diminished prospects for the future.

Clinical Implications

Poorly understood conditions (including somatoform and pain disorders) are by definition complex, challenging, and controversial. Conditions primarily affecting women that are diagnosed and theorized about by men and/or from an ethnocentric position invite therapeutic failure, if not more serious damage. There are no agreed-upon guidelines for therapy, feminist or otherwise, for helping clients who suffer with these conditions. Such being the case, the fallacy of the "expert" who has superior knowledge about another's experience should not interfere with genuine caring and authentic curiosity about how to be helpful. Becoming a student of different perspectives on these phenomena may expand one's awareness of the range of beliefs that have historically and contemporarily influenced ideas about etiology, pathology, prognosis, and treatment. Only by expanding our ideas about human potential and holism can we understand and respect diverse perspectives on health and healing. Therapists may avoid a precipitous rush to judgment by being clear about their own views about the purposes and limits of therapy, the power inequities associated with diagnosing another's experience, and the infinite range of beliefs about health, illness, and the nature of healing. Awareness of our own biases does not guarantee that they will not be imposed on clients, but it may alert us to the sound of our own voices claiming to have answers to unasked questions.

Most importantly, clients who are suffering from poorly understood conditions need to feel that they and their experience are not misunderstood. Pain, exhaustion, fear, and hopelessness are inherently subjective and their manifestations are often interpreted in different contexts than those in which they were initially experienced and named. The therapist's challenges are to be open to clients' own unique perspectives on why they became ill and what they think is likely to be helpful (Epstein, Quill, & McWhinney, 1999; Erickson, Tomlin, & Swain, 1984; Johnson & Webster, 2002), bringing to the therapeutic relationship attitudes of humility, radical acceptance, and hopefulness.

REFERENCES

Alarcon, R., Foulks, E., & Vakkur, M. (1998). *Personality disorders and culture: Clinical and conceptual interactions*. New York: Wiley.
American Psychiatric Association. (1994). *Diagnostic and statistical manual of mental disorders* (4th ed.). Washington, DC: Author.
American Society of Anesthesiologists Task Force on Pain Management. (1997). Practice guidelines for chronic pain management. *Anesthesiology* [Online], 86, 995–1004. Available: http://www.asahq.org/practice/chronic_pain/chronic_pain.html
Ballou, M. (1995). Naming the issue. In E. J. Rave & C. C. Larsen (Eds.), *Ethical decision making in therapy: Feminist perspectives* (pp. 42–56). New York: Guilford Press.
Barsky, A., & Borus, J. (1999). Functional somatic syndromes. *Annals of Internal Medicine, 130*, 910–921.
Bell, I. (1994). Somatization disorder: Health care costs in the decade of the brain [Editorial]. *Biological Psychiatry, 35*, 81–83.
Bennett, R. (1999). Emerging concepts in the neurobiology of chronic pain: Evidence of abnormal sensory processing in fibromyalgia. *Mayo Clinical Proceedings, 74*, 385–398.

Berkley, K. (1997). Sex differences in pain. *Behavioral and Brain Sciences, 20*(3), 371–380.

Biordi, D. (1998). Social isolation. In I. M. Lubkin (Ed.), *Chronic illness: Impact and interventions* (4th ed., pp. 181–204). Boston: Jones & Bartlett.

Blum, H. (1994). Dora's conversion syndrome: A contribution to the prehistory of the Holocaust. *Psychoanalytic Quarterly, 63*(3), 518–535.

Bodnar, R. J. (1998). Pain. In E. A. Blechman & K. D. Brownell (Eds.), *Behavioral medicine and women: A comprehensive handbook* (pp. 695–699). New York: Guilford Press.

Bohman, M., Cloninger, C. R., von Knorring, A., & Sigvardsson, S. (1984). An adoption study of somatoform disorders: III. Cross-fostering analysis and genetic relationship to alcoholism and criminality. *Archives of General Psychiatry, 41*(9), 872–8.

Bohr, T. (1995). Fibromyalgia syndrome and myofascial pain syndrome: Do they exists? *Neurologic Clinical, 13*(2), 365–384.

Brady, K. (1997). Posttraumatic stress disorder and comorbidity: Recognizing the many faces of PTSD. *Journal of Clinical Psychiatry, 58*(Suppl. 9), 12–15.

Brickman, P., Rabinowitz, V., Karuza, J., Coates, D., Cohn, E., & Kidder, L. (1982). Models of helping and coping. *American Psychologist, 37*(4), 368–384.

Brown, L. S., & Ballou, M. (Eds.). (1992). *Personality and psychopathology: Feminist reappraisals.* New York: Guilford Press.

Cassam, N., Stern, T., Rosenbaum, J., & Jellinek, M. (Eds.). (1997). *Massachusetts General Hospital handbook of general hospital psychiatry* (4th ed.). St. Louis, MO: Mosby.

Chapman, C. R. (1998). Psychological interventions for pain: Potential mechanisms. In R. Payne, R. Patt, & C. S. Hill (Eds.), *Progress in pain research and management: Vol. 12. Assessment and treatment of cancer pain* (109–131). Seattle, WA: IASP Press.

Cloninger, C. R. (Ed.). (1999). *Personality and psychopathology.* Washington, DC: American Psychiatric Press.

Cloninger, C. R,, Sigvardsson, S., von Knorring, A., & Bohman, M. (1984). An adoption study of somatoform disorders: II. Identification of two discrete somatoform disorders. *Archives of General Psychiatry, 41*(9), 863–871.

Cook, L. (1997, Fall). The battle to relieve pain: Good news for women. *NIH News and Features* (NIH Publication No. 98–3516), pp. 27–29.

Critser, G. (1996, June). Oh, how happy we will be: Pills, paradise and the profits of drug companies. *Harper's Magazine,* pp. 39–40.

Davidson, J. R. T., & Foa, E. B. (Eds.). (1993). *Posttraumatic stress disorder: DSM-IV and beyond.* Washington, DC: American Psychiatric Press.

Devins, G. (1999). Culturally informed psychosomatic research. *Journal of Psychosomatic Research, 46*(6), 519–524.

Dohrenwend, B. P. (Ed.). (1998). *Adversity, stress and psychopathology.* New York: Oxford University Press.

Duberstein, P. R. , & Masling, J. M. (Eds.). (2000). *Psychodynamic perspectives on sickness and health.* Washington, DC: American Psychological Association.

Ehlert, U., Heim, C., & Hellhammer, D. (1999). Chronic pelvic pain as a somatoform disorder. *Psychotherapy and Psychosomatics, 68*(2), 87–94.

Ehrenreich, B., & English, D. (1978). *For her own good: 150 years of the experts' advice to women.* New York: Doubleday.

Eimer, B. N., & Freeman, A. (1998). *Pain management psychotherapy: A practical guide.* New York: Wiley.

Engleberg, N., & Demitrack, M. (1997). Chronic fatigue syndrome and fibromyalgia. In D. J. Knesper, M. B. Riba, & T. L. Schwenk (Eds.), *Primary care psychiatry* (pp. 259–267). Philadelphia: Saunders.

Epstein, R., Quill, T., & McWhinney, I. (1999). Somatization reconsidered: Incorporating the patient's experience of illness. *Archives of Internal Medicine, 159,* 215–222.

Erickson, E. H. (1994). *Identity and the life cycle.* New York: Norton.

Erickson, H. C., Tomlin, E. M., & Swain, M. P. (1983). *Modeling and role-modeling: A theory and paradigm for nursing.* Englewood-Cliffs, NJ: Prentice-Hall.

Escobar, J. (1995). Transcultural aspects of dissociative and somatoform disorders. *Psychiatric Clinics of North America, 18*(3), 555–569.

Fadiman, A. (1997). *The spirit catches you and you fall down: A Hmong child, her American doctors, and the collision of two cultures.* New York: Farrar, Straus, & Giroux.

Fancher, R. T. (1995). *Cultures of healing: Correcting the image of American mental health care.* New York: Freeman.

Farley, M., & Keaney, J. (1997). Physical symptoms, somatization and dissociation in women survivors of childhood sexual assault. *Women and Health, 25*(3), 33–45.

Felton, D. (1993). The brain and the immune system. In B. Moyers, *Healing and the mind* (pp. 213–238) (B. S. Flowers, Ed.). New York: Doubleday.

Fibromyalgia Health Letter [Arthritis Foundation publication]. (1999, October). 2(5), 3.

Ford, C. (1997). Somatization and fashionable diagnoses: Illness as a way of life. *Scandinavian Journal of Work, Health and Environment, 23*(Suppl. 3), 7–16.

Freud, S. (1990). Selections from "Fragments of an analysis of a case of hysteria." In E. Young-Bruehl (Ed.), *Freud on women: A reader* (pp. 69–88). New York: Norton.

Friedman, M. J., Charney, D. S., & Deutch, A. Y. (Eds.). (1995). *Neurobiological and clinical consequences of stress: From normal adaptation to post-traumatic stress disorder.* Philadelphia: Lippincott-Raven.

Friedman, S. (Ed.). (1997). *Cultural issues in the treatment of anxiety.* New York: Guilford Press.

Gatchel, R. J., & Weisberg, J. N. (Eds.). (2000). *Personality characteristics of patients with pain.* Washington, DC: American Psychological Association.

Gijsbers van Wijk, C., & Kolk, A. (1997). Sex differences in physical symptoms: The contribution of symptom perception theory. *Social Science in Medicine, 45*(2), 231–246.

Gilman, S. (1997). Freud's Dora. In T. Dufresne (Ed.), *Freud under analysis: History, theory, practice: Essays in honor of Paul Roazen* (pp. 1–21). Northvale, NJ: Jason Aronson.

Gosling, F. G. (1987). *Before Freud: Neurasthenia and the American medical community, 1870–1910.* Urbana: University of Illinois Press.

Greenberg, D. (1990). Neurasthenia in the 1980's: Chronic mononucleosis, chronic fatigue syndrome, and anxiety and depressive disorders. *Psychosomatics, 31*(2), 129–137.

Hahn, R. (1997). The nocebo phenomenon. In A. Harrington (Ed.), *The placebo effect: An interdisciplinary exploration* (pp. 56–76). Cambridge, MA: Harvard University Press.

Harrington, A. (Ed.). (1997). *The placebo effect: An interdisciplinary exploration.* Cambridge, MA: Harvard University Press.

Heim, C., Ehlert, U., Hanker, J., & Hellhammer, D. (1998). Abuse-related posttraumatic stress disorder and alterations of the hypothalamic–pituitary–adrenal axis in women with chronic pelvic pain. *Psychosomatic Medicine, 60*(3), 309–318.

Helman, C. G. (1994). *Culture, health, and illness: An introduction for health professionals* (3rd ed.). London: Butterworth-Heinemann.

Hersen, M., & Bellack, A. S. (Eds.). (1999). *Handbook of comparative interventions for adult disorders* (2nd ed.). New York: Wiley.

Hubble, M. A., Duncan, B. L., & Miller, S. D. (1999). *The heart and soul of change: What works in therapy.* Washington, DC: American Psychological Association.

Hunter, D. (1983). Hysteria, psychoanalysis, and feminism: The case of Anna O. *Feminist Studies, 9*(3), 464–488.

Johnson, C., & Webster, D. (2002). *Recrafting a life: Solutions for chronic pain and illness.* New York: Brunner/Routledge.

Johnson, H. (1996). *Osler's web: Inside the labyrinth of the chronic fatigue syndrome epidemic.* New York: Crown.

Johnson, S., DeLuca, J., & Natelson, B. (1999). Chronic fatigue syndrome: Reviewing the research findings. *Annals of Behavioral Medicine, 21*(3), 258–271.

Jonckheere, P., & Stockebrand, B. (1999). The bifocal strategy: A new model for flexible liaison between departments of somatic medicine and psychiatrists or psychologists. *Acta Clinica Belgica, 54*(2), 72–79.

Kaplan, H. I., & Sadock, B. J. (1998). *Synopsis of psychiatry: Behavioral sciences: Clinical psychiatry* (8th ed.). Baltimore: Williams & Wilkins.

Katon, W. (2000). Improvement of outcomes in chronic illness [Editorial]. *Archives of Family Medicine, 9,* 709–711.

Katon, W., & Walker, E. (1998). Medically unexplained symptoms in primary care. *Journal of Clinical Psychiatry, 59*(Suppl. 20), 15–21.

Keefe, F. J., Beaupré, P. M., & Gil, K. M. (1996). Group therapy for patients with chronic pain. In R. J. Gatchel & D. C. Turk (Eds.), *Psychological approaches to pain management: A practitioner's handbook* (pp. 259–282). New York: Guilford Press.

Kellner, R. (1991). *Psychosomatic syndromes and somatic symptoms.* Washington, DC: American Psychiatric Press.

Kendler, R., Thornton, L., & Gardner, C. (2000). Stressful life events and previous episodes in the etiology of major depression in women: An evaluation of the "kindling" hypothesis. *American Journal of Psychiatry, 157*(8), 1243–1251.

Kerns, R., & Payne, A. (1996). Treating families of chronic pain patients. In R. J. Gatchel & D. C. Turk (Eds.), *Psychological approaches to pain management: A practitioner's handbook* (pp. 283–304). New York: Guilford Press.

Kirsch, I. (1999). *How expectancies shape experience.* Washington, DC: American Psychological Association.

Kleinman, A., & Becker, A. (1998). "Sociosomatics": The contributions of anthropology to psychosomatic medicine. *Psychosomatic Medicine, 60,* 389–93.

Klonoff, E. A., & Landrine, H. (1997). *Preventing misdiagnosis of women: A guide to physical disorders that have psychiatric symptoms.* Thousand Oaks, CA: Sage.

Klonoff, E., Landrine, H., & Campbell, R. (2000). Sexist discrimination may account for well-known gender differences in psychiatric symptoms. *Psychology of Women Quarterly, 24*, 93–99.

Kouyanou, K., Pither, C., & Wessely, S. (1997). Iatrogenic factors and chronic pain. *Psychosomatic Medicine, 59*, 597–604.

Kramer, E. J., Ivey, S. L., & Ying, Y.-W. (1999). *Immigrant women's health: Problems and solutions.* San Francisco: Jossey-Bass.

Krieg, K., & Goodwin, J. M. (1993). The Dora syndrome: Attempts to restructure childhood in adult victims of child abuse. In J. M. Goodwin (Ed.), *Rediscovering childhood trauma: Historical casebook and clinical applications* (pp. 169–183). Washington, DC: American Psychiatric Press.

Kroenke, K., & Mandelsdorff, E. (1989). Common symptoms in ambulatory care: incidence, evaluation, therapy, and outcome. *American Journal of Medicine, 86*, 262–266.

Kroenke, K., Spitzer, R., deGruy, F., & Swindle, R. (1998). A symptom checklist to screen for somatoform disorders in primary care. *Psychosomatics, 39*(3), 263–272.

Langer, E. J. (1989). *Mindfulness.* Reading, MA: Addison-Wesley.

Lazarus, R. S., & Folkman, S. (1984). *Stress, appraisal and coping.* New York: Springer.

Leavitt, J. W. (Ed.). (1984). *Women and health in America: Historical readings.* Madison: University of Wisconsin Press.

Lee, S. (1998). Estranged bodies, simulated harmony, and misplaced cultures: Neurasthenia in contemporary Chinese society. *Psychosomatic Medicine, 60*, 448–457.

Lehrer, P. M., & Woolfolk, R. L. (Eds.). (1993). *Principles and practice of stress management* (2nd ed.). New York: Guilford Press.

Lennane, K., & Lennane, J. (1973). Alleged psychogenic disorders in women: A possible manifestation of sexual prejudice. *New England Journal of Medicine, 288*, 288–292.

Lentz, M., Landis, C., Rothermel, J., & Shaver, J. (1999). Effects of selective slow wave sleep disruption on musculoskeletal pain and fatigue in middle aged women. *Journal of Rheumatology, 26*(7), 1586–1592.

Lerman, H. (1986). *A mote in Freud's eye: From psychoanalysis to the psychology of women.* New York: Springer.

Lorig, D. (1996). Chronic disease self-management: A model for tertiary prevention. *American Behavioral Scientist, 39*(6), 676–683.

Lovallo, W. R. (1997). *Stress and health: Biological and psychological interactions.* Thousand Oaks, CA: Sage.

Manu, P. (Ed.). (1998). *Functional somatic syndromes: Etiology, diagnosis, and treatment.* Cambridge, UK: Cambridge University Press.

Maxman, J. S., & Ward, N. G. (1995). *Essential psychopathology and its treatment* (2nd ed.). New York: Norton.

Micale, M. S. (1995). *Approaching hysteria: Disease and its interpretations.* Princeton, NJ: Princeton University Press.

Miller, L. (1998). *Shocks to the system: Psychotherapy of traumatic disability syndromes.* New York: Norton.

Mitchell, J. (1974). *Psychoanalysis and feminism.* London: Lane.

Moldofsky, H. (1995). Sleep, neuroimmune and neuroendocrine functions in fibromyalgia and chronic fatigue syndrome. *Advances in Neuroimmunology.* 5(1), 39–56.

Moldofsky, H. (1994). Chronobiological influences on fibromyalgia syndrome: Theoretical and therapeutic implications. *Baillieres Clinical Rheumatology, 8*(4), 801–810.

Moldofsky, H., & Scarisbrick, P. (1976). Induction of neurasthenic musculoskeletal pain syndrome by selective sleep stage deprivation. *Psychosomatic Medicine, 38*(1), 35–44.

Morrison, J. (1990, October). Managing somatization disorder. *Disease-a-Month,* pp. 539–591.

Morse, D., Suchman, A., & Frankel, R. (1997). The meaning of symptoms in 10 women with somatization disorder and a history of childhood abuse. *Archives of Family Medicine, 6,* 468–76.

National Institute of Allergy and Infectious Diseases. (1997–1998). *Women's health in the U.S.: NIAID research on health issues affecting women.* Rockville, MD: U.S. Department of Health and Human Services, Public Health Service, National Institutes of Health, National Institute of Allergy and Infectious Diseases.

Ornstein, R. (1993). *The roots of the self.* New York: HarperCollins.

Othmer, E., & DeSouza,C. (1985). A screening test for somatization disorder (hysteria). *American Journal of Psychiatry, 142,* 1146–1149.

Paris, J. (1999). *Nature and nurture in psychiatry: A predisposition–stress model of mental disorders.* Washington, DC: American Psychiatric Press.

Parsons, T. (1966). Illness and the role of the physician: A sociological perspective. In W. R. Scott & E. H. Volkart (Eds.), *Medical care: Readings in the sociology of medical institutions* (p. 275). New York: Wiley.

Phillips, J., & Gatchel, R. J. (2000). Extraversion–introversion and chronic pain. In R. J. Gatchel & J . N. Weisberg (Eds.), *Personality characteristics of patients with pain* (pp. 181–202). Washington, DC: American Psychological Association.

Pies, R. (2000). Serious side effects may accompany use of nonprescription antidepressants. *Journal of Clinical Psychiatry, 61,* 815–20.

Post, R., Weis, S., & Smith, M. (1995). Sensitization and kindling: Implications for the evolving neuronal substrates of post-traumatic stress disorder. In M. J. Friedman, D. S. Charney, & A. Y. Deutch (Eds.), *Neurobiological and clinical consequences of stress: From normal adaptation to post-traumatic stress disorder* (pp. 203–224). New York: Lippincott-Raven.

Reilly, J., Baker, G., Rhodes, J., & Salmon, P. (1999). The association of sexual and physical abuse with somatization: Characteristics of patients presenting with irritable bowel syndrome and non-epileptic attack disorder. *Psychological Medicine, 29*(2), 399–406.

Ringel, Y., & Drossman, D. (1999) From gut to brain and back: A new perspective into functional gastrointestinal disorders [Editorial]. *Journal of Psychosomatic Research, 47*(3), 205–210.

Rogers, R. (Ed.). (1988). *Clinical assessment of malingering and deception.* New York: Basic Books.

Rossi, E. L. (1993). *The psychobiology of mind–body healing: New concepts of therapeutic hypnosis.* New York: Norton.

Roth, A., & Fonagy, P. (1996). *What works for whom?: A critical review of psychotherapy research.* New York: Guilford Press.

Ruzek, S. B., Olesen, V. L., & Clarke, A. E. (Eds.). (1997). *Women's health: Complexities and differences.* Columbus: Ohio State University Press.

Sanders, S. (1996). Operant conditioning with chronic pain: Back to basics. In R. J. Gatchel & D. C. Turk (Eds.), *Psychological approaches to pain management: A practitioner's handbook* (pp. 112–130). New York: Guilford Press.

Schwartz, C. E., & Sprangers, M. A. G. (Eds). (2000). *Adaptation to changing health: Response shift in quality-of-life research.* Washington, DC: American Psychological Association.

Schwartz, G. (1990). Psychobiology of repression and health. In J. L. Singer (Ed.), *Repression and dissociation: Implications for personality theory, psychopathology, and health* (pp. 405–434). Chicago: University of Chicago Press.

Shorter, E. (1992). *From paralysis to fatigue: A history of psychosomatic illness in the modern era.* New York: Free Press.

Showalter, E. (1997). *Hystories: Hysterical epidemics and modern media.* New York: Columbia University Press.

Sigvardsson, S., von Knorring, A., Bohman, M., & Cloninger, C. R. (1984). An adoption study of somatoform disorders: I. The relationships of somatization to psychiatric disability. *Archives of General Psychiatry, 41*(9), 853–859.

Silverstein, B., & Perlick, D. (1995). *The cost of competence: Why inequality causes depression, eating disorders and illness in women.* New York: Oxford University Press.

Simon, G., & Von Korff, M. (1992). Somatization and psychiatric disorder in the NIMH Epidemiologic Catchment Area Study. *American Journal of Psychiatry, 148*(11), 1494–5000.

Sims, A. (1995). *Symptoms in the mind: An introduction to descriptive psychopathology* (2nd ed.). London: Saunders.

Smith, G. R. (1990). *Somatization disorder in the medical setting.* Rockville, MD: U.S. Department of Health and Human Services, Public Health Service, National Institutes of Health, National Institute of Mental Health.

Smith-Rosenberg, C. (1985). *Disorderly conduct: Visions of gender in Victorian America.* New York: Knopf.

Sparr, L. (1995). Post-traumatic stress disorder: Does it exist? *Neurologic Clinics, 13*(2), 413–429.

Solomon, S., & Davidson, J. (1997). Trauma: Prevalence, impairment, service use, and cost. *Journal of Clinical Psychiatry, 58*(Suppl. 9), 5–11.

Spector, R. (1996). *Cultural diversity in health and illness* (4th ed.). Stamford, CT: Appleton & Lange.

Stallings, M., Hewitt, J., Cloninger, C., Heath, A., & Eaves, L. (1996). Genetic and environmental structure of the Tridimensional Personality Questionnaire: Three or four temperament dimensions. *Journal of Personality and Social Psychology, 70*(1), 127–140.

Taerk, G. (1998). Psychotherapy of functional somatic syndromes. In. P. Manu (Ed.), *Functional somatic syndromes: Etiology, diagnosis, and treatment* (pp. 237–255). Cambridge, UK: Cambridge University Press.

Tavris, C. (1992). *The mismeasure of woman.* New York: Simon & Schuster.

Taylor, R. L. (1990). *Distinguishing psychological from organic disorders: Screening for psychological masquerade*. New York: Springer.

Teicher, M. (2000). Wounds that time won't heal: The neurobiology of child abuse. *Cerebrum, 2,* 50–67.

Thakker, R., & McCanne, T. (2000). The effects of daily stressors on physical health in women with and without a childhood history of sexual abuse. *Child Abuse and Neglect, 24*(2), 209–221.

van der Kolk, B. A., McFarlane, A. C., & Weisaeth, L. (Eds.). (1996). *Traumatic stress: The effects of overwhelming experience on mind, body and society*. New York: Guilford Press.

Van Hasselt, V. B., & Hersen, M. (Eds.). (1996). *Sourcebook of psychological treatment manuals for adult disorders*. New York: Plenum Press.

Veith, I. (1993). *Hysteria: The history of a disease*. Northvale, NJ: Jason Aronson.

Watkins, A. (Ed.). (1997), *Mind–body medicine: A clinician's guide to psychoneuroimmunology*. New York: Churchill Livingstone.

Webster, D. (2000, April 6). *Nancy Drew meets Sigmund Freud in the mystery of fibromyalgia* [Invited keynote address]. Annual meeting of the Advanced Feminist Therapy Institute, Portland, OR.

Weil, A. (1995). *Health and healing*. Boston: Houghton Mifflin.

Wessely, S., Nimnuan, C., & Sharpe, M. (1999). Functional somatic syndromes: one or many? *Lancet, 354*(9182), 936–939.

White, P. (1989). Fatigue syndrome: Neurasthenia. *British Medical Journal, 298,* 1199–2000.

Williams, B., & Silk, K. (1997). "Difficult" patients. In D. J. Knesper, M. B. Riba, & T. L. Schwenk (Eds.), *Primary care psychiatry* (pp. 61–75). Philadelphia: Saunders.

Wilson, C. P. (1989). Epilogue: Psychotherapeutic techniques. In C. P. Wilson & I. Mintz (Eds.), *Psychosomatic symptoms: Psychodynamic treatment of the underlying personality disorder* (pp. 425–451). Northvale, NJ: Jason Aronson.

Wilson, J. P., & Keane, T. M. (Eds). (1997). *Assessing psychological trauma and PTSD*. New York: Guilford Press.

Wolpert, E., Berman, V., & Bornstein, M. (1999). Efficacy of electroconvulsive therapy in continuous rapid cycling bipolar disorder. *Psychiatric Annals, 29*(12), 679–683.

Worell, J., & Remer, P. (1992). *Feminist perspectives in therapy: An empowerment model for women*. New York: Wiley.

Young, A. (1995). *The harmony of illusions: Inventing post-traumatic stress disorder*. Princeton, NJ: Princeton University Press.

Zborowski, M. (1952). Cultural components in responses to pain. *Journal of Social Issues, 8,* 16–30.

Chapter 7

Raging Hormones?
Feminist Perspectives on Premenstrual Syndrome and Postpartum Depression

JOAN C. CHRISLER
INGRID JOHNSTON-ROBLEDO

The constructs of premenstrual syndrome (PMS) and postpartum depression (PPD) have much in common. Both result from the medicalization of women's experience; were popularized by the British endocrinologist Katharina Dalton; are defined vaguely, which encourages their overuse; represent women's behavior as erratic and potentially dangerous to self and others; have been absorbed into Western (perhaps especially North American) culture as stereotypic caricatures of women; and serve as a form of social control that tells women that some of their emotions are inappropriate, thus silencing them from speaking out about the oppressive conditions of their lives. Premenstrual and postpartum women who do complain find themselves in the awkward position of having their concerns mockingly dismissed by family and friends with jokes that compare them to cultural stereotypes or gently dismissed by medical personnel who tell them that their hormones are imbalanced and that antidepressants will make them feel better.

PMS and PPD provide excellent examples of syndromes that must be theorized and treated from a biopsychosocial perspective. A number of biomedical, psychological, and social causes of PMS and PPD have been

174

theorized, but none has sufficient explanatory power to withstand challenge—perhaps because each hypothesis has been developed in isolation. Causes of such complex phenomena are best assumed to be multifactorial. Furthermore, the "social" aspects must be expanded beyond the usual consideration of quality of intimate relationships and social support. Gendered "psychopathologies" cannot be understood outside of the political, historical, and cultural contexts that shape the expression of the dis-ease.

Cultural beliefs that women are unpredictable, dangerous, and too emotional or fragile for certain social roles date back at least to ancient Greece. Menstruation, pregnancy, and giving birth, as obvious differences between the sexes, were considered the basis of these beliefs long before the scientific discovery of hormones and physician Edgar Berman's infamous worries about the raging hormonal influences on decisions made by women executives. For example, Hippocrates wrote about postpartum emotional problems in 700 B.C.

Feminist scholars (e.g., Chrisler, 1996; Figert, 1996; Houppert, 1999; Martin, 1988; Nicolson, 1995, 1998; Rittenhouse, 1991) have noted ways that political expediency has influenced scientific and cultural interest in PMS and PPD historically. The social construction of PMS is generally agreed to have begun during the Great Depression with the publication of an article by an American gynecologist (Frank, 1931), who described a condition he called *premenstrual tension*. He wrote that women became tense and irritable just prior to menstruation, and he expressed concerns about their tendency to engage in "foolish and ill considered actions" (p. 1054) during that time. Frank's discovery added a modern veneer to the cult of invalidism and Victorian-era concerns about the ill effects that intellectual exertion might have on the menstrual cycle, and it provided a good reason why women should stay out of the workforce and leave what few jobs were available to men. Dalton, who coined the term *PMS*, published her first work on it in the 1950s, when women were being urged to become full-time homemakers and leave their jobs to veterans of World War II. Biomedical and social scientists began to pay serious attention to PMS in the 1970s, after the widespread gains of the women's liberation movement. By the mid-1980s, during the conservative antifeminist backlash in the United States and the United Kingdom and following two sensational murder trials in the United Kingdom in which the courts accepted PMS as a plea of diminished responsibility, PMS was firmly established as a cultural stereotype of women. At the same time, the American Psychiatric Association devised premenstrual dysphoric disorder (PMDD; previously termed "late luteal phase dysphoric disorder") and inserted it in DSM-III-R. Thus, a clear pattern has emerged of professionals reminding women each time they have made gains that they cannot go much further due to their delicate physical and emotional health.

The earliest scientific writings about PPD appeared in the 19th century when the field of obstetrics and gynecology emerged as a medical specialty and male physicians began to restrict and regulate the activities of midwives. Feminist scholars (e.g., Ehrenreich & English, 1979; Showalter, 1978; Wertz, 1983) have described the extent to which physicians have perpetuated the assumption that women's bodies and minds are weak and out of control due to hormonal fluctuations, especially after childbirth. Public acceptance of this assumption was, no doubt, of great help to physicians in securing their economic, political, and professional gains over midwives as the most appropriate obstetrical practitioners. Not only did they have science and professional training on their side; they also had the strength of body and mind that was necessary to "manage" out-of-control women during and after childbirth. The baby blues were referred to as "milk fever" in the 19th century because they occurred at the same time that breast milk was produced in large quantities (Dalton & Holton, 1996). In 1858, Marcé, a French psychiatrist, published one of the first articles that described negative emotional reactions following childbirth (Stern & Kruckman, 1983). He argued for the recognition of "postpartum illness" as a distinct psychiatric disorder that occurs within the first 12 months postpartum (Pitt, 1978, as cited in Nicolson, 1998). In 1939, the British Parliament adopted the Infanticide Act, which protected women who killed their infants within the first 12 months after birth from being charged with murder; instead, they were charged with infanticide and committed to a psychiatric institution (Dalton & Holton, 1996).

Although postpartum affective disturbances are mentioned in various editions of the *Diagnostic and Statistical Manual of Mental Disorders*, none has ever had its own category. "Psychosis with childbirth" appeared in DSM-II (American Psychiatric Association, 1968). In DSM-III (American Psychiatric Association, 1980), postpartum psychosis is listed as one of several types of atypical psychosis, a residual category for disorders that have psychotic features without meeting the criteria for specific disorders. The DSM-IV (American Psychiatric Association, 1994) lists "postpartum depression with or without psychotic features" as a specifier under major depression. Thus, the American Psychiatric Association (1994) recommends that PPD be diagnosed using the same criteria as those for major depression except that the onset of symptoms must occur within 4 weeks of parturition.

DEFINITIONS AND CONCEPTUAL ISSUES

PMS and PPD are defined vaguely and variously (researchers do not even agree on the time of onset), and this vagueness is found in both the professional and the lay literature. Thus, PMS is often confused with PMDD, dysmenorrhea, preexisting conditions, nonproblematic menstrual cycle-related changes, and even with experiences that have nothing to do with the menstrual cycle but coincidentally occur shortly before the menses. PPD is often confused with postpartum psychosis, the baby blues, adjustment to parenthood, preexisting conditions, and any economic, interpersonal, or other experiences that occur around the time a woman gives birth. The concepts of PMS and PPD are so vague and elastic that every woman can see something of her own experience within them. This encourages self-diagnosis, validates the constructs, and enhances the stereotype of the woman driven crazy by her raging hormones.

PMS and PMDD

A variety of physiological and psychological changes have been associated with phases of the menstrual cycle. Those changes that tend to occur premenstrually (usually on days 23 to 28 of the cycle) have been called *premenstrual syndrome* (Dalton, 1977). The most frequently reported premenstrual change is fluid retention, particularly in the breasts and abdomen. Other changes have been classified as follows (Debrovner, 1982): psychological (e.g., irritability, depression, anxiety, lethargy, sleep changes, low morale, crying spells, hostility); neurological (e.g., headaches, vertigo, backaches); gastrointestinal (e.g., nausea, vomiting, constipation, increased cravings for sweet or salty foods); and dermatological (acne). Having difficulty concentrating, feeling out of control, and being easily fatigued or having bursts of energy are among the signs of PMS that women often mention. Over 100 changes have been associated with PMS in the professional and popular literature (Chrisler & Levy, 1990; Figert, 1996; Laws, Hey, & Eagen, 1985), including some so gendered that they would *never* be considered "symptoms" of a disorder in men (e.g., cravings for sweets, increased sex drive) and some that actually occur during the menses (e.g., uterine or pelvic cramps). Hardly anyone ever complains of dysmenorrhea anymore. This is due in part to the discovery that prostaglandins cause uterine cramps, which can be treated successfully in most cases by antiprostaglandin medications, but may have more to do with the fact that the concept of PMS seems to have swallowed up dysmenorrhea; any menstrual cycle-related complaint is now referred to by the general public and the popular press as "PMS-ing."

Although data do indicate that women experience cyclic changes, it is difficult to know how common such changes are. Estimates of the prevalence of premenstrual "symptoms," which depend on how the data were collected, range from 2% (using the strictest criteria of a 30% increase in intensity of selected emotional and physical experience charted daily over at least two menstrual cycles) to 100% (using the loosest criteria: "Have you ever experienced cyclic changes in your physical or emotional state?"). Despite efforts by the Society for Menstrual Cycle Research and the National Institute of Mental Health to produce a standard definition, there is little agreement on how many changes must be experienced or how severe the experience must be in order to be considered PMS. So many different definitions exist in the literature that results cannot easily be compared. Even the timing of the premenstrual phase is unclear. Some researchers have described it as 5 to 7 days prior to the start of the menses; others have described it as the time between ovulation and menstruation (about 2 weeks). The problem of estimates is made more difficult by the fact that premenstrual experience is highly variable and personal. All women do not experience the same changes; moreover, the experience of any given woman may vary from cycle to cycle. In addition, PMS has been so frequently discussed in the last 20 years that the results of surveys have undoubtedly been affected by a response bias in the direction of the stereotype of the premenstrual woman (Chrisler, 1996).

PMDD is defined in DSM-IV (American Psychiatric Association, 1994) as requiring at least five of the following (at least one must be among the first four) symptoms present during most of the week before the menses:

> 1) feeling sad, hopeless, or self-deprecating; 2) feeling tense, anxious, or "on edge," 3) marked lability of mood interspersed with frequent tearfulness; 4) persistent irritability, anger, and increased interpersonal conflicts, 5) decreased interest in usual activities, which may be associated with withdrawal from social relationships, 6) difficulty concentrating, 7) feeling fatigued, lethargic, or lacking in energy, 8) marked changes in appetite, which may be associated with binge eating or craving certain foods, 9) hypersomnia or insomnia, 10) a subjective sense of being overwhelmed or out of control, 11) physical symptoms such as breast tenderness or swelling, headaches, or sensations of "bloating" or weight gain, with tightness of clothing, shoes, or rings. There may also be joint or muscle pain . . . [or] suicidal thoughts. (p. 716)

To distinguish PMDD from other forms of depression that might simply worsen at points during the menstrual cycle, the criteria state that all of the symptoms must be absent during the week after the menses. The DSM-IV description includes the estimation that at least 75% of women report minor or isolated premenstrual changes, but only 3–5% experience symptoms that meet the PMDD criteria. Although it was the stated intent of the psychiatrists who developed PMDD to move away from the general "kitchen sink" diagnostic criteria of PMS and define a subset of women who experienced a unique psychiatric disorder, the symptoms of PMDD virtually overlap with those of PMS as described by Debrovner (1982) and others. For a description of the politics of the development and implementation of this diagnosis, see Caplan (1995) or Figert (1996).

Feminist scholars (e.g., Caplan, McCurdy-Myers, & Gans, 1992; Nash & Chrisler, 1997) have expressed concerns that the presence of PMDD in the DSM will result in more, not fewer, diagnoses and lead to increased bias and discrimination against women. Nash and Chrisler (1997) asked college students to complete a symptom checklist that included the criteria for PMDD and then 2 weeks later to complete it again after having read the diagnostic criteria for PMDD. Half of the 134 students read the criteria as they exist in DSM-IV with the title "PMDD." The others read the criteria with all references to the menstrual cycle removed and the title "episodic dysphoric disorder." They also answered questions about whether they or anyone they knew might be suffering from the disorder. Knowledge of the menstrual "nature" of the diagnosis did not affect women's perceptions of their own menstrual cycle-related changes, but it did increase both men's and women's perceptions that premenstrual changes are a problem for women in general. Participants were willing to suggest that their female friends, relatives, employers, and professors were candidates for the PMDD diagnosis. However, they named both male and female friends and relatives as candidates for episodic dysphoric disorder.

PPD

"Postpartum psychiatric disorders," "puerperal mood disorders," "postpartum depressive reactions," and "postpartum mood disorders" are all terms that have been used to describe psychological "disturbances" that occur in women after they have given birth. Three types of postpartum disorders are recognized (Hopkins, Marcus, & Campbell, 1984). The least common (it affects 0.1–0.2% of new mothers) is postpartum psychosis, which occurs within 2 weeks after birth and is defined by a loss of touch with reality and the experience of hallucinations and delusions that typically involve the baby. PPD and the baby blues, the other types, together affect the largest numbers of women and have received the most attention in the professional literature.

The baby blues (also known as the postpartum or maternity blues) is a transitory reaction that can last up to 2 weeks after birth. It is characterized by irritability, anxiety, and tearfulness, and is believed to occur in 50–80% of new mothers. It is generally regarded as a natural reaction to the sequelae of childbirth; both its "symptoms" and their frequency have caused researchers to liken it to PMS (Dalton & Holton, 1996; Kennerley & Gath, 1989). PPD is thought to be more severe and less common (occurring in 3–17% of new mothers) than the baby blues, to have a later onset (between 4 weeks and 6 months postpartum), and to last longer (as much as 6–12 months) (O'Hara & Swain, 1996; Stowe & Nemeroff, 1995; Whiffen, 1992). PPD is characterized by sadness, crying, self-blame, loss of control, irritability, anxiety, tension, and sleep difficulties (Cox, 1986).

Researchers lack consensus about how and when to assess for PPD, which leads to difficulties in defining it and establishing reliable prevalence rates (O'Hara & Swain, 1996). PPD is most often assessed at about 6 weeks after birth during a routine postpartum visit. Early assessment is likely to underestimate prevalence rates or to confuse PPD with the baby blues. Researchers (Seguin, Potvin, St. Denis, & Loiselle, 1999) who have adopted a longitudinal assessment strategy have reported new cases of PPD that started as late as 6 months postpartum. Different prevalence rates are found when researchers use self-report instruments as opposed to more stringent criteria (e.g., Research Diagnostic Criteria). Self-report measures can result in an underestimation of PPD if women do not report their mood accurately either because they are ashamed to admit they are depressed at a time when they had expected to be happy or because they believe that all new mothers experience depression (Whiffen, 1992). Standardized general self-report measures of depression can overestimate depression if they include somatic symptoms (e.g., appetite change, sleep disturbance) that are influenced by physical recovery from childbirth or include other "symptoms" that even nondepressed new mothers would endorse (e.g., feeling unattractive, difficulty working) (Hopkins, Campbell, & Marcus, 1989).

Researchers also lack consensus on whether PPD can be distinguished from depression experienced at other times and whether PPD can be distinguished from normal postpartum adjustment. Some researchers (e.g., Cox, 1989; Dalton & Holton, 1996) conclude that PPD is an atypical form of depression that requires specialized forms of treatment. However, others

(Nicolson, 1998; Whiffen, 1992) argue that there is little convincing evidence that PPD is a separate clinical entity. After a review of the literature, Whiffen (1992) concluded that PPD is not qualitatively different from other forms of depression, although it is less severe, remits more quickly, and is more likely than major depression to include guilt and agitation. She concluded that PPD should be conceptualized as either a less severe type of major depression or as an adjustment disorder. PPD can also be conceptualized as a generalized stress response similar to that experienced after surgery. In one study (Mandy, Gard, Ross, & Valentine, 1998), women assessed at 6 weeks and at 4 months postpartum were less depressed, anxious, and hostile than women recovering from surgical procedures. The question of differentiating PPD from normal adjustment is more difficult to address, as there are so few data available on "normal" new mothers. Nevertheless, it seems likely that many women who are trying to get used to shortened sleep cycles and a new or heavier work load and thus are irritable, fatigued, and disappointed with their postpartum experience may be labeled with PPD or the baby blues.

ETIOLOGY OF PMS AND PPD

Biomedical Perspectives

Although in recent years most authors have given at least cursory attention to the psychosocial context of women's lives, the biomedical perspective has prevailed in the work on both PMS and PPD. The phases of the menstrual cycle are marked by differing levels of luteinizing hormone, follicle stimulating hormone, estrogen, and progesterone. Pregnancy is marked by increases in progesterone, estrogen, cortisol, and thyroid stimulating hormone. Estrogen and progesterone levels decline abruptly at parturition, and all hormones return to their normal levels in the weeks following birthing. Hormones have been assumed by many to be the causal agents of both PMS and PPD, despite a lack of solid evidence to support the hypothesis.

The major proponent of a hormonal etiology of PMS is Dalton (1964). Her theory is that there is an imbalance in the ratio of circulating progesterone and estradiol. Progesterone is thought to have a calming effect on the nervous system, and estradiol is believed to increase nervous activity. Therefore, a higher ratio of estradiol to progesterone could lead to the tension and irritability reported by women with PMS (Golub, 1992). Dalton has been administering progesterone therapy to her patients for many years, and her success with individual patients has been widely reported in both the scientific and the popular press. However, clinical trials (Rubinow, 1991; Sampson, 1979, 1981) of progesterone therapy have failed to demonstrate its effectiveness, and researchers (O'Brien, Selby, & Symonds, 1980; Reid & Yen, 1981; Sanders, Warner, Backstrom, & Bancroft, 1983) have never convincingly demonstrated differences in progesterone levels between women who do and who do not report PMS.

Other biological etiologies of PMS that have been suggested include excess levels of aldosterone (Janowsky, Berens, & Davis, 1973) or prolactin (Rausch & Janowsky, 1982), melatonin deficits (Parry et al., 1990), prostaglandins (Budoff, 1980), nutritional deficits (Abraham, 1982), and abnormalities in the function of neurotransmitters, such as serotonin, dopamine, and norepinephrine (Golub, 1992). Data to support these theories are scarce and can be described as contradictory at best.

The general consensus among PPD researchers is that data on the relationship between hormones and depression are negative or equivocal (Hendrick, Altschuler, & Suri, 1998; Hopkins et al., 1984; Stowe & Nemeroff, 1995). There is little support for a direct causal link between hormonal fluctuations and PPD (Llewellyn, Stowe, & Nemeroff, 1997; Nicolson, 1998), and no single biological etiology has been identified (Hendrick et al., 1998). Despite these widely recognized conclusions, proponents (e.g., Dalton & Holton, 1996; Epperson, 1999) of a biomedical model continue to insist on the centrality of hormones in the etiology of PPD. For example, Epperson (1999) wrote "that women are at increased risk for mood disorders and are particularly vulnerable at times of hormonal fluctuation (i.e., during premenstruum, postpartum, and perimenopause) suggests that gonadal steroids play an integral role in the pathogenesis of depression in women" (p. 2247). Researchers have also hypothesized estradiol (Hendrick et al., 1998), estriol (Stowe & Nemeroff, 1995), seratonin, and genetics (Dalton & Holton, 1996; Hendrick et al., 1998) as causal agents, and have called for research into their possible connections to PPD.

Psychological Perspectives

PMS and PPD have been studied in relation to personality, psychopathology, and stress and coping. Data on PMS are mixed, due at least in part to the highly variable definitions of the premenstrual phase that have been used by researchers. However, some studies have indicated that women who seek treatment for PMS or PMDD adhere to the feminine gender role (Freeman, Sondheimer, & Rickels, 1987; Stout & Steege, 1985), exhibit higher than average trait anxiety (Giannini, Price, Loiselle, & Giannini, 1985: Halbreich & Kas, 1977; Mira, Vizzard, & Abraham, 1985; Picone & Kirby, 1990), and have a higher than average lifetime incidence of sexual assault and abuse (Taylor, Golding, Menard, & King, 2001) and affective disorders, especially depression and anxiety (DeJong et al., 1985; Dennerstein, Morse, & Varnanides, 1988; Endicott & Halbreich, 1988; Kraaimaat & Veeninga, 1995; Pearlstein et al., 1990; Warner, Bancroft, Dixson, & Hampson, 1991).

A number of researchers (Beck, Gevirtz, & Mortola, 1990; Coughlin, 1990; Gallant, Popiel, Hoffman, Chakraborty, & Hamilton, 1992; Kucz-mierczyk, Labrum, & Johnson, 1992; Maddocks & Reid, 1992; Warner & Bancroft, 1990) have reported that women who describe themselves as suffering from PMS also indicate that they experience high levels of stress, including stress related to marital dissatisfaction, work load and work monotony, hectic schedules, finances, and family conflict. Some data indi-cate that women with PMS (i.e., those with severe symptoms) do not cope as well with stress as asymptomatic women (or those with mild symptoms). Women with PMS, for example, have been found to rely more than other women on avoidance, wishful thinking, appeasement, religion, withdrawal, and focusing on/venting emotions, and to rely less than other women on social support, problem-focused coping, and direct action (Gallant, Popiel, & Hoffman, 1994; Genther, Chrisler, & Johnston-Robledo, 1999; Ornitz & Brown, 1993). Many of the symptoms of PMS (e.g., headaches, backaches, irritability, tension, fatigue, crying) are vague and overlap with physical sensations associated with stress (Chrisler, 1996). Thus, it is not surprising that women with PMS also report high levels of stress. The possibility that the stress of women's busy, and often overburdened, lives contributes as much to the experience of PMS as menstrual cycle-related changes should be acknowledged. Nor is it surprising that women who endorse the femi-nine gender role tend to choose indirect, passive, and self-blaming (e.g., "It's just my PMS") strategies for coping with stress.

Women who were depressed and anxious during pregnancy and women who have experienced psychiatric disorders earlier in life are more vulnerable to PPD than other women (O'Hara & Swain, 1996; Wilson et al., 1996). Neuroticism (as measured by the Eysenck Personality Inventory) has been found to be a significant predictor of both the baby blues and PPD (Kennerly & Gath, 1989; Matthey, Barnett, Ungerer, & Waters, 2000; O'Hara & Swain, 1996). Thus, the stress of labor and birth and the transi-tion to motherhood may be more difficult to manage for women with a history of depression and anxiety. Women who score high on a femininity scale have been found to score low on a depression scale both during pregnancy and at 1 month postpartum (Pfost, Lum, & Stevens, 1989). Perhaps women who identify with the feminine gender role experience fewer conflicts during the transition to motherhood or feel more confident in their nurturing abilities.

Researchers have also applied a stress and coping model to the etiology of PPD. PPD is correlated with marital dissatisfaction, stressful life events, low income, ineffective coping strategies, short maternity leaves, childcare stress, infant temperment, and partner abuse (both physical and psychological) (Cutrona & Troutman, 1986; Gotlieb, Whiffen, Wallace, & Mount, 1991; Hyde, Klein, Essex, & Clark, 1995; Mayberry & Affonso, 1993; O'Hara & Swain, 1996; Steinberg & Bellavance, 1999; Terry, Mayocchi, & Hynes, 1996; Whiffen, 1988; Wilson et al., 1996). Women who are satisfied with the social support they receive during pregnancy, and those whose prenatal expectations for postpartum social support match the levels they actually receive, are less likely to experience PPD (Collins, Dunkel-Schetter, Lobel, & Scrimshaw, 1993; Terry et al., 1996). Homemakers without adequate social support have been found to be more susceptible to postpartum depressive symptomatology than either women who are employed or those who are on maternity leave (Richman, Raskin, & Gaines, 1991). Further evidence of the importance of social support for postpartum adjustment is found in a study (Misri, Kostaras, Fox, & Kostaras, 2000) in which postpartum women who met the DSM-IV criteria for depression were randomly assigned to attend psychoeducational sessions either with or without their partners. Those who attended with their partners experienced a more rapid recovery from depression.

Sociocultural Perspectives

PMS and PPD are little known outside of Western countries, and thus both have been theorized to be culture-bound syndromes (Chrisler, 1996; Stern & Kruckman, 1983). A *culture-bound syndrome* is a constellation of signs, symptoms, or experiences that have been categorized as a dysfunction or disease in some societies but not in others. To say that an illness is culture-bound is not to say that the phenomena that comprise it are illegitimate or imaginary. For example, women in any part of the world may feel tense, sad, or tearful prior to menstruation or after the birth of a baby. However, only in Western societies do they think that their emotions are abnormal and might signify a need for professional intervention. The social construction of femininity and the motherhood mystique tell us that good women, and especially good mothers, are always soft-spoken, patient, receptive, nurturing, and kind. Any woman who is turned inward or otherwise unapproachable must have something wrong with her.

Industrialization may contribute to the belief in modern societies that one can and should exercise self-control in order to feel and behave the same way all the time. U.S. culture encourages people to believe that they have more control over their lives and bodies than is actually possible (Brownell, 1991; McDaniel, 1988). Landers (1988) has suggested that PMS is a metaphor for the common inability of women to control their life situations. Premenstrual and postpartum women often complain of feeling "out of control" because they are irritable, angry, exhausted, craving sweets, or unwilling, even temporarily, to put others' needs ahead of their own. Control is so important to U.S. women that being out of control is frightening (Ritenbaugh, 1982). This impossible need for control contributes not only to PMS and PPD but to other behavior patterns that are related to depression (e.g., perfectionism, eating disorders, compulsive exercise). Furthermore, because of the preference in industrialized societies for control, order, and stability (people should be like well-oiled machines), changeableness, rhythmicity, and emotionality have come to be seen as inherently unhealthy (Koeske, 1983).

The vast majority of participants in studies of PMS and PPD are European American, middle-class, college students (PMS) or married women (PPD). Participants are most often recruited from psychology classes or from private psychiatric or obstetrical/gynecological practices to which lower income women may not have access. This methodological limitation is rarely mentioned in review articles, but it may be important in understanding whose and how experience has been medicalized.

Most of the research on PMS is done by scientists in a few Western countries (Australia, Canada, Germany, Great Britain, the Netherlands, Sweden, and the United States), which share many common cultural beliefs (Chrisler, 1996). World Health Organization surveys indicate that menstrual cycle-related complaints (except cramps) are most likely to be reported by women living in Western Europe, Australia, and North America. Data collected from women in Hong Kong (Chang, Holroyd, & Chau, 1995) and in mainland China (Yu, Zhu, Li, Oakley, & Reame, 1996) indicate that the most commonly reported premenstrual changes are fatigue, water retention, pain, and increased sensitivity to cold. U.S. women do not report cold sensitivity, and Chinese women rarely report negative affect. The results of these studies support the idea that culture shapes which variations in mood and physical sensations are noticed and which are of concern. Further support comes from Paige's (1973) survey of U.S. women. She found that the most severe menstrual complaints came from strict Catholics and Orthodox Jews, both of whom strongly adhered to the feminine gender role.

In their review of the anthropological literature on childbirth, Stern and Kruckman (1983) identified some features that are common across many cultures: a structured postpartum period of up to 40 days, assistance with infant care tasks, social recognition of the transition to motherhood, protection of new mothers' vulnerability, social seclusion, rest, and restriction of normal activities for a time after birthing. Together, these practices provide women with the necessary social support during a major life event, and this support may ultimately protect them from PPD. Although the 40-day period is roughly equivalent to the 6-week postpartum period recognized in the United States, the other practices are not necessarily available to U.S. women. Stern and Kruckman (1983) noted that inadequacies in both social support and social recognition of the mother's new status are factors that may place U.S. women at a higher risk for PPD than women in other countries. In a more recent review of postpartum mood disorders, Zelkowitz (1996) found that most studies from non-Western countries concerned women hospitalized for postpartum psychosis, which is not associated with lack of social support or social recognition.

The theory of PPD as a culture-bound syndrome is also supported by research with immigrant women in the United States. In a recent study (Stewart & Jambunathan, 1996) Hmong women in Wisconsin who had recently given birth were interviewed at 4 months postpartum. They commonly reported a lack of energy, difficulty with normal activities, difficulty making decisions, mood swings, and difficulty concentrating. However, they did not attribute their symptoms to PPD; they believed that their problems were due to living in a different culture, to their limited financial resources, and to increases in childcare responsibilities. Consistent with Stern and Kruckman's (1983) conclusions, the Hmong women cited their social support systems and a 30-day postpartum rest period as most helpful to them in coping during the postpartum.

Feminist scholars (Johnston-Robledo, 2000; Lee, 1997; Mauthner, 1993; Nicolson, 1990, 1997, 1998) have acknowledged the etiological role of sociocultural variables in PPD, and have emphasized the political context in which women experience the transition to parenthood and the institution of motherhood itself. The political climate includes a conspiracy of silence about the realities of motherhood because the patriarchy is well served by cultural images of happy, well-adjusted women who are content with their roles as primary caretakers of their children. These unattainable images, which romanticize and mystify mothers, are supported by a set of unrealistic beliefs that are referred to collectively as the "motherhood mystique" (Hoffnung, 1989; Oakley, 1974). The beliefs most relevant to the conspiracy of silence are that (1) women are naturally equipped with parenting skills, which are part of the maternal instinct (Nicolson, 1998); and (2) good mothers really enjoy motherhood and all the work that accompanies it. Any difficulty with infant care or experiences of ambivalence or conflict with the demands of parenting are therefore unnatural and signs of pathology. These widespread beliefs establish a dichotomy between normal-happy-good-mentally healthy mothers and abnormal-depressed-bad-mentally ill mothers.

This dichotomy is perpetuated by the scientific discourse on PPD. The identification of PPD as a distinct illness, which is qualitatively different from normal postpartum adjustment, implies that women should adjust to parenthood easily and that those who do not must have some underlying pathology. Feminist scholars have argued instead that PPD represents a normal grief reaction for the significant losses in identity and lifestyle that are inherent in the transition to motherhood (Nicolson, 1990) and that it may be more valuable to view PPD as the extreme end of a continuum of postpartum adjustment experiences (Lee, 1997).

Qualitative studies of women's experiences during the postpartum period have revealed categories of stressors that may contribute to depression. Participants in Horowitz and Damato's (1999) study identified stressors related to roles, tasks, resources, and relationships. In her study of new mothers, Nicolson (1990) found that women were coping with four features of the postpartum period: physical adjustment, initial insecurities, support networks, and loss of former identity. Postpartum women have reported being shocked by the difficult realities of motherhood, being surprised that other women they know had not broken the silence to warn them of the difficulties, and feeling guilty about being sad or struggling with the transition to motherhood (Mauthner, 1999; McVeigh, 1997).

Popular Culture

Popular culture plays an important role in establishing and maintaining beliefs such as (1) all women go at least a little crazy just before their menstrual periods and (2) normal mothers are happy and find fulfillment in their role. The images that support these beliefs are ubiquitous in magazines, films, television shows, greeting cards, songs, self-help books, comic strips, and other media; they are easily absorbed into a kind of folk wisdom—things that "everyone knows" about women. Such knowledge leads to self-diagnosis with PMS or PPD and, ultimately, to the perpetuation of stereotypes about women through attributions about self and others.

Results of a content analysis (Chrisler & Levy, 1990) of 78 articles about premenstrual syndrome that were published in the popular press (1980–1987) illustrate the prominence of biological etiologies and the suggestion that hormonal shifts can turn ordinary women into monsters. Journalists referred to the menstrual cycle as the "cycle of misery," a "hormonal roller coaster," "the monthly monster," "the menstrual monster," "the inner beast," the "battle between estrogen and progesterone," and the "war being waged by the body's hormones" (p. 98). The premenstrual and menstrual phases of the cycle are considered "weeks of hell" during which women are "hostages to their hormones," "crippled . . . handicapped"; premenstrual women are described as "raging beasts" and "raging animals" (p. 98). Titles of popular press articles about PMS include "Premenstrual Frenzy," "Dr. Jekyll and Ms. Hyde," "Coping with Eve's Curse," "PMS: The Return of the Raging Hormones," "Premenstrual Misery," "Once a Month I'm a Woman Possessed," and "The Taming of the Shrew Inside of You" (p. 97). These articles were published after the famous criminal trials in the United Kingdom in which PMS was used to argue for diminished responsibility, and the authors of the articles were often obviously influenced by news reports of the trials. The references to Jekyll and Hyde and raging animals may come directly from statements made about his client by one of the lawyers, and the frequent military references (e.g., war, battle, hostages, hell week) may derive from the violence of the crimes (Chrisler, 2002). The image of premenstrual women as enraged, violent, and out of control has spread throughout the culture, and with it has come the implication that all menstruating women (not just those with a diagnosable disorder) are capable of behaving in an erratic, dangerous manner.

The popular press promotes the motherhood mystique through its consistent portrayals of happy, competent mothers. In a content analysis of photographs of mothers in 12 issues of *Parenting* magazine, Molina, Johnston-Robledo, and Babler (2000) found that the images do not reflect the stressful nature of parenting. Situations that could be potentially stressful, such as diapering a wiggling infant or trying to work at a computer with a baby on one's lap, were typically illustrated with photos of mothers who looked happy and composed. Stories of difficult situations were often accompanied by blurry photos or drawings in which the mother's face was turned away, thereby erasing her emotion. Stressful situations and mothers' negative affect were also relegated to humorous cartoons, which trivialize the anger, stress, and frustration inherent in dealing with difficult children or situations. In this way, the magazine's editors promote the conspiracy of silence. Women readers may feel isolated in their distress because they can find no images of mothers who feel the same way they do.

What impact do these images have on women's expectations for and experiences with motherhood? It is difficult to address these questions empirically. However, in their survey of 1,100 pregnant women, Genevie and Margolies (1987) found that most of the women's expectations about motherhood were extremely idealistic. Many women believed that motherhood would be easy and that they would be just like the mothers portrayed in magazines and on television. They expected to be patient, a better mother than others, and able to raise good children. Women who had romantic notions about motherhood during pregnancy later reported more negative feelings about motherhood than did women whose expectations were more realistic.

If women want to compare their postpartum emotional experiences to those of other new mothers, one way they may do so is by reading popular press articles about the postpartum period. A content analysis (Martinez, Johnston-Robledo, Ulsh, & Chrisler, 2000) of magazines articles (1980–1998) was conducted to evaluate the description of postpartum mood disturbances. Only 19 articles on PPD and 8 on the baby blues appeared in North American magazines during the 18-year period covered by the project. The relative absence of coverage of the topic suggests that either everyone already knows that women are depressed after giving birth or that no one should talk about it (a conspiracy of silence). The articles contained a strong bias toward the medical model of PPD, and they contained contradictory information about its definition, prevalence, onset, duration, symptoms, and treatment. Furthermore, the articles often confused PPD, the baby blues, and postpartum psychosis, which could frighten a woman who is feeling sad and irritable into thinking that she is in danger of harming herself or her child. Articles with titles such as "Why Mothers Kill Their Babies" and "When a Mother Kills" (p. 52) build stories around images of postpartum women as murderers, and may lead readers to believe that only "crazy" women experience postpartum depression. When authors do not make it clear that infanticide is a more likely outcome of the much rarer postpartum psychosis than it is of PPD or the baby blues, it is difficult for readers to see the difference between feelings and experiences that are normal and common and those that are abnormal and infrequent.

CONCLUSIONS

Feminist scholars have made important contributions toward an understanding of assumptions about the impact of hormones on women's mood,
cognition, and behavior. These assumptions shape both the scientific and
the popular discourse about PMS and PPD, and they guide research questions, public policy, and treatment models. More could be done to expose
and correct erroneous assumptions, both in print and person to person;
corrections (e.g., hormones don't rage, they circulate) may help women to
understand themselves by putting their personal experiences into a sociopolitical context.

To suggest that PMS and PPD are not necessarily medical conditions is
not to say that women do not experience physical and emotional changes
premenstrually or postpartum, some of which they find disturbing. Women's
experiences should be respected, and they should be given the social and
emotional support they need to cope with their experiences. It is our responsibility as feminist activists, clinicians, and researchers to explain how
hormonal attributions for emotions can undermine women's authority,
trivialize their complaints, and invalidate their anger. For example, it is not
normal to feel the same way everyday—no one does. Change is part of human nature. Why should changes associated with the rhythms of the menstrual cycle be denied or medicated, whereas those associated with the day
of the week or the season of the year are tolerated or even celebrated?

A reliance on the biomedical model to the neglect of psychological and
sociocultural predictors of PPD supports the conspiracy of silence about
women's frustrations with inequalities in the work of parenting and their
difficulties in adjusting to the role of mother. Adjusting to any new role can
be difficult. The adjustment to motherhood may be even more difficult because its negative and challenging aspects are so rarely discussed and thus
unanticipated by many. Childcare is hard work, and new mothers need a
safe forum for discussing their concerns and asking for advice and information. Feminist therapists could sponsor support groups for new mothers or
offer to give public lectures about sociocultural views of postpartum affective disturbances that might provide women with alternative ways of understanding their own experiences.

It is striking that the constructs of PMS and PPD are so widely recognized by physicians, psychotherapists, researchers, popular culture, and
women themselves despite the fact that there is so little consensus about
the exact nature of the conditions. Methodological flaws in research and
theory have contributed to pervasive inconsistencies that are rarely identi-

fied as symptomatic of flawed constructs. Researchers need to do more than acknowledge the limitations of previous work. Studies of more diverse samples of women; interviews with new mothers about their mood fluctuations, fears, and disappointments; and examinations of the usual range of fluctuations of affect, sensation, and behavior across the menstrual cycle may help to elucidate the normal from the abnormal.

Finally, a critical analysis of the parallels between the constructs of PMS and PPD illustrates the value of a contextual, feminist, biopsychosocial approach to understanding women's premenstrual and postpartum experiences. Biomedical and intrapsychic theories of PMS and PPD are insufficient, inaccurate, and inappropriate because the proponents of these approaches ignore the historical, social, cultural, and political contexts of women's lives. Feminist psychologists, on the other hand, recognize the extent to which life circumstances, political ideologies, social institutions, and cultural constructs contribute to the development of women's dis-ease. The feminist approach has proved to be powerful in both validating women's experiences and exposing the extent to which normal physiological events have been pathologized in both professional and popular discourse. It is clear that a variety of factors can contribute to women's experiences of PMS and PPD. The stress and coping model is consistent with both feminist and biopsychosocial approaches, and it may prove to be the most useful way to understand women's experiences and to advise them on how to solve the problems that are the basis for their negative affect.

REFERENCES

Abraham, G. E. (1982). The nutritionist's approach. In C. H. Debrovner (Ed.), *Premenstrual tension: A multidisciplinary approach* (pp. 71–93). New York: Human Sciences Press.

American Psychiatric Association. (1968). *Diagnostic and statistical manual of mental disorders* (2nd ed.). Washington, DC: Author.

American Psychiatric Association. (1980). *Diagnostic and statistical manual of mental disorders* (3rd ed.). Washington, DC: Author.

American Psychiatric Association. (1994). *Diagnostic and statistical manual of mental disorders* (4th ed.). Washington, DC: Author.

Beck, L. E., Gevirtz, R., & Mortola, J. F. (1990). The predictive role of psychosocial stress on symptom severity in premenstrual syndrome. *Psychosomatic Medicine, 52,* 536–543.

Brownell, K. (1991). Personal responsibility and control over our bodies: When expectation exceeds reality. *Health Psychology, 10,* 303–310.

Budoff, P. W. (1980). *No more menstrual cramps and other good news.* New York: Penguin Books.

Caplan, P. (1995). *They say you're crazy: How the world's most powerful psychiatrists decide who's normal.* Reading, MA: Addison-Wesley.

Caplan, P. J., McCurdy-Myers, J., & Gans, M. (1992). Should "premenstrual syndrome" be called a psychiatric abnormality? *Feminism and Psychology, 2,* 27–44.

Chang, A. M., Holroyd, E., & Chau, J. P. C. (1995). Premenstrual syndrome in employed Chinese women in Hong Kong. *Health Care for Women International, 16,* 551–561.

Chrisler, J. C. (1996). PMS as a culture-bound syndrome. In J. C. Chrisler, C. Golden, & P. D. Rozee (Eds.), *Lectures on the psychology of women* (pp. 106–121). New York: McGraw-Hill.

Chrisler, J. C. (2002). Hormone hostages: The cultural legacy of PMS as a legal defense. In L. H. Collins, M. R. Dunlap, & J. C. Chrisler (Eds.), *Charting a new course for feminist psychology* (pp. 238–252). Westport, CT: Praeger.

Chrisler, J. C., & Levy, K. B. (1990). The media construct a menstrual monster: A content analysis of PMS articles in the popular press. *Women and Health, 16*(2), 80–104.

Collins, N. L., Dunkel-Schetter, C., Lobel, M., & Scrimshaw, S. C. M. (1993). Social support in pregnancy: Psychosocial correlates of birth outcomes and postpartum depression. *Journal of Personality and Social Psychology, 65,* 1243–1258.

Coughlin, P. C. (1990). Premenstrual syndrome: How marital satisfaction and role choice affect symptom severity. *Social Work, 35,* 351–355.

Cox, J. L. (1986). *Postnatal depression: A guide for health professionals.* New York: Churchill Livingstone.

Cutrona, C. E., & Troutman, B. R. (1986). Social support, infant temperament, and parenting self-efficacy: A mediational model of postpartum depression. *Child Development, 57,* 1507–1518.

Dalton, K. (1964). *The premenstrual syndrome.* Springfield, IL: Charles C Thomas.

Dalton, K. (1977). *The premenstrual syndrome and progesterone therapy.* Chicago: Yearbook Medical.

Dalton, K., & Holton, W. M. (1996). *Depression after childbirth: How to recognize, treat, and prevent postnatal depression.* New York: Oxford University Press.

Debrovner, C. (1982). *Premenstrual tension: An interdisciplinary approach.* New York: Human Sciences Press.

DeJong, R., Rubinow, D. R., Roy-Byrne, P., Hoban, M. C., Grover, G. N., & Post, R. M. (1985). Premenstrual mood disorder and psychiatric illness. *American Journal of Psychiatry, 142,* 1359–1361.

Dennerstein, L., Morse, C. A., & Varnanides, K. (1988). Premenstrual tension and depression: Is there a relationship? *Journal of Psychosomatic Obstetrics and Gynecology, 18,* 45–52.

Ehrenreich, B., & English, D. (1979). *For her own good: 150 years of the experts' advice to women.* Garden City, NY: Anchor Books.

Endicott, J., & Halbreich, U. (1988). Clinical significance of premenstrual dysphoric changes. *Journal of Clinical Psychiatry, 49,* 486–489.

Epperson, C. N. (1999). Postpartum major depression: Detection and treatment. *American Family Physician, 59,* 2247–2254.

Figert, A. E. (1996). *Women and the ownership of PMS: The structuring of a psychiatric disorder.* New York: Aldine de Gruyter.

Frank, R. T. (1931). The hormonal causes of premenstrual tension. *Archives of Neurology and Psychiatry, 26,* 1053–1057.

Freeman, E. W., Sondheimer, S. J., & Rickels, K. (1987). Effects of medical history factors on symptom severity in women meeting criteria for premenstrual syndrome. *Obstetrics and Gynecology, 72,* 236–239.

Gallant, S. J., Popiel, D. A., & Hoffman, D. M. (1994). The role of psychological variables in the experience of premenstrual symptoms. In N. F. Woods (Ed.), *Mind–body rhythmicity: A menstrual cycle perspective* (pp. 139–151). Seattle, WA: Hamilton & Cross.

Gallant, S. J., Popiel, D. A., Hoffman, D. M., Chakraborty, P. K., & Hamilton, J. A. (1992). Using daily ratings to confirm premenstrual syndrome/late luteal phase dysphoric disorder: II. What makes a "real" difference? *Psychosomatic Medicine, 54,* 167–181.

Genevie, L., & Margolies, E. (1987). *The motherhood report: How women feel about being mothers.* New York: Macmillan.

Genther, A. B., Chrisler, J. C., & Johnston-Robledo, I. (1999, August). *Coping, locus of control, and the experience of premenstrual symptoms.* Poster presented at the annual meeting of the American Psychological Association, Boston.

Giannini, A. J., Price, W. A., Loiselle, R. H., & Giannini, M. D. (1985). Pseudo cholinesterase and trait anxiety in premenstrual tension syndrome. *Journal of Clinical Psychiatry, 46,* 139–140.

Golub, S. (1992). *Periods: From menarche to menopause.* Newbury Park, CA: Sage.

Gotlieb, I. H., Whiffen, V. E., Wallace, P. M., & Mount, J. H. (1991). Prospective investigation of postpartum depression: Factors involved in onset and recovery. *Journal of Abnormal Psychology, 100,* 122–132.

Halbreich, U., & Kas, D. (1977). Variations in the Taylor MAS of women with premenstrual syndrome. *Journal of Psychosomatic Research, 21,* 391–393.

Hendrick, V., Altschuler, L. L., & Suri, R. (1998). Hormonal changes in the postpartum and implications for postpartum depression. *Psychosomatics, 39,* 93–101.

Hoffnung, M. (1989). Motherhood: Contemporary conflict for women. In J. Freeman (Ed.), *Women: A feminist perspective* (4th ed., pp. 157–175). Mountain View, CA: Mayfield.

Hopkins, J., Campbell, S. B., & Marcus, M. (1989). Postpartum depression and postpartum adaptation: Overlapping constructs? *Journal of Affective Disorders, 17,* 251–254.

Hopkins, J., Marcus, M., & Campbell, S. B. (1984). Postpartum depression: A critical review. *Psychological Bulletin, 95,* 498–515.

Horowitz, J. A., & Damato, E. G. (1999). Mothers' perceptions of postpartum stress and satisfaction. *Journal of Obstetric, Gynecologic, and Neonatal Nursing, 28,* 595–605.

Houppert, K. (1999). *The curse: Confronting the last unmentionable taboo.* New York: Farrar, Straus, & Giroux.

Hyde, J. S., Klein, M. H., Essex, M. J., & Clark, R. (1995). Maternity leave and women's mental health. *Psychology of Women Quarterly, 19,* 257–285.

Janowsky, D. S., Berens, S. C., & Davis, J. M. (1973). Correlations between mood, weight, and electrolytes during the menstrual cycle: A renin–angiotensin–aldosterone hypothesis of premenstrual tension. *Psychosomatic Medicine, 35,* 143–154.

Johnston-Robledo, I. (2000). From postpartum depression to the empty nest syndrome: The motherhood mystique revisited. In J. C. Chrisler, C. Golden, & P. D. Rozee (Eds.), *Lectures on the psychology of women* (2nd ed., pp. 128–147). New York: McGraw-Hill.

Kennerley, H., & Gath, D. (1989). Maternity blues: I. Associations with obstetric, psychological, and psychiatric factors. *British Journal of Psychiatry, 155,* 367–373.

Koeske, R. D. (1983). Lifting the curse of menstruation: Toward a feminist perspective on the menstrual cycle. *Women and Health, 8*(2–3), 1–16.

Kraaimaat, F. W., & Veeninga, A. (1995). Causal attributions in premenstrual syndrome. *Journal of Psychology and Health, 10,* 219–228.

Kuczmierczyk, A. R., Labrum, A. H., & Johnson, C. C. (1992). Perception of family and work environments in women with premenstrual syndrome. *Journal of Psychosomatic Research, 36,* 787–795.

Landers, L. (1988). *Images of bleeding: Menstruation as ideology.* New York: Orlando Press.

Laws, S., Hey, V., & Eagen, A. (1985). *Seeing red: The politics of premenstrual tension.* London: Hutchinson.

Lee, C. (1997). Social context, depression, and the transition to motherhood. *British Journal of Health Psychology, 2,* 93–108.

Llewellyn, A. M., Stowe, Z. N., & Nemeroff, C. B. (1997). Depression during pregnancy and the puerperium. *Journal of Clinical Psychiatry, 58,* 26–32.

Maddocks, S. E., & Reid, R. L. (1992). The role of negative life stress and PMS: Some preliminary findings. In A. J. Dan & L. L. Lewis (Eds.), *Menstrual health in women's lives* (pp. 38–51). Chicago: University of Illinois Press.

Mandy, A., Gard, P. R., Ross, K., & Valentine, B. H. (1998). Psychological sequelae in women following either parturition or non-gynecological surgery. *Journal of Reproductive and Infant Psychology, 16,* 133–141.

Martin, E. (1988). Premenstrual syndrome: Discipline, work, and anger in late industrial societies. In T. Buckley & A. Gottlieb (Eds.), *Blood magic: The anthropology of menstruation* (pp. 161–181). Berkeley and Los Angeles: University of California Press.

Martinez, R., Johnston-Robledo, I., Ulsh, H. M., & Chrisler, J. C. (2000). Singing "the baby blues": A content analysis of popular press articles about postpartum affective disorders. *Women and Health, 31*(2–3), 37–56.

Matthey, S., Barnett, B., Ungerer, J., & Waters, B. (2000). Paternal and maternal depressed mood during the transition to parenthood. *Journal of Affective Disorders, 60,* 75–85.

Mauthner, N. (1993). Toward a feminist understanding of "postnatal depression." *Feminism and Psychology, 3,* 350–355.

Mauthner, N. (1999). Feeling low and feeling really bad about feeling low: Women's experiences of motherhood and postpartum depression. *Canadian Psychology, 40,* 143–161.

Mayberry, L. J., & Affonso, D. D. (1993). Infant temperment and postpartum depression: A review. *Health Care for Women International, 14,* 201–211.

McDaniel, S. H. (1988). The interpersonal politics of premenstrual syndrome. *Family Systems Medicine, 6,* 134–149.

McVeigh, C. (1997). Motherhood experiences from the perspectives of first-time mothers. *Clinical Nursing Research, 6,* 335–348.

Mira, M., Vizzard, J., & Abraham, S. (1985). Personality characteristics in the menstrual cycle. *Journal of Psychosomatic Obstetrics and Gynecology, 4,* 329–334.

Misri, S., Kostaras, X., Fox, D., & Kostaras, D. (2000). The impact of partner support in the treatment of postpartum depression. *Canadian Journal of Psychiatry, 45,* 554–558.

Molina, C., Johnston-Robledo, I., & Babler, A. (2000, March). Images of women in *Parenting* magazine. In J. C. Chrisler (Chair), *Sociocultural images of women and their possible effects on life goals, self-esteem, and self-efficacy.* Symposium presented at the annual meeting of the Association for Women in Psychology, Salt Lake City, UT.

Nash, H. C., & Chrisler, J. C. (1997). Is a little (psychiatric) knowledge a dangerous thing?: The impact of premenstrual dysphoric disorder on perceptions of premenstrual women. *Psychology of Women Quarterly, 21,* 315–322.

Nicolson, P. (1990). Understanding postnatal depression: A mother-centered approach. *Journal of Advanced Medicine, 15,* 689–695.

Nicolson, P. (1995). The menstrual cycle, science, and femininity: Assumptions underlying menstrual cycle research. *Social Science and Medicine, 41,* 779–784.

Nicolson, P. (1997). Motherhood and women's lives. In V. Robinson & D. Richardson (Eds.), *Introducing women's studies: Feminist theory and practice* (2nd ed., pp. 375–398). New York: New York University Press.

Nicolson, P. (1998). *Post-natal depression: Psychology, science, and the transition to motherhood.* London: Routledge.

Oakley, A. (1974). *The sociology of housework.* New York: Pantheon Books.

O'Brien, P. M. S., Selby, C., & Symonds, E. M. (1980). Progesterone, fluid, and electrolytes in premenstrual syndrome. *British Medical Journal, 87,* 1161–1163.

O'Hara, M. W., & Swain, A. M. (1996). Rates and risk of postpartum depression: A meta-analysis. *International Review of Psychiatry, 8,* 37–54.

Ornitz, A. W., & Brown, M. A. (1993). Family coping and premenstrual symptomatology. *Journal of Obstetric, Gynecologic, and Neonatal Nursing, 22,* 49–55.

Paige, K. E. (1973). Women learn to sing the menstrual blues. *Psychology Today, 4*(9), 41–46.

Parry, B. L., Berga, S. L., Kripke, D. F., Klauber, M. R., Laughlin, G. A., Yes, S. S. C., & Gillin, C. (1990). Altered wave form of plasma nocturnal melatonin secretion in premenstrual depression. *Archives of General Psychiatry, 47,* 1139–1146.

Pearlstein, T. B., Frank, E., Rivera-Tovar, A., Thoft, J. S., Jacobs, E., & Mieczkowski, T. A. (1990). Prevalence of Axis I and Axis II disorders in women with late luteal phase dysphoric disorder. *Journal of Affective Disorders, 20,* 129–134.

Pfost, K. S., Lum, C. U., & Stevens, M. J. (1989). Femininity and work plans protect women against postpartum dysphoria. *Sex Roles, 21,* 423–431.

Picone, L., & Kirkby, R. J. (1990). Relationship between anxiety and premenstrual syndrome. *Psychological Reports, 67*, 43–48.

Rausch, J. L., & Janowsky, D. W. (1982). Premenstrual tension: Etiology. In R. C. Friedman (Ed.), *Behavior and the menstrual cycle* (pp. 397–427). New York: Marcel Dekker.

Reid, R. L., & Yen, S. S. C. (1981). Premenstrual syndrome. *American Journal of Obstetrics and Gynecology, 139*, 85–104.

Richman, J. A., Raskin, V. D., & Gaines, C. (1991). Gender roles, social support, and postpartum depressive symptomatology. *Journal of Nervous and Mental Disease, 179*, 139–147.

Ritenbaugh, C. (1982). Obesity as a culture-bound syndrome. *Culture, Medicine, and Psychiatry, 6*, 347–361.

Rittenhouse, C. A. (1991). The emergence of premenstrual syndrome as a social problem. *Social Problems, 38*, 412–425.

Rubinow, D. R. (1991). *Models of PMS.* Paper presented at the annual meeting of the Society for Menstrual Cycle Research, Seattle, WA.

Sampson, G. A. (1979). Premenstrual syndrome: A double-blind controlled trial of progesterone and placebo. *British Journal of Psychiatry, 135*, 209–215.

Sampson, G. A. (1981). An appraisal of the role of progesterone in the therapy of premenstrual syndrome. In P. A. van Keep & W. H. Utian (Eds.), *The premenstrual syndrome* (pp. 51–69). Lancaster, UK: MTP Press.

Sanders, D., Warner, P. Backstrom, T., & Bancroft, J. (1983). Mood, sexuality, hormones, and the menstrual cycle: I. Changes in mood and physical state—Description of subjects and method. *Psychosomatic Medicine, 45*, 487–501.

Seguin, L., Potvin, L., St. Denis, M., & Loiselle, J. (1999). Depressive symptoms in the late postpartum among low socioeconomic status women. *Birth, 26*, 157–163.

Showalter, E. (1978). *The female malady: Women, madness, and English culture, 1830–1980.* New York: Pantheon Books.

Steinberg, S. I., & Bellavance, F. (1999). Characteristics and treatment of women with antenatal and postpartum depression. *International Journal of Psychiatry in Medicine, 29*, 209–233.

Stern, G., & Kruckman, L. (1983). Multi-disciplinary perspectives on postpartum depression: An anthropological critique. *Social Science and Medicine, 17*, 1027–1041.

Stewart, S., & Jambunathan, J. (1996). Hmong women and postpartum depression. *Health Care for Women International, 17*, 319–330.

Stout, A. L., & Steege, J. F. (1985). Psychological assessment of women seeking treatment for premenstrual syndrome. *Journal of Psychosomatic Research, 29*, 621–629.

Stowe, Z. N., & Nemeroff, C. B. (1995). Women at risk for postpartum-onset major depression. *American Journal of Obstetrics and Gynecology, 173*, 639–645.

Taylor, D., Golding, J., Menard, L., & King, M. (2001, June). *Sexual assault and severe PMS: Prevalence and predictors.* Paper presented at the meeting of the Society for Menstrual Cycle Research, Avon, CT.

Terry, D. L., Mayocchi, L., & Hynes, G. J. (1996). Depressive symptomatology in new mothers: A stress and coping perspective. *Journal of Abnormal Psychology, 105*, 220–231.

Warner, P., & Bancroft, J. (1990). Factors related to self-reporting of the premenstrual syndrome. *British Journal of Psychiatry, 157*, 249–260.

Warner, P., Bancroft, J., Dixson, A., & Hampson, M. (1991). The relationship between perimenstrual mood and depressive illness. *Journal of Affective Disorders, 23*, 9–23.

Wertz, D. C. (1983). What birth has done for doctors: A historical review. *Women and Health, 8*(1), 7–24.

Whiffen, V. E. (1988). Vulnerability to postpartum depression: A prospective multivariate study. *Journal of Abnormal Psychology, 97*, 467–474.

Whiffen, V. E. (1992). Is postpartum depression a distinct diagnosis? *Clinical Psychology Review, 12*, 485–508.

Wilson, L. M., Reid, A. J., Midmer, D. K., Biringer, A., Carroll, J. C., & Stewart, D. E. (1996). Antenatal psychosocial risk factors associated with adverse postpartum family outcomes. *Canadian Medical Association Journal, 154*, 785–799.

Yu, M., Zhu, X., Li, J., Oakley, D., & Reame, N. E. (1996). Perimenstrual symptoms among Chinese women in an urban area of China. *Health Care for Women International, 17*, 161–172.

Zelkowitz, P. (1996). Childbearing and women's mental health. *Transcultural Psychiatric Research Review, 33*, 391–412.

Chapter 8

Alcohol and Drug Addiction in Women
Phenomenology and Prevention

LYNN H. COLLINS

Despite alleged changes in gender roles, including the double standards that U.S. society holds for women and men, and changes in the way we think about addiction, women who use substances continue to be stigmatized and pathologized (Blume, 1994; Copeland, 1997; Copeland & Hall, 1992; Forth-Finegan, 1991; Garcia, 1997; Gomberg, 1993; Sandmaier, 1992; Woodhouse, 1990). The psychology of substance use and dependence are fraught with gender-related issues from the time of first exposure through the consequences on long-term use. Popular culture and the media still portray substance-using women as criminal, mentally ill, irresponsible, untrustworthy, unloving, hedonistic, poor, child-abusing, promiscuous, whorish, and immoral (Woodhouse, 1990). This contributes both to exaggerated claims of addicted women's incompetence and to under-identification of substance-using women who do not fit this stereotype.

To understand addicted women's lives, we must consider them in the context of gender inequality, cultural influences, socioeconomic status, and situational factors. Women of color, lesbians, older women, and members of other groups may experience additional barriers due to racism, heterosexism, ageism, and other forms of discrimination. Alcohol and substance use are both causes and consequences of the difficulties women face while navigating the course of their lives within this society. Although alcohol, tobacco, and the various substances used by women may have different compositions, effects, and legal consequences, they share the common functions of altering mood, energy, and consciousness. For that reason, this chapter will, like most treatment programs, treat the use of such substances similarly. This chapter describes some of the realities surrounding women's use of drugs and alcohol and suggest ways of changing those realities to create a healthier environment.

HISTORY OF VIEWS OF ADDICTION

In past decades, individuals' problems with alcohol and other drugs were kept secret within families. Indulgence in alcohol, tobacco, marijuana, and heroin for pleasure was viewed very negatively, although use of the same substances in medicinal contexts was deemed acceptable (Erickson, Butters, McGillicuddy, & Hallgren, 2000; Gomberg, 1982). The temperance movement reflected the public belief that drinking was associated with immorality, sin, promiscuity, and weakness (Rathbone-McCuan, Dyer, & Wartman, 1991). The temperance movement, however, drew support from women because it acknowledged that men damaged their families when they spent their wages on alcohol and left their economically dependent wives and children without enough money for sufficient food, housing, and clothing. In 1935 Alcoholics Anonymous (AA) was organized (Hall, 1996). AA addressed drinking problems through the use of social support and spirituality to assist individuals in their quest for abstinence. Members followed a series of 12 steps toward sobriety that involved belief in a higher power, a moral self-inventory, restitution, and helping others attain sobriety (Hall, 1991). Later on, in the 1950s, addiction to alcohol or drugs was reinterpreted as reflecting an underlying psychological problem. It was thought that if you could resolve the individual's psychological problem, his or her drinking or drug use would stop. In 1951 Al-Anon was formed in recognition of the havoc alcoholics wreaked on their families and others around them.

The experimentation period of the 1960s and 1970s may have been more tolerant of drug use than other periods both before and after it. During this time, a new model of addiction was presented that conceptualized addiction as a physical disease process instead of a moral flaw (Baker, 2000; Haaken, 1993). This disease model was formulated by Jellinek (1960; Rhodes & Johnson, 1997). The new view of addiction explained alcoholism in the same manner as other physical diseases and was quickly applied to other addictions as well. This model also directed more attention toward pathology, however. Still, it reduced the moral stigma attached to addictions, neutralized pejorative attitudes toward them to a certain degree, and allowed more opportunities for thinking about addictions diagnostically, psychologically, and therapeutically (Haaken, 1993). The disease model tended to oversimplify addiction problems, however, ignoring the role of societal factors (e.g., sexism, racism, ageism, classism, and attitudes toward the differently abled) in precipitating and maintaining addiction. In doing so, it was less accurate in representing the plight of many groups and therefore interventions structured around this premise were less successful for members of those groups (hooks, 1993).

The 1980s were a time of "Just Say No" campaigns and police pursuit of drug dealers and users (McCrady, 1993). The "War on Drugs" movement during the 1980s criminalized and stigmatized those who used alcohol and other drugs (Baker, 2000). There was an increasingly negative public attitude toward drug use, which was accompanied by longer prison sentences and increases in the legal drinking age. Drunk driving laws became stricter and punishment for violations became more severe. Some states began charging mothers with manslaughter if they ingested cocaine while pregnant because they endangered the lives of their children. The mothers would then be incarcerated, and their children taken away from them (Roberts, Jackson, & Carlton-Laney, 2000). "Three strikes, you're out" laws made consequences even more severe. Crack cocaine and designer drugs were introduced during this time and drug use patterns began to shift. Drug use became increasingly concentrated at the lower economic levels.

During the 1980s the disease model of addiction was embraced and the self-help movement blossomed with groups targeting various subgroups within the addicted population, including specialized groups associated with Alcoholics Anonymous: Alateen, Al-Anon, Narcotics Anonymous, Cocaine Anonymous, Adult Children of Alcoholics, and the like. The *Diagnostic and Statistical Manual of Mental Disorders* (DSM-III; American Psychiatric Association, 1987) criteria were most often used to define disorders involving addiction. Since DSM criteria are largely based on men's experiences with alcohol and other substances, they may not accurately portray the phenomena of addiction in women. Feminists have argued against the destructive labeling of the DSM because of its stigmatizing and potential esteem-damaging effects. They advocated for conceptualizations that include the impact of the environment. Behavioral and cognitive therapists have argued against the emphasis on diagnosis since it serves no therapeutic purpose. Cognitive-behavioral therapists have advocated for a problem-focused approach that takes attention away from the diagnosis and focuses it on patterns of drinking, negative consequences, positive consequences, behavioral deficits, and other facets of the individual's unique experiences with alcohol (McCrady, 1993). The cognitive-behavioral approach, however, still downplays the role of social forces in the etiology of addiction.

During the 1990s there was a proliferation of employee assistance plans (EAPs) and pretrial treatment programs for drug users as well as psychoeducational programs for drunk drivers (McCrady, 1993). These programs were seen as benefiting society by making those addicted to drugs and alcohol more productive members of society. Early detection efforts were launched, and users were introduced to treatment programs before they were even convinced that they had a problem, providing the impetus for studies on the process of change. Most of our models of alcoholism, however, were still developed from white males' experiences (Fraser, 1997).

The addiction literature of the 1980s had characterized women as subordinate and passive participants in the drug world. The 1990s shed a more feminist light on the dynamics behind addiction. Feminists moved away from seeing women as passive victims of social structural forces and emphasized their roles as active agents whose activities were restricted by the dominant social milieu (Baker, 2000). During the 1990s the relationship between trauma and addiction in women was described, and psychologists started to look more at the environmental context in which addiction occurred. Beginning in the 1990s, more people talked about the multiple needs of recovering addicts. Drug and alcohol problems were conceptualized as involving a number of physiological, psychosocial, cultural, and political factors (Hall, 1994). Their use was viewed as a product of the interaction of the addict, those around her or him, and the community. The 1990s saw the beginning of the development of drug treatment programs that provided not only addiction counseling but auxiliary services such as counseling for sexual abuse, physical abuse, and psychiatric illness; parenting skills training; GED programs; independent living skills; domestic violence programs; and medical and other services. Although some "gender-sensitive" programs emerged (Baker, 2000), many more are needed. Most programs were still narrow in the services that they provide.

Today women who drink are still generally seen as more pathological than men who drink because women who drink are violating traditional gender roles by engaging in a male activity and failing to perform their traditional role of maintaining the moral order (Rienzi et al., 1996). Some recent studies of the general population, however, have found that people are not more critical of female than male drinking, intoxication, or aggressive or uncontrolled drinking behavior (Robbins & Martin, 1993). The latter may be related to differences between women and men in the severity of drug- and alcohol-related problems, however.

Drug- and alcohol-using women of color face additional stigmas and consequences because of their color, including having to fight an addiction in the face of even more limited access to resources than white women, heightened levels of violence, divorce, poverty, unemployment, and other problems (McGrath, Keita, Strickland, & Russo, 1990). They are more likely to be punished for their drinking and drug-using behavior and less likely to receive treatment (Taha-Cisse, 1991). African American women also have to fight the stereotypes of Mammy, matriarch, welfare mother, and Jezabel and deal with discrimination (West, 1996). Lesbian women of color face at least quadruple jeopardy as the result of homophobia, racism, sexism, and alcoholism.

GENDER ROLES AND SUBSTANCE USE

Ethnography has shown that greater differences in drinking exist where gender roles are most clearly divided (McDonald, 1994). The magnitude of difference between the drinking patterns of women and those of men mirrored the magnitude of the difference in their positions on the social hierarchy of their country in an international sample (Wilsnack, Vogeltanz, Wilsnack, & Harris, 2000). The more polarized the gender spheres, the greater the differences. For instance, in countries where the division of labor is greatest, where women are most subordinate to men, and where women's movement and activity are most restricted, women's use of alcohol is more restricted. In their general population studies across 10 countries, the International Research Group on Gender and Alcohol (Wilsnack et al., 2000) found that gender roles may also inflate perceptions that biological differences in the impact of alcohol and that gender differences in drinking behavior may be modified by sociocultural factors. They note that even small biological differences seem to justify and contribute to a universal basis for "cultural elaborations" that increase the perception of different patterns of drinking for women and men.

The "convergence hypothesis" holds that as gender roles change and women's and men's lives become more similar, their alcohol and drug use patterns will become more similar as well (Mercer & Khavari, 1990; Mooney & Gilbert, 1999). At this time, the reported annual prevalence of alcohol use by 12th-grade girls and boys is similar (72% and 74%, respectively)

(Johnston, O'Malley, & Bachman, 1995; Lo, 1996). However, adult prevalence rates for alcohol dependence are approximately 2.5–7% for women and 10–20% for men (Dansky, Brewerton, & Kilpatrick, 2000; McLeod, 1995; Nelson & Wittchen, 1998). Women abuse and become addicted to substances at lower rates than men do (McLeod, 1995) and are more likely to be lifelong abstainers (Wilsnack & Wilsnack, 1997). If convergence ever does occur, we can only hope that it will entail men reducing their frequency and quantity of alcohol and drug use to that of women.

For both men and women, the median onset for alcohol abuse and dependence is about 17 years of age. Men and women, but especially women, who used alcohol at age 14 or younger are at increased risk for problematic use later on (Nelson & Wittchen, 1998). Women drink the most and most frequently in their 20s and 30s. Men have the highest rate of consumption in their 20s (Fillmore, 1987). Women's alcohol disorders tend to be of shorter duration than men's, and show higher rates of remission, except during their 30s (Fillmore, 1987). Both women and men drink less as they get older (Fillmore, 1987; Wilsnack et al., 2000), with some international variations in the rate of reduction across age groups. Accurate prevalence rates for illicit drugs are much more difficult to obtain than those for alcohol because of the greater secrecy associated with their use. The most frequently used illicit drugs appear to be marijuana, followed by cocaine, hallucinogens, and heroin.

When women and men drink similar amounts, women may experience stronger effects due to their lighter on average body weight and physiologically different metabolization of alcohol (Lo & Globetti, 1998). For instance, similar doses of alcohol produce higher blood alcohol levels (BAL) in women than in men (Jones & Jones, 1976) due to the lower quantity of bodily fluids and smaller quantities of the enzyme alcohol dehydrogenase (used in metabolizing ethanol) in women's gastrointestinal tracts (Frezza et al., 1990). Lower "first pass" metabolism in women results in greater absorption of alcohol directly into women's bloodstream (Wilsnack et al., 2000). These differences are allegedly related to the greater vulnerability of women to the physical effects of alcohol (Bongars, Van De Goor, Van Oers, & Garretsen, 1998). Short-term physiological and behavioral consequences, however, are actually less severe for women.

Women tend to have fewer negative consequences than men do when they use alcohol and drugs, partly because they tend to use them at lower doses than men (Clayton, Voss, Robbins, & Skinner, 1986; Hughes, Day, Marcantonio, & Torpy, 1997; O'Malley, Johnston, & Bachman, 1995). Women who drink are less likely to report social and health problems

(Nystrom, 1992; Robbins & Martin, 1993). Even when quantities are controlled, women tend to experience equal or fewer negative consequences of drinking at each drinking level (light, moderate, excessive, very excessive) compared to men (Bongars et al., 1998; Nystrom, 1992).

Some have noted that concern about women's drinking seems to increase when women's rights and independence are increasing (Fillmore, 1984; Thom, 1994; Wilsnack et al., 2000). In reality, freedom from oppression and discrimination and increased autonomy were found to be associated with lower levels of substance use and better prognoses in recovery when addiction did occur in a sample of predominantly Caucasian (75%) women (Kelly, Kropp, & Manhal-Baugus, 1995). This chapter examines the influences of socialization and other cultural forces on women's drinking in the United States. It discusses the protective aspects of women's current socialization as well as the negative impact of men's socialization, oppression, and discrimination on women's quality of life.

Protective Aspects of Women's Traditional Socialization

Life is more difficult and stressful for women than for men due in large part to the sexist social structure. Identified risk factors for addiction in women include poverty, homelessness, inadequate education, and inadequate health care during pregnancy. Despite the fact that they live more complicated lives and are more vulnerable to trauma, girls and women become addicted less frequently than men. Although traditional female socialization limits women's experiences in many ways, in other ways it instills a set of values and behaviors that can protect them from addiction or, when addiction occurs, help facilitate their recovery.

Women's socialization encourages self-control, safety, and connection. A heterogeneous sample of girls were found to get intoxicated less frequently than boys. The girls said that they drank less because they had "higher morals" (Warner, Weber, & Albanes, 1999). They also felt pressure to uphold moral standards for sex, aggression, and other behaviors, and to take care of others (Warner et al., 1999). High school women in a predominantly white, working-class sample who drank were less likely than men to act out; fight; encounter law enforcement; cause strain in relationships; experience hangovers, nausea, and vomiting; or have complaints about loss of coordination (Lo & Globetti, 1998). Women learn to control themselves more and have been shown to self-monitor more than men, resulting in less extreme use and intoxication patterns (Caudill, Wilson, & Abrams, 1987; Moore & Lewis, 1989). Girls and women worry that they will engage in irresponsible or inappropriate behavior while intoxicated (32%; Lo & Globetti, 1998), which may serve as a deterrent. Job responsibilities were also important influences on college women's decisions to avoid or discontinue use of alcohol (Traub, 1983).

Parents tend to be more protective of daughters and to set more conservative limits on their behavior (e.g., earlier curfews, insistence on parental supervision, etc.). Parents have been identified as important influences on girls' decisions to avoid or discontinue use of alcohol (Traub, 1983). As a result of parental influence, girls tend to congregate in settings where there is less exposure to drugs and alcohol (Warner et al., 1999). But there is concern that the restriction of girls' activities removes them from needed healthy intellectual and physical experiences in addition to protecting them from danger. The constriction of women's activities may also prevent them from participating in rewarding business and leisure activities. Perhaps in this case we should be taking more steps to limit boys' access to drugs and providing more options for drug- and alcohol-free socializing and networking.

Although the impact of society's emphasis on women's appearance is generally unhealthy, in this case it is protective on the one hand and dangerous on the other. Some adolescent high school girls don't drink because of the impact they fear it will have on their looks (Lo & Globetti, 1998). They also have concerns about how substance use will affect their body, health, aging, memory, and skin (Warner et al., 1999). Alcohol dependence is often associated with problems in the areas of cognition and health, including cardiomyopathy, liver disease, gastritis, ulcers, pancreatitis, and peripheral neuropathies, health practices, and decreased immune response (McCrady, 1993). On the other hand, white girls and women also use substances to help them lose weight and come closer to the media-endorsed ideal body shape for women (Baker, 2000). It is actually more acceptable for Latino and Caucasian girls to use drugs for medicinal purposes, such as taking diet pills to achieve the unrealistic body shape endorsed by U.S. culture, than it is for them to take them to get high and to feel good (Rienzi et al., 1996).

Women worry about the impact of substance use on their children during pregnancy, which can act as a deterrent to use. Any children born during a period of use may manifest fetal alcohol syndrome and birth defects. Women with children may also fear that the children will be taken away from them if they admit to using substances (Bammer & Weekes, 1994; Ettorre, 1994; Preston, 1996). Some people in positions of authority consider medical problems due to substance use during pregnancy a form of child abuse. Lesbian mothers are especially at risk since homophobic authorities may already be inclined to remove their children from their homes due to their lesbian lifestyle (Underhill, 1991).

Early use in girls is in clear conflict with gender-role prescriptions for behavior and may signal that there are circumstances driving them to use, such as neglect, emotional pain, abuse, or threats of abuse (Hawkins, Catalano, & Miller, 1992). Early use can lead to a chain of events that undermine girls' opportunities and therefore their successes. Although the cause-and-effect relationship is difficult to ascertain, it may be that children who refrain from using drugs and alcohol have more opportunities to develop necessary skills while those relying on substances have fewer opportunities.

Although many environments in which substance use takes place are stressful, abusive, and dangerous, an exception may occur within some lesbian communities. Since the 1940s, lesbian bars have been the center of both social and political activity in lesbian communities in the United States (Hall, 1996). I say that the exception occurs in "some" communities because in the 1940s and 1950s some gay bars were allegedly mafia run and often raided, lesbians were harassed by gay males, and "bull dykes" were forced to protect "femmes" (Kennedy & Davis, 1993). The bars were places to meet other lesbians for friendship, love, and political alliances. In some cases, in these bars lesbians felt safer and could more freely express themselves without fear of consequences or rejection (Hall, 1993, 1996). They were a place of refuge within a hostile, heterosexist society (Underhill, 1991). Especially in those early days, alcohol was an unavoidable presence, which was a serious problem for lesbians with alcohol problems. Researchers from within and outside of the lesbian community have found that the rate of alcoholism among lesbians is higher than that among women in general (Hall, 1990, 1996; Lohrenz, Connelly, Coyne, & Spare, 1978; Nicoloff & Stiglitz, 1987; Schilit, Clark, & Shallenberger, 1988). The rate of alcoholism for lesbians has been estimated to be about 25–35%, which is three times as high as that for women in general (Hall, 1996). In response to awareness of this problem, the lesbian community has become very recovery-oriented. Lesbians were one of the first groups to consistently hold alcohol-free events for adults. This was not without controversy, however, since not everyone in the community desires to be abstinent. Fortunately, there are more meeting places and social forums than bars at present, although bars remain important gathering places.

There is a myth (O'Connor, Horwitz, Gottlieb, Kraus, & Segal, 1993; Van Etten, Neumark, & Anthony, 1999a, 1999b) that women's alcohol and drug problems "telescope" or escalate more quickly than men's. *Telescoping* refers to a phenomena in which women allegedly start drinking later, but then speed more quickly than men to the level of problem drinking. It is a way to pathologize the fact that women tend to identify their problems and seek treatment more quickly than do men (O'Connor et al., 1993). In fact, women are more likely than men to seek help for depression and other problems instead of self-medicating with alcohol or drugs and to seek help more quickly when an addiction develops. Furthermore, women are also more likely than men to have the relational skills to do better in self-help groups like Alcoholics Anonymous. They report greater ease than men in connecting with others in the context of groups such as Alcoholics Anonymous, Al-Anon, and Nar-Anon (Rathbone-McCuan et al., 1991). Their socialization helps them to be supportive, empathic group members who can share with others.

Negative Aspects of Women's Traditional Socialization

On the other hand, women are taught behavior control and inhibition to the degree that some become overly submissive and unassertive. They are usually trained to please others rather than to choose what is right for themselves. Consequently, some girls and women attempt to conform by drinking in response to how much peers are consuming. Girls in a sample representative of the U.S. population also drank to increase social assertion (Mooney & Gilbert, 1999). Some girls think that drinking helps them to meet and get closer to other people (Lo & Globetti, 1998). Girls and women are raised to value connection, and when they perceive connection to be difficult, they may drink in order to feel more comfortable and to reduce social inhibition. They are also likely to drink if they perceive their companion to seem tense (Corcoran & Michels, 1999).

Girls are encouraged to take care of others and to put others before themselves. This sends girls the message that they are less important than others. Negative messages about their worth may lead to depression and reduced self-esteem (Desimone, Murray, & Lester, 1994; Hare & Hare, 1986; Rodney, Mupier, & Crafter, 1998; Young, Werch, & Bakema, 1989). In the process of caring for others, girls may lose their identity as individuals and forget about their own needs. First Nations women found that a gender analysis of their lives, including their spirituality, was helpful in sorting out how gender roles and scripts had influenced their lives. It also helped to separate out constructive and destructive aspects of their culture (Herbert & McCannell, 1997). Rather than admitting powerlessness over

alcoholism and taking a moral inventory of themselves as recommended by
the AA 12 steps, girls and women could benefit from empowering themselves, examining the influence of the patriarchy in which most of them
live, and becoming more aware of their thoughts, feelings, competencies,
dreams, values, heritage, strengths, and victories, in addition to any vulnerabilities (Unterberger, 1989). Exploration of one's cultural, ethnic, sexual,
and individual identities can make a difference in how women think about
themselves and can facilitate recovery (Herbert & McCannell, 1997).
Women of color in treatment may benefit from developing a more Afrocentric way of looking at the world. A strong African American identity can
enhance self-esteem and is related to lower levels of drug use (McCreary,
Slavin, & Berry, 1996). First Nation women found support, enhanced
cultural identity, and participation in ceremonies helpful in recovery (Herbert & McCannell, 1997), although at this point in time many of the First
Nation ceremonies are still male-dominated.

    The accuracy of data on women's substance use is questionable
(Rathbone-McCuan et al., 1991). Because of the stigma attached to substance use, and because of the roles endangered by use (such as motherhood), women may be reluctant to admit use. Girls are concerned about
whether others see them as deviant (Warner et al., 1999). In a study of predominantly European American high school students, when the girls used
marijuana, they did so more privately to avoid detection and to reduce risk
of punishment and loss of social status (Lo & Globetti, 1998). Older
woman may feel especially embarrassed and guilty about drinking because
they are more likely to associate drinking with immorality, sin, promiscuity,
and moral weakness (Rathbone-McCuan et al., 1991). Authors of previous
reviews and histories of alcohol concluded that when using alcohol,
women felt that they had failed to meet their responsibilities regarding the
control of the use of alcohol (Lacerte & Harris, 1986; Lender, 1986;
Rathbone-McCuan et al., 1991) and that they would embarrass their families by seeking treatment. Women's lives are more private than men's lives if
they spend most time at home, out of view of others, so their substance use
may go undetected. Family and friends may not want to admit that an older
female family member has a substance-abuse problem and may try to mini-
mize or dismiss substance use as nonproblematic. White family members
may not consider addiction a possibility because it is not consistent with
their perceptions of older women (Beckman & Amaro, 1986).

    The messages women receive about their worth and the consequent
limitations placed on women's control over their environments may lead to
depression and anxiety. Women who use drugs are often diagnosed as de-

pressed (Anthony, Warner, & Kessler, 1994; Brady, Grice, Dustan, & Randall, 1993; McCrady, 1993; Scourfield, Stevens, & Merikangas, 1996). Women of color who use are more likely to be depressed than white women (McGrath et al., 1990). Alcohol use among African American adolescents appears to be associated with feelings of powerlessness, poor interpersonal skills, inadequate social skills, and unsatisfactory relationships with family members (Hare & Hare, 1986). It cannot be determined whether depression causes drinking and drug use or whether use causes depression. It is likely that both are true, especially among clinic populations. Girls and women are more likely than boys to feel guilt, depression, and other negative emotions (34%) after drinking (Lo & Globetti, 1998). Drugs may be used for the purpose of self-medication. Some women use marijuana for its pleasurable effects and alcohol for a feeling of relaxation and physical enhancement (Lo & Globetti, 1998), positive feelings, and affirmation (Preston, 1996). Other women use crack cocaine and crystal methamphetamine for the temporary feeling of euphoria, well-being, and comfort these substances provide (Baker, 2000) to compensate for low self-esteem and depression.

Alternatively, women may turn to food for comfort. The stigma attached to drug use may lead women to turn to food rather than to drugs as a means of relieving anxiety, numbing feelings, and deriving a sense of comfort. Disordered eating and problem drinking share some MMPI profile characteristics and may share predisposing factors (Dansky et al., 2000), such as a common biological pathway (Miller & Gold, 1993), a dysfunctional family (Holderness, Brooks-Gunn, & Warren, 1994), poor self-control (Ricciardelli, Williams, & Kiernan, 1998; Xinaris & Boland, 1990), and poor coping skills (Holderness et al., 1994; Ricciardelli et al., 1998). The choice of eating or drinking in response to depression is related to gender-role expectations. Women with high scores on femininity scales (Hawkins, Turell, & Jackson, 1983; Paxton & Sculthorpe, 1991; Ricciardelli et al., 1998; Ricciardelli, Williams, & Kiernan, 1999; van Strien & Bergers, 1988; Wichstrom, 1995) or low scores on masculinity scales (Johnston et al., 1995) were more likely to exhibit disordered eating, whereas women who scored high on alcohol-dependence measures also scored high on masculinity (Cantrell & Ellis, 1991; Ricciardelli et al., 1998, 1999; Silverstein, Carpman, Perlick, & Perdue, 1990). Women who scored high on both masculinity and femininity displayed greater problems with both eating and drinking. Finally, women with particularly horrific or chronic abuse histories may rely on multiple methods. A population-representative sample of women who exhibited symptoms of both bulimia and alcohol abuse were more likely to have been assaulted, increasing their stress level (Dansky et al., 2000). Higher scores on the masculinity scale suggest an expansion of women's behavioral repertoire into new roles that reject gender-role prescriptions. As women move into other areas they may also expect to receive equal advancement and pay, and therefore become more frustrated and angry, perhaps resulting in increased use of drugs and alcohol.

Negative Consequences of Men's Socialization for Women

The interaction between male socialization and alcohol and drug abuse leads to problematic behavior. Hypermasculinity has been associated with alcohol and drug abuse (Mosher & Sirkin, 1984). Men's drinking appears to be used as a way of proving their masculinity by showing stamina, non-conformity, and bravery (Wilsnack et al., 2000). Spence, Helmreich, and Holahan (1979) found that males with more stereotypically masculine traits had a high frequency of acting-out behaviors, such as drug and alcohol use, fights, misdemeanors, and problems in school. Traditional male socialization may teach that physical violence is a legitimate way to resolve everyday conflicts and get others to comply with ones wishes.

The Male Gateway to Alcohol and Drug Use

It is typically through boys that adolescent girls are introduced to alcohol and drugs. Because male socialization pushes adolescent boys to experiment, be tough, and take risks, boys move in more dangerous circles and have more opportunities to acquire and use drugs. Boys and men may act as intermediaries, "agents of contagion," or gatekeepers regarding drug access (Van Etten et al., 1999a, 1999b; Warner et al., 1999). In adulthood, men typically control access to illicit drugs, which limits women's access to this activity. Heterosexual women who use heroin and other illicit drugs are more likely than men to have tried heroin at the urging of a sex partner addict, whereas men are more likely to try heroin due to pressure from other men (Anglin, Kao, Harlo, Peters, & Booth, 1987). Once an addiction is established, women typically buy drugs from men or barter in another way, for instance, by exchanging sexual favors for drugs, opening the door for their further exploitation.

Even professional men may serve as the gateway to drug use. In the United States, women's concerns are often trivialized and discounted. Women who do not conform to traditional stereotypes and gender roles (e.g., mother, wife, sex object, child) may be considered maladjusted or disturbed. The medical profession is known for its tendency to try to solve problems with pills and may treat "problematic" women with pills as well. Male physicians are more likely to prescribe medication for women than for men (Ashton, 1991; Randolph & Yates, 1993; Verbrugge, 1984; Verbrugge & Steiner, 1985) and for the elderly than for other age groups (Balestrieri, Bortolomasi, Galletta, & Bellantuono, 1997). Physicians may prescribe medications for women upset by events in their lives rather than helping them to find other supports. They are especially likely to prescribe anxiotics and antidepressants (Hohmann, 1989). These differences persist even when the nature and frequency of symptoms are controlled. Abuse of prescription medications by women may appear to be legitimate use and go undetected (Traub, 1983). Physicians may also dismiss legitimate physical problems as psychologically based. In doing so, they prevent the problem from being treated and increase the chance that women may need to find their own means of treatment, including pain reduction. Some women with addictions avoid medical care altogether because of negative past experiences with health professionals (Copeland, 1997).

Public education regarding violence and oppression should be mandated to increase the awareness of the damage done to all as a result of the undersocialization of boys. Current male undersocialization renders boys and men more vulnerable to externalizing (acting-out) and personality disorders, drug and alcohol problems, and poorer academic performance. These problems make it more likely that boys will drop out of high school. Boys and men are also more likely to engage in violent crimes, have legal problems, and be incarcerated. The same undersocialization that results in these behaviors renders them less empathic toward others and more likely to oppress, exploit, and abuse girls and women. If drug and alcohol use as well as coercive behaviors are effectively discouraged among boys and men, then drug and alcohol use will most likely be reduced for all.

If it is closer supervision and keeping girls closer to home that protects them from problems, boys should also be supervised more closely and stricter limits should be set on their behavior. Public pressure and media images should be planned to discourage alcohol and substance use and to reduce the glamorization and "macho" connotations of alcohol and drug use for males. Prosocial behavior should be rewarded and antisocial behavior should be dealt with quickly, firmly, and consistently. Better socialization of boys should include more emphasis on connection, responsibility to the community, and the importance of consulting others when one is having trouble. It should include consciousness-raising regarding the difference between stereotypes of women and reality, including the value and legitimacy of women's perspectives. It should emphasize the virtue of using problem solving rather than physical force and help boys and men employ strategies to resist peer pressure. Efforts to ensure girls' and women's safety until things change through such things as self-defense training will be required.

CULTURAL PERMISSION FOR VIOLENCE AGAINST WOMEN

Violence toward women is a global problem and can lead to and perpetuate alcohol and drug use through the coercion of use and through traumatization. Violence is not caused solely by an individual's pathology; people will abuse others verbally, physically, or sexually when it is tolerated (Amaro, 1995). Women's subordinate status is built into their socialization, as is the idea that it is normal for males to be sexually aggressive (Beneke, 1982; Sanday, 1981). The underlying belief is that women are merely sex objects and possessions rather than equals. Violence against women is exacerbated by men's sexual jealousy and the financial dependency and social isolation of women. In fact, the greater the economic dependence of a woman on a man, the more likely she is to be a victim of rape by him because he feels entitled to sex. The greater the inequity and disorganization within a culture, the higher the rate of domestic violence (Straus, 1994). The situation is exacerbated with drug use.

High rape prevalence has been linked to male dominance in cross-cultural studies. Rape is most common in cultures where a male deity is worshipped, where warfare is celebrated, where sexes are segregated, where women's roles are limited and women hold little or no political or economic power, and where childcare is devalued (Herman, 1990). Sexual assault may preserve the system of male dominance through terror. All men benefit, whether or not they personally commit the assault (Brownmiller, 1975; Groth, 1979; Herman, 1990). Rape-supportive attitudes and beliefs are widely held in the United States (Herman, 1990). Herman (1990) points out that whereas in the case of male pedophiles who victimize boys there is usually a history of the perpetrator having been victimized himself, in the case of male sexual assaults on girls and women normal male socialization is enough. Furthermore, sexual assault of women is rewarding for males. It asserts power, intimidates, and results in pleasure for the perpetrator (Herman, 1990). Alcohol can contribute to the reduction of the inhibition of the desire to rape.

Partner Violence

The problem of partner violence is especially severe for women addicts. Partner violence in a diverse sample of Latina, African American, and European American women included physical abuse and rape (which puts women at risk for HIV), in addition to threats and verbal abuse (El-Bassel, Gilbert, Rajah, Foleno, & Frye, 2000). Drug use heightens conflicts, leading to a greater likelihood of violence, including rape. Lifetime prevalence rates of partner violence reported by women in substance-abuse programs ranges from 60–75% (Bennet & Larson, 1994; El-Bassel et al., 2000). This is at least double the prevalence rate for the general population of women (Browne, 1993). Conversely, many victims of domestic violence are women with substance-use problems. Watson and colleagues (1997) found that 21% of victims of domestic violence in their predominantly white sample of people seeking help with the abuse from programs or psychologists met criteria for alcohol use or dependence.

If women seek treatment against their male partners' wishes, they will encounter resistance from their partners (Beckman & Amaro, 1986; Higgins, Budney, Bickel, & Badger, 1994; McCollum & Trepper, 1995), who are often also substance users (Riehman, Hser, & Zeller, 2000). The resistance may take the form of criticism (Fraser, 1997; McCollum & Trepper, 1995), sexual or physical intimidation, or violence (Amaro & Hardy-Fanta, 1995; Fraser, 1997). The risk of violent retaliation for seeking treatment against partners' wishes is such that women seeking help at treatment facilities should be routinely screened for partner violence. A network of safe housing facilities and other protections from violence should be developed as part of a "safety plan" for women clients. Despite the fact that about 60% of women in a drug treatment center are victims of domestic violence, and about 42% of women in domestic violence programs are drug users, few clinics currently offer women protection from abuse (Bennett & Lawson, 1994). There are even fewer programs designed specifically for lesbians and related lesbian partner abuse.

Heterosexual white (52%), Native Canadian (25%), and black (15%) women receiving methadone treatment reported being raped, sometimes for their partner's needs and at other times simply to humiliate them (Erickson et al., 2000). The myth that drugs such as crack are supposed to enhance women's sex drive and interest raises men's expectations of sex. Cocaine may heighten men's interest in sex while it diminishes men's ability to perform and women's interest in sex, leading to arguments and violence. Men may blame performance problems caused by the drug on the woman instead, and abuse her in response (Erickson et al., 2000). Women who use heroin rely on male drug dealers or partners during use, and are vulnerable to exploitation by them (Marsh, 1982). Men may intentionally administer drugs to women to make them pass out. Women reported that partners and others would try to rape them by having sex with them when the men thought they were high, asleep, or unconscious (El-Bassel et al., 2000). This practice is not confined to men who take illicit drugs. It is also a problem on college campuses and in drinking establishments across the United States (Bohmer & Parrot, 1993).

HIV Risk

Female heroin users face the possibility of contracting HIV from needle sharing, physical and sexual abuse, and prostitution (Rosenbaum, 1981). Heterosexual women addicts are likely to have partners who are addicts and at high risk. These women are often advised to use condoms when having sex. Alcohol and drug use can affect women's judgment, ability, and motivation to use condoms as well as lead to risky behavior during blackouts. Fear of violence, however, is also a major determinant of women's decisions to insist on condom use. Although 87% of non-drug-using Puerto Rican women discussed condom use with their partners and 74% discussed HIV testing with them (Deren, Shedlin, & Beardsley, 2000), some heterosexual women receiving methadone did not ask their partners to use condoms because they feared violent behavior (El-Bassel et al., 2000). Women reported being badly beaten for slipping in a female condom. Partners would become angry and violent when asked to use a condom because they associated condoms with sex workers, distrust, and infidelity. It was also experienced as an attempt to control the partner's behavior, which challenged both his power and his gender role. Violence would be used to regain power. In many cases the priority for these women is immediate survival rather than long-term health, including HIV risk (El-Bassel et al., 2000; Falkin & Strauss, 2000).

The Sex Trade

For many women receiving treatment at methadone clinics and addicted to crack, drug use and economic necessity lead to participation in the sex trade market (El-Bassel et al., 2000; Gilcrest et al., 2001), which increases women's vulnerability to violence, poverty, arrest, and loss of family (Erickson et al., 2000). Because of crack's powerful effects, and the lack of pleasurable substitutes, few women were interested in quitting. For some, crack became the focal point of their lives, often instigating and perpetuating a dangerous lifestyle. Crack use increased women's exposure to violence and sexual abuse: beatings, rapes, knifings, shootings, and murders.

With the introduction of crack cocaine, more women entered the sex trade market, prices for sex service dropped, and violence escalated. Women were turning tricks for as little as $5–10, just enough for another "rock" of crack (Erickson et al., 2000), which meant women had to expose themselves to even more risk to support themselves. Participation in the sex trade may also result in jealous reactions by partners, even in cases where the partner had encouraged the woman to enter the sex trade to enhance his own income (El-Bassel et al., 2000). Women who are sexually active with more than one male weaken the control any one male has over them (Warner et al., 1999). Jealousy and fear of losing control of a woman may result in violence (Browning & Dutton, 1986; El-Bassel et al., 2000). Violence may be used to reinstate the man's power in the relationship.

Women often reported that they would stop hooking if they did not have to support their habit, although some said they would still need the money for necessities (Gilcrest et al., 2001). Perhaps this reality needs to be acknowledged and policies developed that are aimed at encouraging safe use. Some have suggested that if drugs were provided free or prices were reduced, women would cease their involvement in the sex trade and be less frequent victims of violence. However, since few non-drug-using men are interested in relationships with ex-addicts, most heterosexual women would continue to be involved with drug-using men. Heterosexual women addicts reported that drug use made partners unpredictable, irrational, and paranoid (El-Bassel et al., 2000). The greater availability of drugs might cause their partners to be intoxicated more often and to be more violent as a result.

Cycle of Trauma

Physical abuse, sexual abuse, and other forms of victimization used in an effort to control women's behavior play a significant role in the development of posttraumatic stress disorder (PTSD) and the perpetuation of substance-use disorders (American Psychiatric Association, 2000; Bollerud, 1990; Rohsenow, Corbett, & Devine, 1990). Women substance users are more likely to be victims of sexual assault than men users (Grice, Brady, Dustan, Malcolm, & Kilpatrick, 1995; Taubman, 1986) and often report that they use drugs to numb the pain resulting from neglect, trauma, self-hate, and anger, as well as physical and sexual abuse perpetrated by intimate, substance-using partners (Erickson et al., 2000; Woodhouse, 1990). First Nation women may use substances to anesthetize their feelings of powerlessness, pain, and emptiness resulting from oppression and abuse (Herbert & McCannell, 1997). Women may use illicit drugs to cope with trauma, to dull the pain of anticipated abuse, or to escape during partner rape (Copeland, 1997; El-Bassel et al., 2000; Falkin & Strauss, 2000). They continue to use it because it makes them feel normal, high, good, happy, relaxed, or numb (Erickson et al., 2000).

The lack of awareness of abused women's experiences and needs in the recovery movement contributes to their vulnerability and addiction. Fear of more abuse keeps women quiet and compliant. Women who have experienced the above may turn to substances in an attempt to modulate their symptoms of hypervigilance, emotional reactivity, and physiological reactivity (de Loos, 1990; Grice et al., 1995; van der Kolk & Greenberg, 1990). Unfortunately, although alcohol and drugs offer temporary symptom relief, they may make recovery and the transition to learning to cope without using alcohol and drugs more difficult. Self-medicating the consequences of trauma may both interfere with the processing of the trauma and exacerbate PTSD symptoms (Grice et al., 1995). Substance use also increases the likelihood of future victimization and traumatization (Cottler, Compton, Mager, & Spitznagel, 1992; Dansky, Brewerton, & Kilpatrick, 2000; Resnick, Kilpatrick, Dansky, & Saunders, 1993). For instance, cocaine users had significantly higher rates of sexual and physical assault than those using alcohol, perhaps because of the contacts required to obtain the drug (Grice et al., 1995).

CULTURAL DEVALUATION OF WOMEN AND ITS CONSEQUENCES

Both men and women are socialized to devalue women's work and worth. The resulting differences in financial resources gives men more power in both the private and the public sectors. This gives most men the upper hand financially in addition to physically, so women may hesitate to challenge them about poor treatment and exploitation. Heterosexual women reported being dominated by men and depending on men for money, drugs, and sex (Woodhouse, 1990). In addition to fearing retaliation, economically challenged women may lack independent access to transportation, childcare, or health benefits, putting them at the mercy of their male partners and other men. Their lack of financial resources can be a barrier to re-

covery (Copeland, 1997; Rathbone-McCuan et al., 1991). Women are freer
to move forward when they are more financially independent and not opposed by their partners. More problem recognition and motivation were
present when women provided at least half of their own financial support.
This suggests that helping women to achieve greater financial independence may help their recovery.

Given that women's access to economic resources is already limited,
women are especially hesitant to take days or other time off from work for
treatment (Copeland, 1997). Although some companies offer employee assistance plans, women worry that company awareness of the problem may
jeopardize their employment. Women who do not work outside of the
home or who work at companies with poor benefits may not be able to afford treatment (Blume, 1994). Thus, there may be considerable reluctance
to both admit there is a problem and to seek treatment (Thom, 1986).

Offering women ways to stabilize their employment status and related
incomes, such as providing educational opportunities, is important to the
maintenance of sobriety (Kelly et al., 1995) and predicts mental (Kessler,
1982) and other health statuses (Liberatos, Link, & Kelsey, 1988; Winkleby, Jatulis, Frank, & Fortmann, 1992), as well as protects against addiction (Curran et al., 1999). Involvement in aftercare plans, GED programs,
and vocational and educational programs are all associated with increased
length of sobriety (Kelly et al., 1995). Skills enhancement (assertiveness,
communication, cognitive coping, parent training, and problem solving)
would help to expand women's repertoire and options. Further development of specific life and work skills, including money management, job
interviewing, job success, accessing the legal system, and how to locate
resources, would be helpful. Timing and pacing are important, however, because many of these women may be struggling with feelings of being overwhelmed and unable to cope. It is therefore important not to contribute to
these feelings by taking on too many issues at one time (Copeland, 1997).

Social Support

Unsupportive family of origin, family violence (physical and sexual, often
related to parental alcoholism), often related to parental alcoholism and
substance abuse (Bassuk & Weinreb, 1993; Curran et al., 1999; Janlert &
Hammarstrom, 1992; Rutherford, 1992), and lack of community support
are all associated with adolescents' choices to use drugs and alcohol
(Hawkins et al., 1992). A family history of alcoholism is an especially
strong predictor among women with low incomes.

Women tend to receive less support from men than men do from women for entering treatment (Beckman & Amaro, 1986). Women are less likely to recover when they cohabitate with actively drug-using partners, who may not recognize their use as problematic (Riehman et al., 2000). Women are more likely to recognize and recover from addiction when their cohabitating partner is in treatment. It is difficult for women addicts to find partners who have never been addicts. Nonaddicted men are usually wary of becoming involved with a formerly addicted or addicted woman (Rosenbaum, 1981), so most women have partners who are current or former addicts. Even when both heterosexual partners are in treatment, it is difficult to get the woman to focus on her own treatment and recovery rather than on how to help her male partner to manage. If a male partner who had been in treatment left the program, his female partner would often do the same. Women, on the other hand, have little impact on male partners' drug and alcohol use (Leonard & Das Eiden, 1999). Addicted women do receive some support from other women, however. Crack-addicted women provide some constructive support for each other in the forms of social support (e.g., encouraging them to get drug treatment) and day-to-day support (helping them to get drugs and food, helping them to get to the doctor). Addicts' mothers may also provide love and support, but may be experienced as controlling (Falkin & Strauss, 2000).

"Electronic bars" (Correll, 1995) provide an additional source of support. These online meeting places have been created for a variety of purposes. They may provide many of the same things as a real bar, with the exception of eye-to-eye and physical contact. Electronic forums are "always open," although the number of participants at any one time may vary. Access is limited by financial considerations (one needs a computer, unless one can use a public-access computer), but these "bars" do provide a way for some geographically isolated, housebound, and other women who have difficulty meeting others to connect. Although absolute confidentiality is difficult to assure (as it is with AA groups), electronic bars may provide a meeting place that is not limited geographically. Electronic bars alone may not be enough for some because of the lack of actual, physical human contact, but for those with few other opportunities for community, those located in remote areas or areas without lesbian bars, bookstores, or community centers, or those reluctant to go public with their problems, electronic support forums may provide a sense of community not otherwise available (Correll, 1995). They are a place where identities can be developed, community and resources can be publicized, and recovery can happen.

SUMMARY

If lower levels of anxiety, stable relationships, financial stability, education, skills training, occupational security, health care, access to medical treatment, a violence-free environment, and community support are associated with positive addiction treatment outcomes (Gibbs & Flanagan, 1977), then perhaps they can prevent the onset of addiction. The expansion of social policies and programs such as family leave policies, worksite childcare, living wage, vocational training, access to health care, and freedom from violence, aggression, and oppression would create a healthier environment for all, which would contribute to the likelihood of a stable home life and supportive family of origin. Parent training can help addicts manage their children more effectively, thereby reducing addicts' stress levels and facilitating their recovery (Baker, 2000). The latter would provide a better environment for children that could offer more support, encourage education, and respond more effectively to their needs. A social environment that encourages and rewards children's adaptive coping skills such that children develop a good social problem-solving repertoire, as well as believe in their ability to cope and to problem solve, is protective against the initiation of substance use (Hawkins et al., 1992).

Perhaps the best tack to take is to provide such opportunities to all women, with special attention to those who, lacking them, are suffering from addiction at this point. In essence, the fewer women who are deprived of resources, the greater women's chances for healthy functioning and recovery. The use of mobile units to provide house calls, telephone counseling services, and even Internet counseling resources (accessed through public computers) could improve access. Information about community resources (Alcoholics Anonymous, Narcotics Anonymous, community support groups, community centers, grants for education, etc.) need to be publicized widely, perhaps including on a national website. Nonaddicted women also lead complicated lives. Such facilities could provide services that would benefit all women.

Education

A key part of change will require ending the oppression of women and the violence that enforces it. The traditional values, beliefs, behaviors, and systems that contribute to male oppression of and violence against women need to continue to be challenged. Issues of power and exploitation should be discussed openly and messages that adults communicate through their behavior monitored. We need early education and consciousness-raising about sociopolitical realities (oppression, discrimination, specific dynamics of racism, classicism, and sexism, impact and prevention of physical and sexual violence) (Herman, 1990). All children could benefit from accurate information about these issues. Children should be taught and encouraged to treat others with respect, and to respect others' privacy, opinions, and choices.

There also needs to be a public education campaign regarding the images of women addicts that stigmatize them in a way that harms them and their chances for recovery. More people need to be aware of the complexity of addiction and the wide diversity of addicts in terms of age, ethnicity, race, culture, class, religion, and other factors. The empowerment of women and the broadening of previously sex-typed behavioral repertoires are critical to the prevention and treatment of addiction.

Herman (1990) has suggested the circulation of "early warning signs" regarding boys and men who may be sexual predators. Although she made these recommendations over 10 years ago, they have yet to be widely distributed. We need to take immediate action when violations occur, so that the unacceptability of violence is unambiguous. Since perpetrators rarely have the internal motivation to change their behavior, in addition to education, punitive measures such as legal sanctions, radical behavior modification, pharmacological interventions, close supervision or incarceration, and other measures may be required (Herman, 1990). Studies have suggested that adolescence is a critical period in the development of sexually assaultive behavior (Groth, Longo, & McFadin, 1982). Immediate, consistent, and appropriate sanctions are required for first rape offenses, even those perpetrated by adolescents. A substitute behavior, support, and sources of hope and self-esteem are also required for rape abstinence, as with other addictions (Herman, 1990). Groups fostering misogynist views (teams, clubs, the military) should be targeted for intervention, since such attitudes are associated with sexual exploitation. We also need to understand how to block the male-to-female drug gateway so that women are not coerced into using drugs and alcohol. We need to better predict physical and sexual violence so that there can be early intervention to prevent the violence that leads to coerced alcohol and drug use, trauma, HIV infection, oppression of women, and prevention of recovery.

Topics for Further Study

Much early research was based on inaccurate stereotypes of women substance users (Woodhouse, 1990) or tended to focus on the effects of drinking and drug use on women's biological and traditional gender roles, such as mother and caretaker. For instance, research on women who use cocaine increased in the 1980s not out of concern for them, but out of concern for their children (Humphries, 1999; Murphy & Rosenbaum, 1999). Researchers rarely examine women's perceptions of and experiences with drugs and alcohol. Many research protocols have ignored women, or, at best, have underrepresented them (Garcia, 1997; McCrady & Raytek, 1993). Currently, the representation of women in self-treatment studies ranges from 6–50% (Copeland, 1997; Kropp, Menhal-Baugus, & Kelly, 1996), with most studies falling at the lower end of this range. The number of studies with diverse samples (in terms of ethnicity, class, or other specific characteristics) or samples of members of minority groups are even more rare. They are virtually nonexistent when the question being asked is at odds with contemporary stereotypes. There are no studies regarding the reasons that African American girls and women choose to abstain from drug or alcohol use or of factors predicting nonpathological use. Even when women are included in studies, bias is likely to influence the interpretation of the results. Connor, Williams, and Ricciardelli (1999) found that men drank more than women did, drank in more contexts, and that a principle component analysis of their responses to restraint measures resulted in two factors for men and one factor for women. They interpreted their results as meaning that because women were less experienced drinkers, they had never had the opportunity to learn to make more sophisticated, refined assessments of their cognitions about drinking. They stopped short of recommending that women should drink more so that they could achieve men's insights about drinking!

A more feminist approach to addiction would shift attention away from the search for internal deficits and look instead at the multiple environmental and cultural influences on addiction. Alcohol and drug problems are not the direct results of the pharmacological properties of substances and individual responses to them, but should be studied in the context of the users' social role, norms, and the situation in which they are used, with the well-being of women as a priority. A more feminist approach would focus efforts on creating a healthier environment as well as providing resources to undo the damage caused by unhealthy environments. Treatment would include undoing the internalized aspects of the original damaging negative environment (Rhodes & Johnson, 1997).

Recent studies have made some progress in understanding girls' and women's experiences regarding alcohol and drug use, but more studies are needed. Much can be learned about the impact of substances on women's lives from the treatment literature (Copeland, 1997; Woodhouse, 1990), including the small, qualitative studies cited in this chapter. It is from conversations with women in treatment programs that we can learn about specific problems associated with abuse and dependence for women. Therapists working in the field hear about women's struggles at firsthand and have been proactive in trying to uncover the reasons women leave treatment and how they recover from addiction on their own (Copeland, 1997).

If we consider women as the ultimate experts on themselves and their needs, then their requests should give us clues to the causes and prevention of problems, as well as lead us to ideas for larger scale, more representative studies. We need to revise assessment instruments to reflect women's experiences and behaviors resulting from alcohol. Instruments might include questions about guilt, embarrassment, shame, confidence, enlightenment, reputation, sexual activity, feeling closer to others, regrets about drinking, increased interpersonal tension, and negative mood. Such measures may also help women decide whether they have a problem with drugs and alcohol by developing criteria that are relevant to their own experiences.

Activism

Sobriety has the potential to sharpen women's thinking and allow them to have more of a political impact. The AA step that directs members to carry the feminist AA message to other addicts and to practice these principles in all our affairs could lead to empowerment by helping addicts like themselves. Underhill (1991) believes that recovery should involve admitting powerlessness regarding addiction while simultaneously embracing control of other aspects of life, resulting ultimately in empowerment and allowing them to "Take charge" (Fraser, 1997). Women need to focus on themselves: their identity, their health, their needs, and their own recovery. Women should be encouraged to find opportunities to take action and make a difference in contributing to changes that could contribute to a more women-friendly environment (Rhodes & Johnson, 1997). Empowerment would then replace powerlessness and provide opportunities for women to take control (Fraser, 1997).

REFERENCES

Amaro, H. (1995). Love, sex, and power: Considering women's realities in HIV prevention. *American Psychologist, 50,* 437–447.

Amaro, H., & Hardy-Fanta, C. (1995). Gender relations in addiction and recovery. *Journal of Psychoactive Drugs, 27,* 325–337.

American Psychiatric Association. (1987). *Diagnostic and statistical manual of mental disorders* (3rd ed.). Washington, DC: Author.

Anglin, M. D., Kao, C., Harlow, L. L., Peters, K., & Booth, M. W. (1987). Similarity of behavior within addict couples: I. Methodology and narcotics patterns. *International Journal of the Addictions, 22,* 497–524.

Anthony, J. C., Warner, L. A., & Kessler, R. C. (1994). Comparative epidemiology of dependence on tobacco, alcohol, controlled substances, and inhalants: Basic findings from the National Comorbidity Survey. *Experimental and Clinical Psychopharmacology, 2,* 244–268.

Ashton, H. (1991). Psychotropic-drug prescribing for women. *British Journal of Psychiatry, 158,* 30–35.

Baker, P. L. (2000). I didn't know: Discoveries and identity transformation of women addicts in treatment. *Journal of Drug Issues, 30,* 863–880.

Balestrieri, M., Bortolomasi, M., Galletta, M., & Bellantuono, C. (1997). Patterns of hypnotic drug prescription in Italy: A two-week community survey. *British Journal of Psychiatry, 170,* 176–180.

Bammer, G., & Weekes, S. (1994). Becoming an ex-user: Insights into the process and implications for treatment and policy. *Drug and Alcohol Review, 13,* 285–292.

Bassuk, E. L., & Weinreb, L. (1993). Homeless pregnant women: Two generations at risk. *American Journal of Orthopsychiatry, 63,* 348–357.

Beckman, L. J., & Amaro, H. (1986). Personal and social difficulties faced by women and men entering alcoholism treatment. *Journal of Studies on Alcohol, 47,* 135–145.

Beneke, T. (1982). *Men on rape: What they have to say about sexual violence.* New York: St. Martin's Press.

Bennett, L., & Larson, M. (1994). Barriers to cooperation between domestic violence and substance abuse programs. *Families in Society, 75,* 277–286.

Blume, S. B. (1994). Gender differences in alcohol-related disorders. *Harvard Review of Psychiatry, 2,* 7–13.

Bohmer, C., & Parrot, A. (1993). *Sexual assault on campus: The problem and the solution.* New York: Lexington Books.

Bollerud, K. (1990). A model for the treatment of trauma-related syndromes among chemically dependent inpatient women. *Journal of Substance Abuse Treatment, 5,* 83–87.

Bongars, I. M. B., Van De Goor, L. A. M., Van Oers, J. A. M., & Garretsen, H. F. L. (1998). Gender differences in alcohol-related problems: Controlling for drinking behaviour. *Addiction, 93,* 411–421.

Brady, K. T., Grice, D. E., Dustan, L., & Randall, C. (1993). Gender differences in substance use disorders. *American Journal of Psychiatry, 150,* 1707–1711.

Browne, A. (1993). Violence against women by male partners: Prevalence, outcomes, and policy implications. *American Psychologist, 48,* 1077–1087.

Browning, J., & Dutton, D. (1986). Assessment of wife assault with the Conflict Tactics Scale: Using couple data to quantify the differential reporting effect. *Journal of Marriage and the Family, 48,* 375–379.

Brownmiller, S. (1975). *Against our will: Men, women, and rape.* New York: Simon & Schuster.

Cantrell, P. J., & Ellis, J. B. (1991). Gender role and risk patterns for eating disorders in men and women. *Journal of Clinical Psychology, 47,* 53–57.

Caudill, B. D. G., Wilson, T., & Abrams, D. B. (1987). Alcohol and self-disclosure: Analyses of interpersonal behavior in male and female social drinkers. *Journal of Studies on Alcohol, 48,* 401–409.

Clayton, R. R., Voss, H. L., Robbins, C., & Skinner, W. F. (1986). Gender differences in drug use: An epidemiological perspective. In B. A. Ray & M. C. Braude (Eds.), *Women and drugs: A new era for research (National Institute for Drug Abuse Research Monograph 65,* pp. 80–99). Rockville, MD: Department of Health and Human Services, National Institute on Drug Abuse.

Connor, J. P., Williams, R. J., & Ricciardelli, L. A. (1999). Gender differences in drinking restraint. *Journal of Studies on Alcohol, 60,* 643–646.

Corcoran, K. J., & Michels, J. L. (1999). Interpersonal perception and alcohol expectancies predict beverage selection in opposite sex dyadic interactions. *Journal of Child and Adolescent Substance Abuse, 9,* 29–38.

Copeland, J. (1997). A qualitative study of barriers to formal treatment among women who self-managed change in addictive behaviours. *Journal of Substance Abuse Treatment, 14,* 183–190.

Copeland, J., & Hall, W. (1992). A comparison of women seeking drug and alcohol treatment in a specialist women's and two traditional mixed-sex services. *British Journal of Addiction, 87,* 883–890.

Correll, S. (1995). The ethnography of an electronic bar: The lesbian cafe. *Journal of Contemporary Ethnography, 24,* 270–298.

Cottler, L. B., Compton, W. M., Mager, D., & Spitznagel, E. (1992) Post-traumatic stress disorder among substance users from the general population. *American Journal of Psychiatry, 149,* 664–667.

Curran, G. M., Stoltenberg, S. F., Hill, E. M., Mudd, S. A., Blow, F. C., & Zucker, R. A. (1999). Gender differences in the relationship among SES, family history of alcohol disorders and alcohol dependence. *Journal of Studies on Alcohol, 60,* 825–832.

Dansky, B. S., Brewerton, T. D., & Kilpatrick, D. G. (2000). Comorbidity of bulimia nervosa and alcohol use disorders: Results from the National Women's Study. *International Journal of Eating Disorders, 27,* 180–190.

de Loos, W. S. (1990). Psychosomatic manifestations of post-traumatic stress disorder. In M. E. Wolf & A. D. Mosniam (Eds.), *Post-traumatic stress disorder: Etiology, phenomenology, and treatment* (pp. 94–105). Washington, DC: American Psychiatric Press.

Deren, S., Shedlin, M., & Beardsley, M. (2000). *The therapeutic community: Theory, model, and method.* New York: Springer.

Desimone, A., Murray, P., & Lester, D. (1994). Alcohol use, self-esteem, depression, and suicidality in high school students. *Adolescence, 29,* 939–942.

El-Bassel, N., Gilbert, L., Rajah, V., Foleno, A., & Frye, V. (2000). Fear and violence: Raising the HIV stakes. *AIDS Education and Prevention, 12,* 154–170.

Erickson, P. G., Butters, J., McGillicuddy, P., & Hallgren, A. (2000). Crack and prostitution: Gender, myths, and experiences. *Journal of Drug Issues, 30,* 767–788.

Ettorre, E. (1994). Women and drug abuse with special attention to Finland. *Women's Studies International Forum, 17,* 83–94.

Falkin, G. P., & Strauss, S. M. (2000). Drug-using women's communication with social supporters about HIV/AIDS issues. *Journal of Drug Issues, 30,* 801–822.

Fillmore, K. M. (1984). "When angels fall": Women's drinking as cultural preoccupation and as reality. In S. C. Wilsnack & L. J. Beckman (Eds.), *Alcohol problems in women: Antecedents, consequences, and intervention* (pp. 7–36). New York: Guilford Press.

Fillmore, K. M. (1987). Women's drinking across the adult life course as compared to men's. *British Journal of Addiction, 82,* 801–811.

Forth-Finegan, J. L. (1991). Sugar and spice and everything nice: Gender socialization and women's addiction—A literature review. In C. Bepko (Ed.), *Feminism and addiction* (pp. 19–48). New York: Haworth Press.

Fraser, J. (1997). Methadone clinic culture: The everyday realities of female methadone clients. *Qualitative Health Research, 7,* 121–139.

Frezza, M., Di Padova, C., Pozzato, G., Terpin, M., Baraona, E., & Lieber, C. S. (1990). High blood alcohol levels in women: The role of decreased gastric alcohol dehydrogenase activity and first-pass metabolism. *New England Journal of Medicine, 322,* 95–99.

Garcia, S. (1997). Ethical and legal issues associated with substance abuse by pregnant and parenting women. *Journal of Psychoactive Drugs, 29,* 101–111.

Gibbs, L., & Flanagan, J. (1977). Prognostic indicators of alcoholism treatment outcome. *International Journal of the Addictions, 12,* 1097–1141.

Gilcrest, G., Taylor, A., Goldberg, D., Mackie, C., Denovan, A., & Green, S. T. (2001). Behavioural and lifestyle study of women using a drop-in center for female street sex workers in Glasgow, Scotland: A 10 year comparative study. *Addiction Research and Theory, 9,* 43–58.

Gomberg, E. S. L. (1982). Historical and political perspective: Women and drug use. *Journal of Social Issues, 38,* 9–23.

Gomberg, E. S. L. (1993). Women and alcohol: Use and abuse. *Journal of Substance Abuse, 3,* 211–219.

Grice, D. E., Brady, K. T., Dustan, L. R., Malcolm, R., & Kirkpatrick, D. G. (1995). Sexual and physical assault history and posttraumatic stress disorder in substance dependent individuals. *American Journal on Addictions, 4,* 297–305.

Groth, A. N. (1979). *Men who rape: The psychology of the offender.* New York: Plenum Press.

Groth, A. N., Longo, R. E., & McFadin, J. D. (1982). Undetected recidivism among rapists and child molesters. *Crime and Delinquency, 28,* 102–106.

Haaken, J. (1993). From Al-Anon to ACOA: Codependence and the reconstruction of caregiving. *Signs: Journal of Women in Culture and Society, 18,* 321–345.

Hall, J. M. (1990). Alcoholism recovery in lesbian women: A theory in development. *Scholarly Inquiry for Nursing Practice: An International Journal, 4,* 109–122.

Hall, J. M. (1991). Recovery in Alcoholics Anonymous: Three nursing theory perspectives. *Perspectives on Addictions Nursing, 2,* 3–6.

Hall, J. M. (1993). What really worked?: A case analysis and discussion of confrontational intervention for substance abuse in marginalized women. *Archives of Psychiatric Nursing, 7,* 322–327.

Hall, J. M. (1994). How lesbians recognize and respond to alcohol problems: A theoretical model of problematization. *Advances in Nursing Science, 16,* 46–63.

Hall, J. M. (1996). Lesbians' participation in Alcoholic Anonymous: Experiences of social, personal, and political tensions. *Contemporary Drug Problems, 23,* 113–138.

Hare, N., & Hare, J. (1986). *The endangered black family: Coping with the unisexualization and coming extinction of the black race.* San Francisco: Black Think Tank.

Hawkins, J. D., Catalano, R. F., & Miller, J. Y. (1992). Risk and protective factors for alcohol and other drug problems in adolescence and early adulthood: Implications for substance abuse prevention. *Psychological Bulletin, 112,* 64–105.

Hawkins, R., Turell, S., & Jackson, L. (1983). Desirable and undesirable masculine and feminine traits in relation to students' dieting tendencies and body image dissatisfaction. *Sex Roles, 9,* 705–718.

Herbert, E., & McCannell, K. (1997). Talking back: Six First Nations women's stories of recovery from childhood sexual abuse and addictions. *Canadian Journal of Community Mental Health, 16,* 51–68.

Herman, J. L. (1990). Sex offenders: A feminist perspective. In W. L. Marshall, D. R. Laws, & H. E. Barbaree (Eds.), *Handbook of sexual assault: Issues, theories, and treatment of the offenders* (pp. 177–193). New York: Plenum Press.

Higgins, S. T., Budney, A. J., Bickel, W. K., & Badger, G. J. (1994). Participation of significant others in outpatient behavioral treatment predicts greater cocaine abstinence. *American Journal of Drug and Alcohol Abuse, 20,* 47–56.

Holderness, C. C., Brooks-Gunn, J., & Warren, M. P. (1994). Co-morbidity of eating disorders and substance abuse: Review of the literature. *International Journal of Eating Disorders, 16,* 1–34.

Hohmann, A. A. (1989). Gender bias in psychotropic drug prescribing in primary care. *Medical Care, 27,* 478–490.

hooks, b. (1993). *Sisters of the yam: Black women and self-recovery.* Boston: South End Press.

Hughes, T. L., Day, E., Marcantonio, R. J., & Torpy, E. (1997). Gender differences in alcohol and drug use among young adults. *Substance Use and Misuse, 32,* 317–342.

Humphries, D. (1999). *1999 crack mothers: Pregnancy, drugs, and the media.* Columbus: Ohio State University.

Janlert, U., & Hammarstrom, A. (1992) Alcohol consumption among unemployed youths: Results from a prospective study. *British Journal of Addiction, 87,* 703–714.

Jellinek, E. M. (1960). *The disease concept of alcoholism.* New Haven, CT: Yale University Press.

Johnston, L. D., O'Malley, P. M., & Bachman, J. G. (1995). *National survey results on drug use from the Monitoring the Future Study, 1975–1994* (Vol. I). Rockville, MD: National Institute on Drug Abuse.

Jones, B. M., & Jones, M. K. (1976). Male and female intoxication levels for three alcohol doses, or do women really get higher than men? *Alcohol Technical Report, 5,* 11–14.

Kelly, V. A., Kropp, F. B., & Menhal-Baugus, M. (1995). The association of program-related variables to length of sobriety: A pilot study of prognostic indicators of successful treatment for chemically dependent women. *Journal of the Addictions and Offender Counseling, 15,* 42–50.

Kennedy, E. L., & Davis, M. D. (1993). *Boots of leather, slippers of gold: The history of a lesbian community.* New York: Routledge.

Kessler, R. C. (1982). A disaggregation of the relationship between socioeconomic status and psychological distress. *American Sociological Review, 47,* 752–764.

Kropp, F. B., Menhal-Baugus, M., & Kelly, V. A. (1996). The association of personal-related variables to length of sobriety: A pilot study of chemically dependent women. *Journal of the Addictions and Offender Counseling, 17,* 21–34.

Lacerte, J., & Harris, D. L. (1986). Alcoholism: A catalyst for women to organize. *Affilia: Journal of Women in Social Work, 1,* 41–52.

Lender, M. E. (1986). A special stigma: Women and alcoholism in the late 19th and 20th centuries. In D. L. Stug, S. Piryadarsini, & M. M. Hyman (Eds.), *Alcohol interventions: Historical and sociocultural approaches* (pp. 41–58). New York: Haworth Press.

Leonard, K. E., & Das Eiden, R. (1999). Husband's and wife's drinking: Unilateral or bilateral influences among newlyweds in a general population sample. *Journal of Studies on Alcohol, 60,* 130–138.

Liberatos, P., Link, B. G., & Kelsey, J. L. (1988). The measurement of social class in epidemiology. *Epidemiology Review, 10,* 87–121.

Lo, C. C. (1996). Are women heavier drinkers than we thought they were? *Journal of Studies on Alcohol, 57,* 531–535.

Lo, C. C., & Globetti, G. (1998). Gender differences in the consequences of alcohol use among adolescents. *Sociology of Crime, Law, and Deviance, 1,* 263–276.

Lohrenz, L., Connelly, J., Coyne, L., & Spare, K. (1978). Alcohol problems in several midwestern homosexual communities. *Journal of Studies on Alcohol, 39,* 1959–1963.

Marsh, J. (1982). Public issues and private problems: Women and drug use. *Journal of Social Issues, 38,* 153–165.

McCollum, E. E., & Trepper, T. S. (1995). "Little by little, pulling me through"— Women's perceptions of successful drug treatment: A qualitative inquiry. *Journal of Family Psychotherapy, 6,* 63–82.

McCrady, B. S. (1993). Alcoholism. In D. H. Barlow (Ed.), *Clinical handbook of psychological disorders: A step-by-step treatment manual* (pp. 362–395). New York: Guilford Press.

McCrady, B. S., & Raytek, H. (1993). Women and substance abuse: Treatment modalities and outcomes. In E. S. L. Gomberg & T. D. Nirenberg (Eds.), *Women and substance abuse* (pp. 314–338). Norwood, NJ: Ablex.

McDonald, M. (1994). Introduction: A socioanthropological view of gender, drink and drugs. In M. McDonald (Ed.), *Gender, drink, and drugs* (pp. 1–31). Providence, RI: Berg.

McGrath, E., Keita, G., Strickland, B., & Russo, N. (1990). *Women and depression: Risk factors and treatment issues.* Washington, DC: American Psychological Association.

McLeod, J. D. (1995). Social and psychological bases of homogamy for common psychiatric disorders. *Journal of Marriage and Family, 57,* 201–214.

Mercer, P. W., & Khavari, K. A. (1990). Are women drinking more like men?: An empirical examination of the convergence hypothesis. *Alcoholism: Clinical and Experimental Research, 14,* 461–466.

Miller, N. S., & Gold, M. S. (1993). A hypothesis for a common neurochemical basis for alcohol and drug disorders. *Psychiatric Clinics of North America, 16,* 105–117.

Mooney, D. K., & Gilbert, B. O. (1999). Predicting alcohol consumption: The influences of perceived opposite-sex peer expectancies and drinking behavior. *Journal of Child and Adolescent Substance Abuse, 9,* 73–84.

Moore, N. P., & Lewis, G. R. (1989). Substance abuse and the physician. In G. W. Lawson & A. W. Lawson (Eds.), *Alcoholism and substance abuse in special populations* (pp. 131–137). Rockville, MD: Aspen.

Mosher, D. L., & Sirkin, M. (1984). Measuring a macho personality constellation. *Journal of Research in Personality, 18*, 150–163.

Murphy, S., & Rosenbaum, M. (1999). *1999 women in recovery: Combating stereotypes and stigma.* New Brunswick, NJ: Rutgers University Press.

Nelson, C. B., & Wittchen, H. (1998). DSM-IV alcohol disorders in a general population sample of adolescents and young adults. *Addiction, 93*, 1065–1077.

Nicoloff, L. K., & Stiglitz, E. A. (1987). Lesbian alcoholism: Etiology, treatment, and recovery. In Boston Lesbian Psychologies Collective (Eds.), *Lesbian psychologies: Explorations and challenges* (pp. 283–293). Urbana: University of Illinois Press.

Nystrom, M. (1992). Positive and negative consequences of alcohol drinking among young university students in Finland. *British Journal of Addiction, 87*, 715–722.

O'Connor, P. G., Horwitz, R. I., Gottlieb, L. D., Kraus, M. L., & Segal, S. R. (1993). The impact of gender on clinical characteristics and outcomes in alcohol withdrawal. *Journal of Substance Abuse Treatment, 10*, 59–61.

O'Malley, P. M., Johnston, L. D., & Bachman, J. G. (1995). Adolescent substance abuse: Epidemiology and implications for public policy. *Pediatric Clinics of North America, 42*, 241–260.

Paxton, S. J., & Sculthorpe, A. (1991). Disordered eating and sex role characteristics in young women: Implications for sociocultural theories of disturbed eating. *Sex Roles, 24*, 587–598.

Preston, L. (1996). Women and alcohol: Defining the problem and seeking help. *International Journal of Sociology and Social Policy, 16*, 52–72.

Randolph, M. J., & Yates, W. R. (1993). Antisocial personality in alcohol and drug dependent individuals. *The American Journal on Addictions, 2*, 9–17.

Rathbone-McCuan, E., Dyer, L., & Wartman, J. (1991). Double jeopardy: Chemical dependence and codependence in older women. In N. Van Den Bergh (Ed.), *Feminist perspectives on addictions* (pp. 101–113). New York: Springer.

Resnick, H. S., Kilpatrick, D. G., Dansky, B. S., & Saunders, B. E. (1993). Prevalence of civilian trauma and posttraumatic stress disorder in a representative national sample of women. *Journal of Consulting and Clinical Psychology, 61*, 984–991.

Rhodes, R., & Johnson, A. (1997). A feminist approach to treating alcohol and drug-addicted African-American women. *Women and Therapy, 20*, 23–37.

Ricciardelli, L. A., Williams, R. J., & Kierman, M. J. (1998). Relation of drinking and eating to masculinity and femininity. *Journal of Social Psychology, 138*, 744–752.

Ricciardelli, L. A., Williams, R. J., & Kiernan, M. J. (1999). Bulimic symptoms in adolescent girls and boys. *International Journal of Eating Disorders, 26*, 217–221.

Riehman, K. S., Hser, Y., & Zeller, M. (2000). Gender differences in how intimate partners influence drug treatment motivation. *Journal of Drug Issues, 30*, 823–838.

Rienzi, B. M., McMillin, J. D., Dickson, C. L., Crauthers, D., McNeill, K. F., Pesina, M. D., & Mann, E. (1996). Gender differences regarding peer influence and attitude toward substance abuse. *Journal of Drug Education, 26*, 339–347.

Robbins, C. A., & Martin, S. S. (1993). Gender, styles of deviance, and drinking problems. *Journal of Health and Social Behavior, 34*, 302–321.

Roberts, A., Jackson, M. S., & Carlton-Laney, I. (2000). Revisiting the need for feminism and Afrocentric theory when treating African-American female substance abusers. *Journal of Drug Issues, 30,* 901–918.

Rodney, H. E., Mupier, R., & Crafter, B. (1998). Predictors of alcohol drinking among African American adolescents: Implications for violence prevention. *Journal of Negro Education, 65,* 434–444.

Rohsenow, D. J., Corbett, R., & Devine, D. (1990). Molested as children: A hidden contribution to substance abuse? *Journal of Substance Abuse Treatment, 7,* 13–18.

Rosenbaum, M. (1981). *Women on heroin.* New Brunswick, NJ: Rutgers University Press.

Rutherford, S. (1992). Reproductive freedom and African-American women. *Yale Journal of Law and Feminism, 4,* 225.

Sanday, P. R. (1981). *Female power and male dominance: On the origins of sexual inequality.* New York: Cambridge University Press.

Sandmaier, M. (1992). *The invisible alcoholics: Women and alcohol* (2nd ed.). Blue Ridge Summit, PA: TAB Books.

Schilit, C. L., Clark, W. M., & Shallenberger, E. A. (1988). Social supports and lesbian alcoholics. *Affilia, 3,* 27–40.

Scourfield, J., Stevens, D. E., & Merikangas, K. R. (1996). Substance abuse, comorbidity, and sensation seeking: Gender differences. *Comprehensive Psychiatry, 37,* 384–392.

Silverstein, B., Carpman, S., Perlick, D., & Perdue, L. (1990). Nontraditional sex role aspirations, gender identity conflict, and disordered eating among college women. *Sex Roles, 23,* 687–695.

Spence, J. T., Helmreich, R. L., & Holahan, C. K. (1979). Negative and positive components of psychological masculinity and their relationships to self-reports of neurotic and acting-out behaviors. *Journal of Personality and Social Psychology, 37,* 1673–1682.

Straus, M. A. (1994, Spring). State-to-state differences in social inequality and social bonds in relation to assaults on wives in the United States [Part of a special issue on family violence]. *Journal of Comparative Family Studies, 25,* 7–24.

Taha-Cisse, A. H. (1991). Issues for African American women. In P. Roth (Ed.), *Alcohol and drugs are women's issues: Vol. 1. A review of the issues* (pp. 54–60). Metuchen, NJ: Women's Action Alliance/Scarecrow Press.

Taubman, S. (1986, January–February). Beyond the bravado: Sex roles and the exploitive male. *Social Work,* pp. 12–18.

Thom, B. (1986). Sex differences in help-seeking for alcohol problems: 1. The barriers to help-seeking. *British Journal of Addiction, 81,* 777–788.

Thom, B. (1994). Women and alcohol: The emergence of a risk group. In M. McDonald (Ed.), *Gender, drink, and drugs* (pp. 33–54). Providence, RI: Berg.

Traub, S. H. (1983). Characteristics of female college student drug use. *Journal of Drug Education, 13,* 177–186.

Underhill, B. L. (1991). Recovery needs of lesbian alcoholics in treatment. In N. Van Den Bergh (Ed.), *Feminist perspectives on addictions* (pp. 73–86). New York: Springer.

Unterberger, G. (1989, December 6). Twelve steps for women alcoholics. *Christian Century,* p. 1150.

van der Kolk, B. A., & Greenberg, M. S. (1990). The psychobiology of the trauma response. In B. A. van der Kolk (Ed.), *Psychological trauma* (pp. 63–88). Washington, DC: American Psychiatric Press.

Van Etten, M. L., Neumark, Y. D., & Anthony, J. C. (1999a). Male–female differences in the earliest stages of drug involvement. *Addiction, 94,* 1413–1419.

Van Etten, M. L., Neumark, Y. D., & Anthony, J. C. (1999b). Initial opportunity to use marijuana and the transition to first use: United States, 1979 to 1994. *Drug and Alcohol Dependence, 49,* 1–7.

van Strien, T., & Bergers, G. P. (1988). Overeating and sex-role orientation in women. *International Journal of Eating Disorders, 7,* 89–99.

Verbrugge, L. M. (1984). How physicians treat mentally distressed men and women. *Social Science and Medicine, 18,* 1–9.

Verbrugge, L. M., & Steiner, R. P. (1985). Prescribing drugs to men and women. *Health Psychology, 4,* 79–98.

Warner, J., Weber, T. R., & Albanes, R. (1999). "Girls are retarded when they're stoned": Marijuana and the construction of gender roles among adolescent females. *Sex Roles, 40,* 25–43.

Watson, C. G., Barnett, M., Nikunen, L., Schultz, C., Randolph-Elgin, T., & Mendez, C. M. (1997). Lifetime prevalence of nine common psychiatric/personality disorders in female domestic abuse survivors. *Journal of Nervous and Mental Disease, 185,* 645–647.

West, C. M. (1996). Mammy, Sapphire, and Jezebel: Historical images of black women and their implications for psychotherapy. *Psychotherapy, 32,* 458–456.

Wichstrom, L. (1995). Social, psychological and physical correlates of eating problems: A study of the general adolescent population in Norway. *Psychological Medicine, 25,* 567–579.

Wilsnack, R. W., & Wilsnack, S. C. (1997). *Gender and alcohol: Individual and social perspectives.* New Brunswick, NJ: Rutgers Center of Alcohol Studies.

Wilsnack, R. W., Vogeltanz, N. V., Wilsnack, S. C., & Harris, T. R. (2000). Gender differences in alcohol consumption and adverse drinking consequences: Cross-cultural patterns. *Addiction, 95,* 251–265.

Winkleby, M. A., Jatulis, D. E., Frank, E., & Fortmann, S. P. (1992). Socioeconomic status and health: How education, income, and occupation contribute to risk factors for cardiovascular disease. *American Journal of Public Health, 82,* 816–820.

Woodhouse, L. D. (1990). An exploratory study of the use of life history methods to determine treatment needs for female substance abusers. *Response, 13,* 12–15.

Xinaris, S., & Boland, F. J. (1990). Disordered eating in relation to tobacco use, alcohol consumption, self-control, and sex-role ideology. *International Journal of Eating Disorders, 9,* 425–433.

Young, M., Werch, C. E., & Bakema, S. (1989). Area-specific self-esteem scales and substance abuse among elementary and middle-school children. *Journal of School Health, 59,* 251–254.

Chapter 9

The Chrysalis Program
Feminist Treatment Community for Individuals Diagnosed as Personality Disordered

MARGO RIVERA

Four days a week 20 individuals stream into a 19th-century limestone building on the shore of Lake Ontario to engage in an intensive program of group psychotherapy. Many of them have experienced histories of childhood neglect and abuse, about half of them suffer from a high degree of dissociative symptomatology, and they have all been diagnosed in the psychiatric system with severe personality disorders. They have a history of engaging in self-destructive behaviors, such as multiple suicide attempts and self-mutilation; a range of addictive behaviors; severe eating disorders; and volatile personal relationships. They are a group of people who use emergency health and mental health services with great frequency and little positive effect. When they are hospitalized in response to suicidal actions and/or threats, self-mutilation, or complaints of severe depression, they are frequently unable to make constructive use of the inpatient service. Most of these individuals have participated in regimens of individual outpatient psychotherapy, and many of them have been followed in psychiatric treatment for years with little significant amelioration of their suffering.

The majority of them make substantial changes in their lives through participation in the Chrysalis Day Program. This chapter describes the program that has been designed to help these people build on their strengths, contain and understand their turbulent symptomatology, and eventually build constructive lives.

The Chrysalis Program started in May 1995 as part of the Kingston Psychiatric Hospital's Personality Disorders Service, in Kingston, Ontario, Canada. It is staffed by a multidisciplinary team including two nurses, a social worker, and a clinical dietician full time and a physiotherapist, a psychiatrist, and a psychologist part time (the director also serves part time). One hundred and fourteen people have participated in the Chrysalis Program since its inception for an average of 267 days (at 4 days a week, 66 weeks). Seventy percent of the participants remained in the program for more than 3 months.

The program was created in response to the Kingston medical, mental health, and social service community's expressed need for a specialized service that would offer intensive and effective treatment to individuals suffering from borderline and other personality disorders who were utilizing crisis lines, general hospital beds, emergency room services, and family doctors' support for crisis intervention—all with little positive effect. It also evolved out the Personality Disorders Service staff's frustration with the limitations of the ways in which we were able to help our clients make deep and lasting changes while we had only two treatment options to offer them, weekly outpatient sessions or psychiatric hospitalization.

Many mental health professionals have noted the difficulties the staff of the Chrysalis Program and Kingston professionals encountered in offering helpful service to this group of people. Personality disorders have proven to be particularly difficult to define, diagnose, treat, and trace eti ologically by psychiatry and psychology (Gunderson, 1983; Livesley, 1987; Paris, 1994; Widiger, 2001; Zimmerman, 1994). People with this primary diagnosis frequently present with numerous additional psychiatric or psychological problems (Andreoli, Gressot, Aapro, Tricot, & Gognalons, 1989; Dolan-Sewell, Krueger, & Shea, 2001), such as depression (Ferro, Klein, Schwartz, Kasch, & Leader, 1998; Klein, Wonderlich, & Shea, 1993), eating disorders (Beckman & Burns, 1990) and suicidal and self-mutilatory behaviors (Kernberg, 1988; Paris, Nowlis, & Brown, 1989; Stone, 1990).

Some personality disorder labels (borderline, histrionic, dependent) also imply that, while the behaviors may be ego-syntonic and are not always distressing to the individual so labeled, other people will be annoyed and troubled by them. This is carried to an extreme when certain personality disorder labels are commonly used as punitive epithets by mental health practitioners rather than as scientifically based signposts to compassionate and helpful treatment (e.g., "She is a bad borderline").

If indeed personality disorders represent stable and enduring traits, as designated by the DSM-III introduction to Axis II psychopathology, this implies that expectations for treatment outcome should be minimal at best. The diagnosis of borderline personality disorder, in particular, has frequently been defined by treatment failure (Sanislow & McGlashan, 1998) and has become synonymous with "the difficult patient" (Kernberg, Selzer, Koenigsberg, Carr, & Applebaum, 1989). Encounters with such individuals are often perceived by frontline mental health professionals as "formidable, frustrating, and fruitless" (Links, 1998).

Though this view of personality pathology as intractable has been widespread, there have been some systematic attempts to understand, effectively treat, and document therapeutic outcome, particularly for individuals diagnosed with borderline personality disorder. A manualized treatment protocol, *dialectical behavioral therapy* (DBT), has been developed by Marsha Linehan (1993). DBT combines behavioral, cognitive, and supportive interventions within an individual and group format. Three behavioral goals are priorized: reduction of life-threatening behaviors, reduction of behaviors that interfere with therapy, and reduction of behaviors that reduce quality of life. A series of research studies have demonstrated the impact of this treatment program on reducing suicidal behaviors and inpatient hospitalizations, as well as demonstrating significantly better global functioning in the participants' lives.

Hassan Azim, William Piper, and their colleagues (Piper, Rosie, Joyce, & Azim, 1996) in Edmonton, Alberta, have developed a day treatment program that includes 60% of personality disorder participants. This program, which has operated continuously since 1973, is based on psychodynamic group therapy within a milieu in which behavioral and cognitive skill building is combined with an interpersonal orientation.

Paul Links (1993) argues that a rehabilitation model—focusing on skill development and environmental change to further better functioning rather than psychotherapy of any sort—is often more appropriate for some individuals with borderline personality disorder.

Otto Kernberg and his colleagues (Kernberg et al., 1989; Koenigsberg et al., 2000) have delineated an approach to psychodynamic psychotherapy for individuals with borderline psychopathology that they call *transference-focused psychotherapy* (TFP). This treatment model differs from conventional psychodynamic therapy in that it is based on a more specific treatment contract, allows for deviations from technical neutrality, prescribes a more active role for the therapist, and is more dependent on nonverbal channels of communication. A recent study suggests that this structured psychodynamic treatment is effective for individuals diagnosed with borderline personality disorder (Clarkin et al., 2001).

Joel Paris (1996, 1998) prescribes an eclectic therapy process, combining both cognitive-behavioral and dynamic methods that educates the personality disordered client to modify extreme personality traits (impulsivity and affective instability in borderline personality disorder) and develop alternative coping strategies.

These approaches differ significantly from each other. What they have in common is the recognition that effective treatment or rehabilitation for individuals suffering from severe personality disorders will be long term, and because there are a range of affective, cognitive, and behavioral symptoms to target for change, no narrow treatment approach is likely to meet their diverse needs (Links, 1998). The *Practice Guidelines for the Treatment of Patients with Borderline Personality Disorder* (Work Group on Borderline Personality Disorder, 2001) notes that substantial improvement may not occur until a full year of psychotherapeutic intervention has been provided and that many individuals require much longer treatment than that. In the *Handbook of Personality Disorders* (2001), Livesley frames personality disorders as involving multiple domains of psychopathology and concludes that comprehensive treatment requires a combination of interventions tailored to the particular biopsychosocial problems of each individual client.

THE DILEMMA OF DIAGNOSIS

As part of the Chrysalis preadmission process, applicants are given a thorough psychiatric interview and a battery of psychological tests. Collateral information from other caregivers and/or institutions is sought as part of creating a diagnostic picture of each individual.

Axis I

Seventy-seven percent of the participants qualified for a diagnosis of posttraumatic stress disorder; 74% of them were currently suffering from a major depressive episode; 81% had suffered from major depression in the past; 94% of them currently suffered from panic disorder; 94% suffered from social phobia, and 74% suffered from at least one specific phobia. Though none of these individuals were chronically psychotic, their thinking was unusual enough that 81% qualified for a diagnosis of delusional disorder, and 77% of them suffered from obsessive–compulsive disorder. Half of them had a dissociative disorder; 69% of them had an eating disorder; 77% had experienced serious problems with drug and/or alcohol dependence. The average number of Axis I diagnoses per participant was 14.2, with a range from 6 to 19.

Axis II

The computer-assisted SCID II interview served to refine and confirm Axis II diagnoses. The most common diagnosis in this group was that of border-line personality disorder, followed by depressive personality disorder, then avoidant and obsessive–compulsive personality disorders. The mean number of Axis II diagnoses per participant was 2, with a range from 1 to 7.

Psychometric testing can be helpful in unearthing and systematically documenting the range of personal, social, psychological, and physiological problems that bring individuals suffering from personality disorder to treatment and that therefore must be targeted for change. However, adding together both Axis I and Axis II diagnoses is cumbersome, and at present, unfortunately, there is no officially sanctioned way to describe the particular group of consumers of mental health services served by the Chrysalis Program, except to assign them multiple diagnoses from an array of DSM categories. This undermines the utility of the diagnostic process, as listing more than a dozen separate labels does not offer an evocative and parsimonious description of the set of difficulties the person is experiencing—for example, where they came from, why they adopted particular self-destructive strategies, and how they interact with other problems and affect the individual's capacity to lead a stable and satisfying life. Phenomenological diagnosis does not begin to capture the subtleties and complexity of the ways in which people respond over the life span with their characteristic personality traits and coping styles. Most problematically, it does not point to effective treatment.

Diagnosis and Trauma History

Sixty percent of Chrysalis participants report experiences of childhood sexual abuse; 75% report physical abuse; 89% report emotional abuse. Twenty-five percent of the participants suffered from severe physical, sexual, and emotional abuse from earliest childhood through adolescence, as reported on the Trauma Antecedents Questionnaire and frequently documented in medical history and child welfare and/or legal records.

Many clinicians who work with survivors of prolonged and repeated trauma have identified the need for a new diagnostic category that takes into account both the etiology of their difficulties and the profound personality changes that frequently result from their experiences. Judith Herman (1992) proposed identifying a syndrome—complex posttraumatic stress disorder—that would document the details of the areas of personality damage and disorganization, while at the same time acknowledging the etiology of these difficulties and their complex interrelations.

The working group for the DSM-IV examined the category "posttraumatic stress disorder"—a diagnosis based on the trauma prototypes of combat, natural disaster, and rape—for its applicability to the experiences of survivors of prolonged interpersonal trauma. They recommended that a new DSM category, disorders of extreme stress, be included in DSM-IV to replace the fragmented type of diagnosis that such individuals now tend to receive with a category that reflects the range of debilitating problems and the connections among them that need to be acknowledged, understood, and resolved if the individual's treatment is to be effective (van der Kolk, Roth, Pelcovity, & Mandel, 1993). The DSM-IV task force did not support the proposal, compromising by including a recognition of the range of complex adaptations to trauma (disturbed affect regulation, aggression against self and others, dissociation, somatization, and altered relationships with self and others) in the "Associated Features and Disorders" section of the DSM-IV's entry on posttraumatic stress disorder (American Psychiatric Association, 1994, p. 425).

The World Health Organization's classification of mental disorders (ICD-10), used in many countries outside North America, recognizes the connections among posttraumatic stress symptoms in a way the DSM does not. It places a range of "reactions to severe stress and adjustment disorders" (F43) side by side with "dissociative disorders" (F44), "somatoform disorder" (F45), and "enduring personality changes following a catastrophic stress" (F62) (World Health Organization, 1992).

Challenge to Categories of Pathology

Feminist-informed practitioners (Brown, 1994; Brown &, Ballou 1992; Chesler, 1972; Hare-Mustin & Marecek, 1990; Lerman, 1996) have critiqued the notion of pathology and disorder as a construction of distress that locates the source of the problem in the distressed individual, often reifying normative expressions of gender, race, or class as pathological. Feminism, conversely, frames as disordered the forces of patriarchal societies, including racism, sexism, classism, heterosexism, and all the other ideologies and practices that justify and maintain power differentials, exclusion, and oppression. In commenting on the use of the term "disorder" to label her, one woman suffering from severe posttraumatic dissociation protested:

> Words are powerful symbols. I cringe each time I hear the term "disorder." I struggle to accept the means I used to survive absolutely horrendous sexual, physical and emotional abuse by my father and other family members. I struggle to celebrate the fact that I found a way to deal with the chaos without going crazy. Our language does not enlighten my struggle, it increases it. I am fully aware that what was once adaptive is now rather messy, to put it mildly. But I am not crazy. I am not ill. I am not a disorder. I am a human face who had to survive in a home that was totally crazy, very sick and constantly disordered. Please do not define me in terms of their behavior. (quoted in Rivera, 1996, p. 4)

There is a reasonable argument to be made for challenging any type of mental illness or psychopathology model of posttraumatic responses (Root, 1992). If extreme distress and the psychological and physiological responses that follow upon such distress (e.g., pervasive mistrust, hyperarousal, numbing, dissociation, emotional lability, and many others) were understood to be the normal self-protective reactions of the traumatized person—elaborated and reinforced when the trauma is not acknowledged and the individual not tended to properly—rather than framed as a medical syndrome, perhaps more focus would be directed on the prevention of the traumatic events, rather than stigmatizing individuals for having experienced these events and their aftermath as traumatic (Brown, 2000).

PREVIOUS TREATMENT

As well as a wide range of problems, participants in the Chrysalis Program also share a history of unsuccessful treatment. Most of them have engaged in at least one course of individual psychotherapy—often many more—and have tried a range of other therapeutic modalities as well. They tended to use community crisis services from suicide lines to hospital emergency departments, sometimes daily during times of great stress.

As is common among individuals diagnosed with personality disorders

(Paris, 1998), these participants often collected a pharmacopeia of psycho-tropic drugs and painkillers, each directed at a discreet symptom, most with weak and marginal effects. The pharmacological interventions some-times offered a temporary easing of the intensity of some symptoms, but they were rarely helpful in the long run and frequently led to serious and debilitating side effects and prescription drug dependency that exacerbated rather than ameliorated their problems.

Hospitalizations on psychiatric wards, though frequently requested or demanded, have often been stressful for these clients and everyone in-volved in their inpatient treatment, and such hospitalizations were usually counterproductive. Again their experiences were reflected in the research of inpatient hospitalization treatment of borderline personality disorder. Hos-pitalizations have been demonstrated to be counterproductive, leading to regression and exacerbating suicidal behaviors (Dawson & MacMillan, 1993; Linehan, 1993), with no empirical evidence supporting the assump-tion of the admitting physicians that hospitalization prevents completion of suicide (Paris, 1994).

Some of the individuals participating in the Chrysalis Program found practitioners and agencies that became committed to supporting them and did so for many years, earning the respect and sometimes the dependent at-tachment of the client, who usually felt alone in her suffering. Though these sincere attempts to help have often been greatly appreciated, they did not en-able them to overcome their difficulties and lead stable, productive lives.

The Chrysalis Program has been successful in helping many of these individuals steadily and gradually to contain the behaviors that created such chaos in their lives, and eventually—and again gradually—to use their considerable strengths to build constructive lives in which they contribute to their communities, rather than seeing themselves as continually victim-ized by others and/or taking from them.

The program offers a resource for individuals with less extensive histo-ries of trauma and more limited damage to personality organization, as well as to those with histories of more severe and earlier-onset childhood trau-ma and the deeply rooted adaptations that enabled them to survive these circumstances. Most of the participants make the changes they desire and then go on to use less intensive therapeutic support (either from program staff or from therapists in their own communities) to consolidate these gains. A minority of those with profound and extensive difficulties make significant changes and then return periodically, and usually part time, to deal with further problems that emerge in response to the demands of jobs, relationships, or some form of retraumatization.

HOW DOES THE CHRYSALIS PROGRAM WORK?

In order to qualify for admission to the Chrysalis Program, individuals must have the ability to express a few concrete changes that they wish to make in their lives. This represents the starting point for each person to begin the process of moving through a series of therapeutic stages, predominantly in groups, to address those specific problems identified by them.

The first group of the program week is the Goals Group, in which participants report on the progress they have made with the previous week's goals and make new goals for the upcoming week. Each individual signs her individual goals and keeps a copy, while another copy goes into the program files. As well as serving as a useful reminder of what she wants most urgently and immediately to change in her life (and many participants carry their goals with them throughout the week or post them in a prominent place in their homes), these self-generated records of progress constitute the principle way in which each participant's involvement in the program is officially documented. This practical policy of framing both problems and solutions in participants' own words creates a frame of reference about their difficulties and the ways they are attempting to overcome them that is meaningful to them.

Although this is empowering, it often creates an initial sense of unease, because it challenges the ways in which individuals who have been involved in the mental health system for a long time have learned to think about themselves and their behaviors. The DSM diagnostic system and how it is frequently applied has created the illusion for many of the people in the Chrysalis Program that they have many separate illnesses, rather than a complex pattern of cognitive distortions, a limited capacity to tolerate strong feelings, and physiological reactions that are disruptive and demoralizing—all of which are characteristic ways they have learned to respond to their life experiences. When the illness frame of reference is challenged, individuals begin to evolve a more complex perspective on why they behave the way they do, think the way they do, and experience somatic responses that radically interfere with their stable functioning.

For example, it is common for participants to declare that they have missed a day at program because they have depression, and that one of the symptoms of their depressive illness is that they can't get up some mornings. This tautological reasoning usually gets a chuckle from more experienced group members, who point out that depression does not mean you have broken your legs. It simply means that you feel very bad and staying in bed is easier than coming to group and using all the varied treatment modalities the program offers to build up tolerance for how miserable you feel, both physically and emotionally, and to develop more adaptive responses to your dysphoria than staying in bed all day.

Many individuals arrive at the Chrysalis Program clutching their favorite diagnosis to them as a replacement for a robust sense of themselves, dropping psychiatric terminology into every other sentence. Eventually they become clear as to why they are attached to such an inadequate characterization of themselves, when they begin to recognize the level of responsibility that is incurred by understanding that they have developed their own style (cognitive, emotional, physiological) of functioning to enable them to survive. When acknowledged and increasingly understood, some of that style is changeable; even in the short run, much of that style is manageable. The gradual awareness of oneself as a complex coping creature, whose problems have been solutions in disguise, can be daunting, but for many of the participants of the Chrysalis Program that awareness is eventually the core of their empowerment. They no longer have to struggle to be "treatment-compliant," but rather to be increasingly honest about who they are, what they want, and how they cope. From that basis, they can then create new beliefs to replace outmoded ones and expand their capacities to feel deep and often disturbing feelings, rather than creating increasingly complex and dysfunctional ways of avoiding such feelings. They can learn to care for themselves with rigor, kindness, and common sense, rather than continually recapitulating the ways they learned to treat themselves and others throughout the course of their lives.

The Chrysalis Program uses the following three basic modalities to create a milieu in which personal change in coping capacities can be created by participants:

1. Dynamic psychotherapy, with particular focus on the therapeutic alliance(s).
2. Specialized groups encompassing different therapeutic modalities, including cognitive and behavioral skill-building groups; physical, recreational, and life skills programming; and expressive therapies.
3. Therapeutic community.

Each aspect of the program is essential to its successful functioning. The rest of this chapter focuses on the third modality and describes the advantages of surrounding an intensive therapeutic process with a challenging and supportive community based on feminist values.

As part of the process of developing treatment strategies that would enable our clients to cope more creatively, we could not avoid noticing the many ways in which their life experiences, past and present, were influenced by the social, political, and cultural forces that shape all our lives. We observed the ways in which they incorporated the oppressive practices to which they were subjected—in homes and in religious, educational, and medical institutions—and how they struggled against being destroyed, physically, mentally, emotionally, and spiritually.

There are many ways in which the Chrysalis community is a living theater of the feminist postulate that the personal is political. Examples of how feminist values are central to the program's identity and functioning could be gleaned from almost everything staff and participants do each day. The rest of this chapter describes a few of the ways we understand our efforts to reach out to the participants in the Chrysalis Program and engage them in a therapeutic process that is empowering and transformative to be quintessentially feminist.

A THERAPEUTIC COMMUNITY
BASED ON FEMINIST VALUES

The vast majority of the participants of the Chrysalis Program are women. In fact, in the 6 years of the program's operation, only three biological males and one transgendered male participated in the program for more than a few weeks. Very few men are referred to the program, and those who are often exhibit their disturbance in ways (wife beating, physical and sexual assault, child abuse) that exclude them from participation with a group of women, many of whom have been physically and sexually abused, frequently by men, both in childhood and adulthood. Our service has developed two adjunctive programs that are more likely to meet the needs of some men who are referred to us: a highly structured cognitive therapy group and a program of short-term individual therapy, both of which focus on learning to understand and control powerful emotions. Even in these programs, women far outnumber men in terms of both referrals and attendance, but men participate successfully.

Because of its location in Kingston, Ontario, a small Canadian city that is more culturally and racially homogeneous than larger Canadian urban centers, and because it serves a very large surrounding rural area, which is even less heterogeneous, 90% of the participants have been white, with more Aboriginal participants (4%) than members of any other racial group.

Medical coverage is universal in Canada. Because the Chrysalis Pro-

gram is part of a psychiatric hospital service, there is no cost to the participants. Lunch is provided each day, and individuals who need assistance for
transportation or childcare can often access it. Because it is financially accessible, a large majority of the participants are extremely poor. Some come
from poverty-stricken backgrounds, others from working-class homes. Some
come from middle-class families, but their own severe social and psychological difficulties have made it impossible for them to support a middle-
class lifestyle themselves. In general, the only participants who live a
middle-class life in the present are those who are married to husbands who
make a substantial income. Even very young participants have been cut off
from their families of origin, at least in terms of financial support. There is a
wide range of educational levels among the participants, from individuals
who did not finish elementary school to those with a postsecondary education. The majority of the participants are heterosexual, but individuals who
identity as lesbian (14%), bisexual (3%), gay male (1%), and transgendered
(2%) have participated in the Chrysalis Program.

The program is accessible to people with physical disabilities, and
women who are moderately to severely physically disabled participate. Both
seeing-eye and special skills dogs have been ongoing and much-loved program participants. A participant with a severe physical disability com-
mented on how she learned to deal with her particular challenges in the
context of the Chrysalis Program:

"My previous experiences of therapy tried to address the affect my disability had on my life. But the practical issues I talked about were not really the source of my serious problems. The helplessness I felt as a child
undergoing so many medical procedures and being different from other
children—those things were affecting me all the time. In the Chrysalis
Program, I got to talk about what it was like to be a person with a severe
and obvious disability. But I also learned to see that some of the problems
I had were common to most of the able-bodied participants. For instance, I had a lot of trouble asking for help.

"In my life, I have always needed a lot of assistance, but, before my participation in the Chrysalis Program, most of the people who helped me were
either family or professionals. I did not have to ask for the help I needed;
I could just expect them to know. I used to avoid any setting that forced
me to acknowledge directly my differences and my needs. When I first
joined the Chrysalis Program, I refused to leave the room during a group,
even when I needed to, explaining that I have trouble opening the door

and my wheels squeak, which would disturb the group. When I was challenged to be more respectful to myself and take care of my basic needs, I realized that nobody minded accommodating me in small ways, like opening a door, and the issue was whether I believed I had a right to be in the group like everyone else. My disability was not seen in the Chrysalis Program as a reason to bar me from day trips or overnight camping, but as there was no specialized assistance available, I was expected to take the lead in planning how to accommodate my practical needs. Negotiating with others, both staff and participants, about what they were able and willing to do for me, was not easy, but eventually I learned to ask directly for help and to be open to the person's genuine response. This has made it possible to expand my activities, to go to college, for example, where I encounter all kinds of physical, emotional, and intellectual challenges, new ones each day."

Challenge to Middle-Class Assumptions and Values

There is a conscious effort on the part of the staff (who are all middle class in terms of education level and current lifestyle) to ensure that there is not an assumption of the superiority of middle-class values and that when this assumption arises, it is challenged. This issue is addressed directly, for example, when participants express their own assumptions that making improvements in their emotional well-being will necessarily lead to making lots of money or that the material trappings of a middle-class life are a sign of mental health. Participants are often reminded—and remind each other—that many well-educated and wealthy people are as miserable as they are and create their own materially comfortable lives in ways that are harmful to others. Most of the participants know such people, and though many of them, over the course of the program, go back to school or join the workforce to improve the material conditions of their lives, they rarely buy completely into the assumption that a middle-class lifestyle should be an overarching goal that, when reached, will prove their superiority to those who are poorer or less educated. They are much more likely to appreciate the perspectives and the strengths they have gained through their participation in the margins of our culture, and while looking forward to shedding some of the most onerous of its oppressions, like grinding poverty, they are unlikely to be willing to shape themselves to meet the requirements of the dominant middle-class culture.

There is also an atmosphere of ongoing challenge to the assumption that certain ways of expressing oneself, through clothing or language style, for example, are superior to others. Though cleanliness and personal hygiene are valued as a means of showing respect toward oneself and others, participants (and staff for that matter) embrace a range of sartorial styles and a wider range of language than is usually permissible in a professional treatment milieu. Excessive use of psychiatric jargon is discouraged, as it is seen both as an ineffective way of expressing the degree of distress and disturbance the participants experience and has often been used, from the participants' perspective, to reinforce power differentials between themselves and professionals. So one participant may describe herself as being "fucked up," another may note that the excuses she had been concocting for certain behaviors are "bullshit," and a staff member may reflect to a frantic participant, "It sounds like you are having a really shitty day."

Both staff and participants can, when they choose, use polysyllables to express themselves, but complex and/or constrained language is not privileged. Though it is an upper- and middle-class truism that vulgar language is used only by those who are not capable of finding more sophisticated synonyms, it is the experience of both participants and staff that the inclusion of the type of street language that is comfortable and evocative for the majority of the participants is generally helpful in undercutting pretense and deemphasizing class and educational differences among participants and between participants and staff. The atmosphere created through the use of varied, emotion-filled, and sometimes salty language also subverts the assumption that the professionals' points of view and middle-class styles and values underlie the process (and consequently the outcomes) of psychotherapy.

Assessment of the Treatment Process: A Joint Responsibility

It is a basic value of feminist therapy that assessment is not only the prerogative and the responsibility of the professional. Therapy is always a partnership. Unless clients respect their own role, as well the role of the mental health professional, the process is likely to undermine their strengths rather than contribute to their growth (Brown, 1994; Rivera, 1996).

When individuals are initially introduced to the Chrysalis Program, they are encouraged to spend 4 full days a week there. The purpose is to immerse themselves in the community enough so that they can decide, within the first month, whether the program matches their needs and their values. The staff make it clear in the intake interview, the program orientation, and in the informed consent that is signed prior to attending the program that the Chrysalis Program has a specific philosophical base and offers a particular kind of therapy that does not work for everyone. There is a strong emphasis on the participant's responsibility to attempt to understand the treatment and to assess whether or not it suits her. Often, usually in the initial psychiatric assessment or the intake interview with the director, applicants decide that the program is not for them, but sometimes the need for some form of help is so intense that such a decision does not seem to them to be an option.

The first month of the program participation is framed as a trial period, during which time participants are reminded that they have both the right and the responsibility to leave the program if they truly think it does not meet their needs, and staff have a similar responsibility to let new participants know if they think the program will not help them. In this case, staff will do their best to make an appropriate referral, if the client wishes them to do so.

This way of framing participation in the program emphasizes the participant's expertise regarding her own life, including her right and her responsibility to decide what form of psychological treatment serves her best interests. Each participant in the Chrysalis Program—no matter how volatile her behavior and how helpless she may see herself and present herself to others—is understood to be a competent adult, with all the rights and responsibilities that accrue to such adults. Part of the intake process is a determination that the applicant is not currently psychotic or suffering from a mental illness in which she is likely to become psychotic periodically (though she may exhibit behavior now and then that appears psychotic, or, due to active dissociative symptomatology, she may be disoriented occasionally or even frequently) and that she wants to take more control over her own life than she has in the past.

The treatment of each individual as a competent adult is not only core to the philosophy of the program but is a practical tool to prevent counterproductive power struggles. Ongoing and fruitless arguments about aggressive acting out toward oneself or others on the program site or about whether the program should accept responsibility for an individual's life decisions and hospitalize her if she mentions suicide, engages in self-harm behavior, or even feels really bad, for example, are avoided by referencing the initial agreement and pointing out the demonstrable reality that there are a range of treatment venues with radically different philosophies, most of which are willing to take over responsibility for an individual's behavior and life course under certain circumstances. If, indeed, a Chrysalis participant truly believes she is not capable of managing her own life responsibly, according to the norms set out in the consent form, and does not want a

therapy process that guides her in that direction, she does have other options. One participant noted the importance of these guidelines regarding
self-care and responsible behavior.

> "Prior to being in the Chrysalis Program decisions such as where I should
> live and what I needed medically were not being made by me. How I felt
> or what I wanted was not particularly relevant. Nobody helped me be re-
> sponsible for my destructive behavior, or for my refusal to take basic care
> for myself. I did feel some guilt over my destructive behaviors and my
> stays in hospital, and I was aware at some level that these actions were
> not necessary, yet the professionals I was involved with treated me as
> though I had no choice in these behaviors, and I did take advantage of
> this view. The Chrysalis Program's view that I was responsible for myself,
> in spite of my inner struggles, allowed me to see clearly the choices I was
> making and to see that being self-destructive was in fact a choice. This
> enabled me to stop behaving in harmful ways and to start making deci-
> sions for myself in regards to my life. The result is that I gained a sense of
> self-respect, which I was greatly lacking previously."

This framework of personal responsibility is an ongoing aspect of the
therapeutic process. There are usually many occasions over the course of
treatment when participants experience staff as unsympathetic, overly
confrontative, and stubbornly unwilling to agree with their interpretation
of self-destructive behavior or harmful actions toward others as uncontrol-
lable and an inevitable result of a history of victimization or of psychiatric
illness. It is an expected part of a grueling therapeutic enterprise that participants sometimes experience their therapists as insensitive or downright
hurtful. It is the professionals' responsibility to consider these accusations
for any truth they may contain. If staff members cannot agree that they
should change their point of view or approach, they encourage the participant to engage in the same process of self-examination. "If indeed after serious consideration, you really think I [or we, or the program] am truly
harmful to you, then you need to think seriously about whether or not to
participate in this program." Participants are encouraged to state their disagreements openly and clearly, and then to decide for themselves whether
the process, in balance, is helping or harming them. Though the program is
open to clear and even volatile expression of frustration and/or disagree-
ment, an ongoing pattern of tantrumous rage followed by sullen compliance (familiar to many of these individuals in their relationships with
mental health practitioners) is not understood as responsible behavior for

either participant in the interaction (client or professional) and is not indulged in the Chrysalis Program.

Though this challenge to engage responsibly in their therapeutic project can seem onerous, particularly in the initial stage, it creates the basis of respect and equality upon which the program is grounded. When asked, in follow-up interviews after discharge, to reflect on why they made the changes they made in the context of the Chrysalis Program, participants almost always reference, first and foremost, the respect for them as people who have a right to make their own choices, before they go on to list the therapeutic tools they were offered to help them accomplish their goals, as the following comments by a Chrysalis Program participant demonstrate:

"Coming from a background where silent compliance, rigid conformity, and selfless caretaking were among the only real values I knew, collapsing into 'depression' was considered a major disgrace. Coming to terms with my weakness and climbing back up to resume my place seemed an impossibility. So, being the obedient, compliant woman I had been taught to be, I handed complete control of my life over to the mental health professionals. After 8½ months of cooperating in psychiatric hospital wards, undergoing a variety of treatments including endless ECT, I seemed no closer to being capable of resuming responsibility for myself, let alone my two small children. Although I readily went along with what I was told, I wasn't particularly interested in what the doctors had to say about what was wrong nor the prescribed treatment of the week. I knew that my problem was me—my life—36 years of bottled-up emotions and internal conflict.

"I had been shaped and molded as a child to believe that I was worthless as a human being and all the more so because I was a female. My purpose in life was to be an obedient, subservient daughter first, wife and mother second. There was no room to question my role or my value; my place was set. I had no right to balk at or complain about the sexual abuse I endured for years as a child because after all he couldn't help himself and as a girl it was my place to accede. This I carried over to my marriage. I couldn't escape my husband's unwanted sexual advances; my duty was to serve him regardless of the fact that his touch made me recoil. It never occurred to me that I had a right to question the many beliefs and values I had been taught; those beliefs were reinforced at every turn in our culture, society, schools, and religion. If I was unhappy with my life then I knew that it was because there was something inherently wrong with me. Then a day came where I could no longer hold in my anger; I wanted out of the confines of the hospital, and so I left the inpatient unit and, with very little trust or hope, decided to give the Chrysalis Program a try. From day 1 the staff made it clear that plenty of resources were available for me to use but that I was responsible for how I used them. I was challenged at every turn to take control of my life, my personal safety, and the choices I made every minute of every day. Having responsibility put back in my lap in a way it never quite had before was both terrifying and empowering. Within 3 months of starting the program I had regained control of my life. I had stayed out of hospital, was no longer on any medications, and was ready to resume full responsibility for my family. Once I had stabilized my life to some degree, I had room to start really exploring what was going on, what had gone wrong, what I believed, where the conflicts were, who I really was, and what I really wanted. I had never before been asked to think about or question anything I had been taught and yet a lot of what I had been taught was destroying me."

Incorporation of the Treatment of Dissociative Disorders

Some of the applicants to the Chrysalis Program present with a dissociative disorder as part of their original complaint, and others are completely unaware that dissociative mechanisms are part of the reason they have no recollection of their childhoods; they can injure themselves severely without experiencing physical pain; they can create radically different relationships with different people, including professionals; and they have severe memory deficits. As with all of the other disorders and diagnoses that Chrysalis participants carry, dissociative identity disorder (and other forms of extreme dissociative adaptations) are not seen as mental disorders to be treated in isolation from their social context, the ways in which these symptoms worked for them in the past and continue to provide solutions that both protect and limit them in their present-day lives.

Both in our assessment and treatment protocols, the Chrysalis Program neither denies, discounts, nor privileges dissociation as a coping strategy. All Chrysalis participants suffering from Axis I dissociative disorders also struggle with significant Axis II symptomatology, and the Chrysalis Program emphasizes resolving floridly dysfunctional behaviors and stabilizing day-to-day life. Only once significant stabilization is achieved and consolidated is more systematic treatment of dissociation undertaken in individual sessions.

In the group programming, severely dissociative individuals are taught to speak about themselves in a language that acknowledges more cohesion and unity than they actually experience. For example, though a dissociative individual may experience the thoughts, feelings, and behaviors that emerge from alternate aspects of herself as completely ego-dystonic and "not me," she is encouraged to use the language of parts of the self when describing these beliefs and behaviors in the group. This language they share with all the other group members, including those who do not suffer from dissociative disorders.

The rationale for the policy of not allowing "multiple personality talk" is that it sets the individual apart from the group and exaggerates her differences from the other participants. Almost all the significantly dissociative clients have experienced scapegoating in peer groups throughout their lives and are willing to learn to speak about their experiences in a way that does not set them apart from the group. The few clients who have received secondary gains in previous treatment through an emphasis on their dissociative symptoms, though they may rebel initially at not being able to insist that their alter personalities be called by name and acknowledged as separate people, soon either become accustomed to a different approach or leave the program quickly to return to a type of treatment in which there is more to be gained from being seen as special because of a floridly dissociative symptom picture.

Many of the participants in the Chrysalis Program see a staff member or a community psychotherapist for an hour of individual therapy a week as a supplement to their participation in groups. Within this context, there is much more leeway for dissociative individuals to explore distinct ego states, acknowledging openly just how much they do not experience themselves as unified and how little ownership and responsibility they take for their beliefs, feelings, and behaviors when they are in an altered state of consciousness. This combination of freedom to explore the depth of their dissociation and the demand that they challenge their rigid cognitions about not being who they are seems to be an effective balance of validation and challenge for severely dissociative clients, as well as a check against factitious presentations and symptom contagion that could be a potential danger in a therapeutic community. In fact, some clients who present at intake with a questionable dissociative disorder diagnosis and/or an unhealthy investment in dissociative symptoms soon shift their focus to their very real problems when they discover there is nothing to be gained from staff through a histrionic presentation and when other participants make it clear they have little tolerance for what they see as distracting and annoying behavior.

Challenging Stereotypical Sex-Role Gender Socialization and Constructions of Sexuality

The Chrysalis Program offers, both in the general attitude of the staff and in structured groups, a challenge to the socialization re gender and sexuality that is imposed on women and men in our society. Most—if not all—of the participants have been socialized to stereotypical norms of gender and sexual expression by their upbringings. Some of them have made great efforts to conform to these norms, usually at a high cost to their sense of personal authenticity and their empowerment in intimate relationships, and some have rebelled constantly and angrily and generally see themselves as outsiders who will never be able to construct a life in which they feel secure and accepted for who they are.

The program offers two groups on the topics of gender and sexuality. The participants select either "Heart and Soul: Exploring Heterosexuality" or "Heart and Soul: Alternative Experiences of Gender and Sexuality" (Rivera & Wachob, in press) to help them develop an authentic sense of themselves as gendered and sexual people.

Challenging Chronic Patterns of Disordered Eating

Many feminists (e.g., Bordo, 1990; Chernin, 1986; Orbach, 1979; Szekeley, 1988; and Wolf, 1990) have drawn the connection between the evolution of the second wave of the women's movement and the consequent breaking down of social barriers that excluded women from participating in the public sphere and the weight-loss cult that not only sickens and destroys the many women who suffer from the extremes of clinically diagnosable eating disorders (like the majority of the participants in the Chrysalis Program) but most Western women who are fixated on food consumption and body size. They see the public passion about female weight as a counterbalance to the dangers posed to the status quo of institutional patriarchy by the economic and reproductive freedom women have achieved in the last four decades of the 20th century.

The majority of Chrysalis participants suffer from eating disorders, many of them serious enough to undermine their physical health and sometimes their cognitive capabilities. Some of these participants have engaged in specialized individual and group treatment for eating disorders with limited success in terms of developing and sustaining patterns of healthy nutrition.

As with other specific problems, such as severe dissociation, disordered eating patterns are seen in the Chrysalis Program as one part of a symptom constellation that enables people to cope with a pervasive sense of threat and dyscontrol. It is also understood that widespread social messages prescribing a correlation between thinness, sexual desirability, and basic worth are incorporated by all women in our culture, and a great deal of effort is made to counteract this destructive socialization through readings, discussions, and practical projects as well. A cognitive group on the topic of disordered eating facilitated by a clinical dietician is attended by all individuals suffering from eating disorders to ensure that they have basic information about the deleterious physical effects of restricting food intake for long periods of time, binge eating, bulimia, and excessive dieting. This group also offers readings and structured discussions to help participants—who frequently do not see that there is anything wrong with their drive for extreme thinness and all of the ways in which they try to achieve that goal—challenge this incorporation of some of society's most destructive values about women and their bodies.

A project called "Collective Kitchen" (Scott, 1999, 2000) creates a milieu in which the values that are taught by the program about the importance of healthy eating to the building and sustaining of an empowered lifestyle are enacted practically. Participants meet monthly to decide what dishes they wish to make and how many servings of each dish they want to take home. They each contribute a share of the money that will be spent for the ingredients, shop for the food, and then spend one morning cooking a variety of dishes, which they then divide up and take home to freeze and eat over the course of the month. Many of the disagreements, cognitive distortions, and fears around food and eating that are encountered in the disordered eating discussion group are faced in Collective Kitchen as well. However, the pressure to cook approximately six different meals in a morning gives an urgency to surmounting these obstacles, and even women who refuse to agree that there is anything wrong with their patterns of unhealthy eating are often influenced by participating in this communal experience of nurturing oneself and others to expand their beliefs and their behaviors regarding food.

Another group, entitled "Body Image," focuses more broadly on the many ways in which women in our culture are taught to see our bodies as objects for others' use, and to examine the ways in which practices based on this profoundly undermining value can be challenged and replaced with other healthier and more personally and socially empowering practices. The Body Image group includes assigned readings, homework assignments to write personal reflections about the readings, discussion about these reflections, and three periods a week of physical exercise with the goal of gaining strength, flexibility, and physical awareness and confidence.

Chronic eating disorders are one of the most difficult problems for Chrysalis participants to overcome. Though this reality is undoubtedly overdetermined, one of the reasons is that women attempting to transform a lifestyle centered around severely restrictive eating and/or binge eating and purging not only have to engage in their own personal battles to change these deeply rooted coping styles but also have to fight the general social prescription of a mature, successful women as one who denies her hunger and her natural female shape. It is painful to observe the horror with which participants who make changes in their self-destructive eating patterns experience the gradual growth of a normal female body. It is only through participating intensively in a community that continually challenges this equation of any female body fat with ugliness and starvation with self-discipline and power—a community that encourages the participants to celebrate the bodies they develop as a result of healthy self-care and self-appreciation—that some of the participants are able to transform their relationship to the way they nourish themselves and live in their bodies.

Incorporating Ethics and Spirituality into a Psychological Treatment Program

In general, mainstream mental health practice excludes existential issues related to the meaning of life that are often framed as religious or spiritual. For many of the participants of the Chrysalis Program, these issues are in the foreground of their struggle to live rather than to die, to challenge the destructive values they were taught as children and create for themselves ones they understand as reasonable and ethical, and to choose, as they express it, good over evil, in their relationships with others, even when the respectful engagement with someone else is much more difficult than using that person as an object to relieve pressure or meet needs.

There are two different ways in which the Chrysalis Program undertakes the project of responding to its participants' felt and expressed need to address these issues directly as part of their therapeutic process. The first is to challenge the assumption that every issue raised in therapy is a psychological one, ignoring the ethical dimensions of our clients' quest for a more meaningful life.

I became aware that I had begun engaging more consciously in this realm when, at the early stage of the program's development, a client said that she had been up all night thinking about something I had said when I walked into a room in which she was speaking to two vulnerable women in a way that was increasing their sense of shame and stupidity. "You said to me," she declared, " 'What I see going on here makes me sick.' "

She went on to say that she had been in one therapy after another for 20 years, and though she had been offered much insight about the source of her problems and much advice about solving them, no one had ever told her before that she was often a nasty person who was skilled at making other people feel bad when she wanted some relief from her own pain. "That I can do something about, if you all continue to let me know when I am doing it."

From this perspective two new groups developed. The Values Group addresses a range of topics suggested each semester by the participants, for example, My Rights, Control, Forgiveness, Trust, Prejudice, Guilt, Pleasure, Purpose and Meaning, and Life, Death, Relationships, and Work.

A series of questions are posed under each heading, and participants struggle to understand and articulate their beliefs. This always involves much wrestling with contradictions and rarely results in easy certainties. Values is considered one of the most challenging groups in the program, but participants invariably grow measurably in their ability to question their values, to question their questions, and finally to begin to develop a mature and conscious belief system that is a helpful guide to behavior. As part of this group, the participants created the statement depicted in Figure 9.1, in which they expressed their view of what they were agreeing to in terms of their rights and the rights of others when they joined the Chrysalis Program. They consider it to be their own informed consent.

Everyone participates in the Values group; it is now core to the program. About half the participants choose to attend the second group that evolved out of discussions about what brings moments of peace and hope to the participants' tumultuous and frequently despair-filled lives. Though Chrysalis group members are diverse in religious/cultural backgrounds and current religious beliefs, they were readily able to identify common sources of grounding and strength, including music, nature, relationships with animals and/or children, quiet reflection/meditation, and poetry and other inspirational writings. We decided to come together once during the week to read aloud, sing, and sit a while in silence—a time dedicated to focusing on these sources of peace and connecting with a level of existence that is deeper than the agitated anguish most participants experience more often than not. This has led to the ongoing creation of a book of readings and songs from a range of cultures and a shelf full of natural objects that hold

Show respect for myself and others':

- Differences
- Confidentiality
- Struggles
- Privacy
- Opinions
- Space
- Beliefs
- Property

Take responsibility for:

- Being aware of how my actions and words affect others.
- Not judging others based on race, religious, or cultural beliefs and backgrounds or sexual orientation.
- Not acting out destructive and self-destructive behaviors in program, that is, no physical violence toward others, no verbal lashing out at others, no self-harm.
- Learning how to speak about my experiences in groups in a way that does not upset or scare other participants (e.g., no graphic details of traumatic experiences, past or present); instead, focusing on my feelings and my struggles.
- Not dumping my problems on the laps of others; not asking that others rescue me from myself.
- Encouraging others to be responsible for themselves rather than rescuing them.
- Being rigorous about confidentiality; not disclosing any information from the program to nonparticipants.
- Sharing food, computer time, telephone access, and other program resources fairly with others.
- Being open in group about my own struggles and also bringing grievances and disagreements with others out directly in the group.
- Cleaning up after myself both in program space and on hospital property, indoors and out.
- Asking for help when I need it, rather than waiting for someone else to notice.
- Doing my share to create a clean and pleasant physical environment.
- Being willing to listen with an open mind, even when what is being said is difficult to hear.
- Being open to challenge and/or constructive criticism.
- Meeting weekly goals whenever possible and acknowledging openly when this is not happening rather than waiting for someone else to point it out.
- Arriving at groups on time with homework completed.
- Paying attention to what others have to say in groups, rather than fidgeting, doodling, sleeping, etc.
- Understanding that anger and power struggles with staff and other participants are to be learned from, not suppressed or acted out.
- Not engaging in any sexual behavior with other program participants.
- Showing tolerance, knowing that everyone's struggle is difficult.
- Bringing back to group anything I am concerned about that occurs or is said in social situations with other program participants.
- Not gossiping or spreading rumors.
- Being discrete about taking medications.
- Eating a healthy lunch each day at program and not wasting food.
- Being kind to any animals who are at the program, not feeding them, and when taking them out, picking up after them.
- Attending all groups for which I have signed up.
- Notifying the program anytime I have to be absent, so that others do not worry about me.

FIGURE 9.1. Chrysalis Day Program covenant.

254

great meaning for the clients who choose to participate in the group called "Reflections." Frequently, clients who have been part of this group request, on graduation, a copy of the book of readings and songs, so they can incorporate them into their ongoing life. Two participants expressed their views about the difference the values component of the program made to their growth:

"Being a part of a group of people struggling with some issues the same as mine, some very different, has not been easy for me. I had little tolerance for people who were gay, who were not white, or who came from different countries and had different customs. I was taught these prejudices in my family and didn't even think to challenge them as an adult. Because of wanting to be in this group so as to change my life I have worked hard to be open to people who are different from me—both in the program and in the community I live in. We have two groups that are based on what our beliefs and values are and these have helped me to look at my beliefs, to understand how I developed them, and to ask myself if I still want to hold on to them. For the first time, I can feel what another person is feeling and care about that, rather than walking around in a rage, not aware of anything or anyone except my anger. I know that the prejudices I learned as a child are ignorant, and I am trying to change the ways I judge people."

"Before I came to the Chrysalis Program I had very little sense of right and wrong and not much conscience about harmful actions. In my family, people went to church on Sunday and beat and starved their children every day of the week. I learned to be scornful of any values people talked about, thinking they were deceitful. Now I am trying to discover what my beliefs are and to treat people (including myself) according to them. It is very hard to turn around 50 years of thinking, but I have a little hope that I can make my life different if I do this."

TREATMENT OUTCOME

There are many ways in which the Chrysalis program participants demonstrate the benefits that accrue from their intensive treatment regimen. Each week, every Chrysalis participant records both her goals regarding specific changes she wishes to make ("No self-harm"; "Eat one healthy meal and one snack each day"; "Leave the room and do an emotion sheet when I feel a strong impulse to scream at my son") and her degree of success in meeting the previous week's goals. These weekly goals and achievements are systematically entered into her chart. At the end of each semester, she summarizes the changes she has made in her life over the preceding 4 months and reads these accomplishments aloud in the community group. The summary is then also entered into her chart. The chart entries provide a clear record of each participant's progress both weekly and by semester.

A quantitative measure of the effectiveness of the Chrysalis program as a whole is the reduced number of psychiatric inpatient days required by participants during treatment and after discharge. Although many individuals diagnosed with severe personality disorders are regular consumers of hospital inpatient services, research suggests that they do not benefit from their frequent or prolonged hospitalizations; in fact, their symptoms are often exacerbated in the hospital (Dawson & MacMillan, 1993; Linehan, 1993; Paris, 1994). We have had similar clinical experiences with Chrysalis participants. Many of them have spent long periods of time on psychiatric wards or in psychiatric hospitals, and they have rarely benefited from these treatments.

We started keeping track of psychiatric hospitalization records in 1998. We were able to gather complete information on 40 participants, who have been discharged for more than 1 year since that date. The data (Table 9.1) demonstrate that the program enables participants to decrease significantly their dependence on psychiatric hospitalization, both while they engage in treatment and 1 year after discharge. This enhances the quality of participants' lives and cuts health care system costs.

CONCLUSION

Throughout history, there have been individuals in every society who have not conformed to social norms about how people should behave. Which

TABLE 9.1. Forty Clients Discharged for More Than 1 Year, 1998–2001

	No. clients admitted to psychiatric hospital/ward	Avg. no. admissions per client admitted	Avg. length of admission
Five years before entry	26 (65.0%)	3.3	47 days
During program	8 (20.0%)	1.3	19 days
One year after leaving	5 (12.5%)	1.8	12 days

behaviors are framed as pathological (or criminal or sinful) depends on their threat to the particular social order within which they live. Psychiatry and psychology rarely analyze or challenge the norms we prescribe. Practitioners and researchers in the area of mental health are mainly concerned with what we understand as pathology, and we rarely concern ourselves with questioning our epistemological frameworks and our values. Along with most other mental health professional programs, particularly those in a mainstream institution, the Chrysalis Program incorporates categories of pathology that are extremely problematic. We speak and write about our clients in language that is limited at best and frequently stigmatizing and oppressive. At the same time and in the same context, we offer a therapy process to these same clients that encourages them to rebel against these oppressive frameworks. Such contradictions are part of our everyday functioning, and we are willing to live with them in order to offer the services we do to people who could not ordinarily afford them. What we are not willing to do is pretend that these contradictions do not exist.

Though it is clear that the people who participate in the Chrysalis Program have a great deal of trouble "creating stable lives in the community," as the program pamphlet states, it is an extremely narrow explanation of this phenomenon to say that this is because they have personality disorders. But it is the explanation the mental health system offers again and again, through its emphasis on psychometric testing, psychodiagnosis, and our tautological explanations about why people behave in the distressing ways they do: "She cuts her body up because she has borderline personality disorder; we know she has borderline personality disorder because she cuts her body up."

The framework of the Chrysalis Program conforms to contemporary psychological and psychiatric norms to as great a degree as any other program operating out of a university hospital. Though we buy into many limited and limiting practices of mainstream mental health ideology, we also challenge the norms every day of the Chrysalis Program's operation. It's the best we can do, as far as we can see, if we are to offer practical help that our clients can access and afford. As Hanna Lerman (1996) has observed, if a treatment model is not clinically useful, it may not be feminist. The ability to live with uncomfortable contradictions in order to make ourselves as useful as possible to our clients is a particularly feminist feat. Refined and rarefied therapeutic models may be theoretically satisfying to construct, but they rarely encompass the very real and pressing needs of the people who have been and continue to be most damaged by the oppressive culture in which they live.

The process of both buying into mainstream mental health ideology and practice and alternately and often simultaneously disrupting it is reflective of all our personal and social struggles with living in the social context we do. Learning to survive and even thrive within a patriarchal society, conforming to many of its restrictive dictates while at the same time challenging them, is a social skill worth passing on to the participants in the program, whose material circumstances make it unlikely that they will be able to create an alternative lifestyle for themselves that is radically independent of mainstream culture and its demands.

Many of the Chrysalis participants have always rebelled against the norms of the dominant culture, sometimes directly, most often through what are understood as their symptoms. They do not cut and burn themselves, scream and yell at authority figures, repeatedly attempt suicide, starve themselves, and forget huge chunks of their life experience because they have a disease or a dozen diseases. They do so mostly to say "No." No, I won't carry the burden of our secrets. No, I won't pretend it is alright to live the way I do. No, no, no—something about the way things are has to change.

These are generally not very effective protests. They are antiestablishment, but they are conservative as well. These women revolt, but they are destroyed. They display the cracks in the smooth surface of the system, but the system almost always closes in on them, and its power is reinforced by the destruction of those who dare to expose its underbelly. Their protests end up reinforcing the walls of the prisons that they are attempting to break out of, prisons that were created by many others—and indeed by all of us at some level—and to which they eventually contribute themselves. But they are protests more than they are symptoms of a disease, and it is the goal of the Chrysalis Program not to cure them of a disorder, but to enable them to protest more creatively and effectively for the rest of their lives, as well as to live in some personal peace within the culture that both nurturers and diminishes us all. One of the participant's response to the question, "How has the Chrysalis Program made a difference in your life?", reflects her appreciation of a feminist therapeutic community that fosters both protest and peace:

"I have found a safe place I never dreamed existed—a place where I've been given permission to acknowledge the rage I carry and to use that rage constructively to really explore and question the beliefs that regulate my life minute by minute. I'm being encouraged and challenged each and every day to feel, question, and think beyond the boundaries of conformity. I am being shown that it is okay to have a voice of my own, that I can decide for myself what matters, what is important, what I want. For the first time in my life, I now know that I have both the right and the power to make my own choices."

REFERENCES

American Psychiatric Association (1994). *Diagnostic and statistical manual of mental disorders* (4th ed.). Washington, DC: Author.

Andreoli, A., Gressot, G., Aapro, L., Tricot, L., & Gognalons, M. Y. (1989). Personality disorders as a predictor of outcome. *Journal of Personality Disorders, 3*(4), 307–320.

Beckman, K. A., & Burns, G. L. (1990). Relation of sexual abuse and bulimia in college women. *International Journal of Eating Disorders, 9*(5), 487–492.

Bordo, S. (1990). Reading the slender body, In M. Jacobus, E. F. Keller, & S. Shuttleworth (Eds.), *Body/politics: Women and the discourses of science.* New York: Routledge.

Brown, L. S. (2000). Discomforts of the powerless: Feminist constructions of distress. In R. A. Neimeyer & J. D. Raskin (Eds.), *Constructions of disorder: Meaning-making frameworks for psychotherapy* (pp. 287–308). Washington, DC: American Psychological Association.

Brown, L. S. (1994). *Subversive dialogues: Theory in feminist therapy.* New York: Basic Books.

Brown, L. S., & Ballou, M. (Eds.). (1992). *Personality and psychopathology: Feminist reappraisals.* New York: Guilford Press.

Chernin, K. (1986). *The hungry self: Women, eating and identity.* London: Virago Press.

Chesler, P. (1972). *Women and madness.* Garden City, NY: Doubleday.

Clarkin, J. F., Foelsch, P. A., Levy, K. N., Hull, J. W., Delaney, J. C., & Kernberg, O. F. (2001). The development of a psychodynamic treatment for patients with borderline personality disorder: A preliminary study of behavioral change. *Journal of Personality Disorders, 15*(6), 487–495.

Dawson, D., & MacMillan, H. L. (1993). *Relationship management of the borderline patient: From understanding to treatment.* New York: Brunner/Mazel.

Dolan-Sewell, R. T., Krueger, R. F., & Shea, M. T. (2001). Co-occurrence with syndrome disorders. In W. J. Livesley (Ed.), *Handbook of personality disorders: Theory, research, and treatment* (pp. 84–104). New York: Guilford Press.

Ferro, T., Klein, D. N., Schwartz, J. E., Kasch, K. L., & Leader, J. B. (1998). 30-month stability of personality disorder diagnoses in depressed outpatients. *American Journal of Psychiatry, 155*(5), 653–659.

Gunderson, J. (1983). DSM-III diagnoses of personality disorders. In J. P. Frosch (Ed.), *Current perspectives on personality disorders* (pp. 20–39). Washington. DC: American Psychiatric Press.

Hare-Mustin, R., & Mareck, J. (Eds.). (1990). *Making a difference: Psychology and the construction of gender.* New Haven, CT: Yale University Press.

Herman, J. (1992). *Trauma and recovery: The aftermath of violence from domestic abuse to political terror.* New York: Basic Books.

Kernberg, O. F., (1988). Clinical dimensions of masochism. *Journal of the American Psychoanalytic Association, 36,* 1005–1029.

Kernberg, O. F., Selzer, M., Koenigsberg, H., Carr, A., & Appelbaum, A. (1989). *Psychodynamic psychotherapy of borderline patients.* New York: Basic Books.

Klein, M. H., Wonderlich, S., & Shea, M. R. (1993). Models of relationships between personality and depression: Toward a framework of theory and research. In M. H. Klein, D. J. Kupfer, & M. T. Shea (Eds.), *Personality and depression: A current view* (pp. 1–54). New York: Guilford Press.

Koenigsberg, H., Kernberg, O. F., Stone, M. H., Appelbaum, A. H., Yeomans, F. E., & Diamond, D. (2000). *Borderline patients: Extending the limits of treatability.* New York: Basic Books.

Lerman, H. (1996). *Pigeonholing women's misery: A history and critical analysis of the psychodiagnosis of women in the twentieth century.* New York: Basic Books.

Linehan, M. M. (1993). *Cognitive-behavioral treatment of borderline personality disorder.* New York: Guilford Press.

Links, P. (1993). Psychiatric rehabilitation model for borderline personality disorder. *Canadian Journal of Psychiatry, 38*(Suppl.), 5358–5385.

Links, P. (1998). Developing effective services for patients with personality disorders. *Canadian Journal of Psychiatry, 43,* 251–259.

Livesley, W. J. (1987). A systematic approach to the delineation of personality disorders. *American Journal of Psychiatry, 144,* 772–777.

Livesley, W. J. (2001). A framework for an integrated approach to treatment. In W. J. Livesley (Ed.), *Handbook of personality disorders: Theory, research, and treatment* (pp. 570–600). New York: Guilford Press.

Orbach, S. (1979). *Fat is a feminist issue.* London: Hamlyn.

Paris, J. (1994). *Borderline personality disorder: A mutidimensional approach.* Washington, DC: American Psychiatric Press.

Paris, J. (1996). *Social factors in the personality disorders: A biopsychosocial approach to etiology and treatment.* New York: Cambridge University Press.

Paris, J. (1998). *Working with traits: Psychotherapy of personality disorders.* Northvale, NJ: Jason Aronson.

Paris, J., Nowlis, D., & Brown, R. (1989). Predictions of suicide in borderline personality disorder. *Canadian Journal of Psychiatry, 34,* 8–9.

Piper, W., Rosie, J., Joyce, A., & Azim, H. (1996). *Time-limited day treatment for personality disorders: Integration of research and practice in a group program.* Washington, DC: American Psychological Association.

Rivera, M. (1996). *More alike than different: Treating severely dissociative trauma survivors.* Toronto: University of Toronto Press.

Rivera, M., & Wachob, S. (in press). The darkness rainbow: Treating child sexual abuse survivors who are lesbian, gay, bisexual, and transgendered. In L. Walker (Ed.), *Handbook of the treatment of child sexual abuse* (2nd ed.). New York: Springer.

Root, M. P. P. (1992). Reconstructing the impact of trauma on personality In L. S.

Brown & M. Ballou (Eds.), *Personality and psychopathology: Feminist reappraisals* (pp. 229–265). New York: Guilford Press.

Sanislow, C., & McGlashan, T. (1998). Treatment outcome of personality disorders. *Canadian Journal of Psychiatry, 43*, 237–250.

Scott, L. (1999, Fall). Chrysalis Day Program collective kitchens. Washington, DC: *Mental Health Network Newsletter, 3*.

Scott, L. (2000, Spring). Chrysalis Day Program collective kitchens satisfaction survey. Washington, DC: *Mental Health Network Newsletter, 4*.

Stone, M. H. (1990). *The fate of borderline patients: Successful outcome and psychiatric practice*. New York: Guilford Press.

Szekeley, E. (1988). *Never too thin*. Toronto: Women's Press.

van der Kolk, B., Roth, S., Pelcovity, D., & Mandel, F. (1993). *Disorders of extreme stress: Results of the DSM-IV field trials for PTSD*. Washington, DC: American Psychiatric Association.

Widiger, T. A. (2001). Official classification systems. In W. J. Livesley (Ed.), *Handbook of personality disorders: Theory, research, and treatment* (pp. 60–83). New York: Guilford Press.

Wolf, N. (1990). *The beauty myth: How images of beauty are used against women*. London: Vintage.

Work Group on Borderline Personality Disorder. (2001). Practice guidelines for the treatment of patients with borderline personality disorder. *American Journal of Psychiatry, 158*(Suppl.), 1–52.

World Health Organization. (1992). *International statistical classification and diseases and related health problems* (10th rev.). Geneva: Author.

Zimmerman, M. (1994). Diagnosing personality disorders: A review of issues and research methods. *Archives of General Psychiatry, 51*, 225–242.

Chapter 10

Contextual and Developmental Frameworks in Diagnosing Children and Adolescents

NATALIE PORTER

The medical model in general and the DSM classification system in particular do not represent the mental health realities of women or children. Medical models have been critiqued by feminists as pathology driven, individualistically oriented (Sherwin, 1992), concentrated on power hierarchies, disregarding of social context, and applying medical disease models to social problems, including those created by oppression (Liburd & Rothblum, 1995). Much of this volume has elaborated on feminist critiques and analyses of the problems and limitations of mental health diagnosis and personality assessment as they are commonly applied to women. The critiques offered generally are applicable to the issues surrounding mental health diagnoses for children and adolescents as well. In this chapter I specifically critique the mental health diagnostic issues confronting children and adolescents. I will not reiterate much of the feminist critique provided in previous chapters, although they set the context for this chapter.

Children are ill served by contemporary diagnostic systems and practices in the following ways:

1. Development is insufficiently addressed and adult diagnoses do not fit childhood problems.
2. Context is ignored or not addressed in meaningful ways.

3. Power and control issues often contribute to the misdiagnosis and mistreatment of children and adolescents.
4. Victimization, trauma, and loss are too infrequently addressed.
5. Pathology is emphasized while strengths are ignored or minimized.
6. Long-term costs of mental health diagnoses and treatment are frequently overlooked or unknown.
7. Sexism, classism, racism, and homophobia clearly contribute to children's mental health problems, but rarely are considered in their diagnoses or in diagnostic nomenclature.

DEVELOPMENT IS INSUFFICIENTLY ADDRESSED IN DIAGNOSTIC SCHEMAS

Adult diagnoses do not fit childhood disorders, behaviors, or experiences and, as many of the previous chapters demonstrate, the diagnostic system is all too often irrelevant and ill suited for women. In the case of children and adolescents, it is derivative as well. An adult-centered diagnostic system has been handed down with relatively little attention paid initially to its pertinence or usefulness. For the most part, the diagnostic nomenclature and categories developed to describe symptoms and disorders experienced by adults were adapted or expanded to include children. There have been improvements and refinements in these categories over time, evidenced by the differences between the original DSM and the DSM-IV, as attempts to address these limitations were made. Nevertheless, the improvements are more akin to altering the suit of an adult man to fit a 5-year-old boy than to tailoring an appropriate outfit for the boy from new cloth. The DSM remains an exercise of fitting the child to the category rather than beginning with a system that is developmental in nature and takes a holistic approach in understanding and describing children's experiences and behaviors within a broader social, economic, and familial framework.

Although in theory Western clinical psychology is swinging back from describing human beings solely from an individualist perspective, practice has not kept pace, especially in mental health and diagnostic areas. A developmental perspective, by definition, would attend to children within the context of their families, cultures, and environments. The developmental principle of adaptation affirms that children are shaped by and adapt to the environmental contexts in which they live. Thus, these contexts do more than inform us about the child's experience, they form the child.

POWER AND CONTROL ISSUES BIAS DIAGNOSIS AND TREATMENT OF CHILDREN AND ADOLESCENTS

"Children have traditionally been at the bottom of the hierarchy in terms of status, power, control, and/or decision-making" (Conoley & Larsen, 1995, p. 203) and have historically been labeled with the same adjectives as women: "dependent, intellectually inferior, physically weak, and with limited roles potential" (Conoley & Larsen, 1995, p. 202). However, the comparison between children and adult women is complex. Children do require support and protection to develop fully or to achieve their potential. The challenge is to develop a policy and a diagnostic perspective about children and adolescents that takes into account their needs, vulnerabilities, and developmental levels while promoting growth and increasing self-determination. Policy should make the child's needs the priority rather than adult self-interest or self-promotion. Feminists have advocated for and supported child protection legislation in several areas because we consider children and adolescents more vulnerable and easily exploited than adults. Sexual abuse legislation is an example of a protection generally viewed as necessary by feminists and child advocates. At the same time, feminists have supported increased self-determination for adolescents in areas such as medical decision making, where research has demonstrated their capacity to understand the issues and make sound decisions by the age of 14 (Melton, 1983).

Childhood mental health symptoms are most commonly defined through children's relationships with adults. The range of behaviors addressed in formal diagnostic schema is limited, and nuance is distinctly lacking in how symptoms are viewed or described. From this adult-oriented perspective, what appears to be noticed most often is whether children comply with rules and avoid disrupting others. Children are referred for treatment when their behavior is annoying to adults, particularly to their caretakers and teachers. On the one hand, these adults may be best equipped to observe a child's difficulties. On the other hand, behaviors that are annoying may be disproportionately reported. The result may be overattention to "misbehavior" and lack of attention to the environmental contexts that are either causing or exacerbating the expression of the positive symptom ("acting out") or suppressing the expression of other, more prosocial behaviors. These "children should be seen but not heard" biases are built into the DSM and related diagnostic systems. The result is often the tendency to overlook the more "silent" disorders such as depression and to give children and adolescents diagnoses of attention deficit, conduct, and oppositional defiant disorders when the behaviors manifested fall into the realm of "misbehavior." The same symptoms of misbehavior may also be symptomatic of posttraumatic stress disorder, anxiety disorders, or depression. The section below that discusses the physical and sexual victimization of children elaborates further on this problem.

Children diagnosed with oppositional defiant disorder represent a significant proportion of the children and adolescents in the mental health system. Estimates of prevalence rates range from 8.7 to 34% (Finney, Riley, & Cataldo, 1991). However, many research studies have confirmed that acting-out behaviors are common in children who are depressed or anxious. Brumback, Dietz-Schmidt, and Weinberg (1977) found that anger and irritability are common symptoms among depressed children and adolescents. So too are "negativism, uncooperativeness, sulking, a belligerent attitude . . . [and] . . . decreased academic performance, social withdrawal, antisocial behavior, increased drug and alcohol use (Stark, Dempsey, & Christopher, 1993, p. 116). Relationships among depression, aggression or conduct disorder, and suicidal behavior have also been found (Apter, Bleich, Plutchik, & Mendelsohn, 1988; Cairns, Peterson, & Nickerman, 1988).

A more fundamental problem may be the failure to evolve a diagnostic system that adequately takes developmental research into account by differentiating "misbehavior" that is the result of conduct problems (e.g., intentional, planned behavior) from a child or adolescent's failure to develop particular abilities or skills. For example, the abilities to self-regulate and control impulses require both biological maturation and social conditions that promote learning control, such as caretaker expectations. Interference with development may mean interference with the development of these abilities. For example, stress and anxiety may interfere with the developmental of self-regulation because they prevent the consolidation of learning. Given the individualistic and goal orientations of U.S. society, the distinction between a problem behavior that represents interference with development or victimization from one that represents "intentional misbehavior" is often considered irrelevant by the public, even to those who work with children. However, there are clear implications for mental health interventions and prevention, and mental health nomenclature would be more useful if developmental distinctions were made. As the system currently operates, the diagnoses of conduct and oppositional defiant disorders are such nonspecific categories that they provide insufficient information to be of much use in treatment or prevention. But they do provide a rationale for punishment and control of adolescents via juvenile justice venues rather than in mental health settings, particularly for children and adolescents of color (Valdez, 1994). Feminists have been less visible in advocating for children's mental health issues, particularly in working to ensure positive interventions rather than incarceration for children and adolescents who are poor or of color.

VICTIMIZATION, TRAUMA, AND LOSS ARE INSUFFICIENTLY ADDRESSED IN CURRENT SCHEMAS

As with adult women, the prevalence of physical and sexual abuse in children and adolescents is substantial. Diagnoses that do not address this victimization directly are just as problematic for children and adolescents as they are for adult women. Sexual abuse and severe physical abuse in infants and children have been found to result in aggressive behavior on the part of the child or adolescent as well as in serious depression (Egeland, Sroufe, & Erickson, 1983). What is unclear is whether the behavioral problems found in abused children are the result of their depression and stigmatization rather than a conduct disorder or oppositional defiant disorder per se. Just as in adult women, a category of trauma-related disorders would better serve children and adolescents because they would result in less stigmatization and guide treatment in more appropriate directions. Furthermore, one can conceptualize the behavioral disorders in abused children as symptoms of distress. Yet, when the diagnosis of conduct or oppositional defiant disorder is given to the child, she or he becomes the focus of the intervention, which may not allay the true problem.

Some researchers have suggested that conduct disorder is a depressive reaction to physical abuse (Lakey, Hartdagen, Frick, & McBurnett, 1988; Wishik, Bachman, & Bertch, 1989). Physical abuse occurring in infancy, childhood, or adolescence, appears to result in both higher levels of acting-out problems in adolescents (Deykin, Alpert, & McNamarra, 1985; Livingston, 1987) and depression (Kazdin, Moser, Colbus, & Bell, 1985). Coercive parent–child interactions have been found to lead to the development of conduct disorders in children (Horne, Norsworthy, Forehand, & Frame, 1990; Patterson, Reid, Jones, & Conger, 1975). The research by Patterson and colleagues (1975) suggests that what is interpreted as antisocial behavior in children is actually made up of many different symptom clusters. They argue that the child's clinical picture can only be understood by examining the behavior in the context of the situation. Reeves, Werry, Elkind, and Zametkin (1987) studied 108 children with diagnoses related to behavioral problems, including conduct disorder (CD), oppositional defiant disorder (ODD), and attention deficit disorder (ADD). They concluded that ODD and CD may actually be the same disorder, with CD diagnosed in boys and ODD in girls. The hallmarks of both diagnoses were negative childrearing contexts and poor interpersonal relationships. Children with two of the diagnoses, typically ADD and CD, were found to have a much greater frequency of adverse family backgrounds, usually having fathers with alcoholic or antisocial personalities and lower educational levels. Depression scores have also been found to correlate with family dysfunction (Kaslow, Rehm, & Siegel, 1984) and to be moderately associated with the number of conflicts with parents (Forehand et al., 1988). What is less clear from research, but supported anecdotally, is whether the ODD and CD diagnoses take precedent over those of depression in children suffering from abuse and conflict-ridden family environments because they are more obvious and disruptive.

As with physical abuse, sexual abuse produces significant variations in symptom constellations. Sexually abused girls exhibit greater behavior and emotional difficulties than girls who had not been abused (Einbender & Friedrich, 1989; Friedrich, Beilke, & Urquiza, 1987; Mannarino, Cohen, & Gregor, 1989), and some of these differences fall into the area of problem behaviors. Ten percent of children known to have been sexually abused receive diagnoses of CD and ODD, and an additional 3–5% are diagnosed as ADD (Cohen & Mannarino, 1993; Sirles, Smith, & Kusama, 1989). Sexually abused girls have been found to have higher scores on the Child Behavior Checklist on the total behavior problem scale, the internalization scale, the externalizing scale, and on seven of nine subscales at the initial evaluation and at 6- to 12-month follow-up (Mannarino, Cohen, Smith, & Moore-Motily, 1990). Sexually abused children tend not to endorse specific symptoms such as depression on checklists, but instead endorse items that express their feeling of being stigmatized, such as that they feel "different," possess less trust, feel responsible for negative events and disbelieved by others (Cohen & Mannarino, 1993). Sexually abused children also exhibit significantly greater rates of "sexually inappropriate" behaviors (Friedrich et al., 1987; Mannarino et al., 1989).

Diagnosis does matter when the diagnosis given refers to a serious behavioral disorder. As Ballou (1995) has pointed out, "naming is a powerful act. In naming we clinically define and direct attention to certain things and away from other things" (p. 42). For example, consider the difference between labeling an adolescent who as a child had been routinely sexually abused by her grandfather and made to witness him strangling her cat, with a diagnosis of posttraumatic stress disorder (PTSD) versus ODD, when her rage and confusion emerged. Or consider the outcome of diagnosing an adopted child who is not establishing relationships with her new parents, whose history included witnessing her parents being killed by the army of her country of origin, as severe reactive attachment or with PTSD stemming from severe loss or dislocation. A child whose diagnosis connotes poor prospects for developing interpersonal relationships and leaves bewildered parents and other caretakers with a sense of hopelessness and powerlessness may experience significantly different outcomes than a child with a diagnosis that promotes concern and empathy and carries hope for change.

CONTEXT IS IGNORED OR NOT ADDRESSED IN MEANINGFUL WAYS

The failure to address context in all of its forms is problematic with diagnostic systems for both children and adults. Other authors in this volume have addressed this issue comprehensively. Their analyses pertain to children and adolescents as well; diagnosis cannot occur without understanding the child or adolescent holistically and taking into account all aspects of her or his "environment" and all it encompasses (Koss-Chioino & Vargas, 1999). The tendency to diagnose abused children with CD or ODD is one such failure. Although the latest revisions of the DSM have attempted to incorporate context in diagnosing children, particularly through the use of V-codes and global scales of stress and functioning, this approach is insufficient. It fails to recognize that behavior (symptoms), their meaning, their severity, one's experiences (antecedents), and the environment (stressors) represent an interactive, reciprocal, dynamic process, not a summative, static process. Contexts cannot be viewed as "auxiliary information" about a child or adolescent that can be linearly tacked on to a diagnostic impression. Such is the case with current diagnostic systems. When contexts are considered, they rarely are viewed as integral to one's understanding of the whole picture of the child and fundamental to grasping what "psychopathology" means for any particular individual in any specific context.

The mental health reimbursement system exacerbates this diagnostic dilemma. When the more interactive diagnoses that connote family conflict or abuse or poverty are given as primary diagnoses, they are not accepted by mental health insurers as sufficient for payment for treatment. Children diagnosed with "adjustment disorders," for example, are not viewed as having serious difficulties, when, from a developmental and contextual perspective, the environmental issues may interfere substantially with the child's capacity to develop cognitively and emotionally. From a developmental perspective, psychological interventions should be available when developmental interruptions occur and not only when serious consequences have emerged. Some circumstances, such as adverse poverty, may actually disqualify children and adolescents from receiving treatment because they are viewed as sociocultural rather than "psychological" problems.

COSTS OF MENTAL HEALTH DIAGNOSES AND TREATMENT MAY OUTWEIGH THE BENEFITS

The effect of mental health diagnoses is a serious consideration for the feminist psychologist. As mental health professionals, we would like to think that diagnosis has positive or at least benign consequences. Ideally, a child or adolescent who receives an accurate diagnosis would be better understood by her or his caretakers, receive more appropriate treatment in social and community settings such as school systems, and receive supports through the mental health system. As feminist psychologists, we are all too aware of the reality versus the ideal.

Stigmatization is a serious consequence of mental health diagnoses. Selekman (1997) has eloquently argued that the diagnostic label a child receives will become the only way of thinking about her or his problem, not only in the present but also in the past and future as well. Historically, diagnosis was considered less valuable in the field of child mental health, but began to increase two decades ago as reimbursement standards required it (Lonigan, Elbert, & Johnson, 1998). Clinicians cannot receive payment for services without diagnoses, but children with diagnoses may experience long-term financial, educational, emotional, and social jeopardy. Families of children with mental health diagnoses increasingly report that they are denied insurance coverage and are unable to change insurance carriers, or that their children must report mental health or substance abuse treatment on college and employment application forms. Children and families feel increasingly stigmatized by a system that forces labeling to receive services and then denies services and restricts one's future opportunities because of the label that connotes a stable affliction rather than a developmentally and socially based period of difficulty.

The relationship of medical model diagnoses to the growing reliance on psychopharmacological treatments is another concern. The *Report of the*

Surgeon General on Children's Mental Health (1999) described the "dramatic" (p. 140) rise in the use of psychotropic medications in children and adolescents despite the "dearth of research" (p. 141). The report summarizes the lack of studies or evidence in three areas specifically: (1) the long-term safety or efficacy of medications, and in many cases even short-term efficacy; (2) pediatric pharmacokinetics; and (3) the efficacy of medication when combined with other interventions. Although recent research has not found that attention-deficit/hyperactivity disorder (ADHD) is overdiagnosed or overmedicated (Jenson et al., 1999), when prevalence rates are compared to treatment rates, the Surgeon General's report suggests that some of the substantial increase in stimulant prescriptions in the past decade could be the result of misdiagnosis and inappropriate treatment. Angold and Costello (1998), for example, found that most of the children receiving stimulants do not meet the criteria for the diagnosis of ADHD. Jenson and colleagues (1999) found that most of the stimulants are prescribed by family practitioners who are less likely than pediatricians or psychiatrists to perform comprehensive evaluations, offer mental health interventions, or follow-up care.

I would argue that medications are increasing as other resources for children are declining. Teachers faced with increasingly larger numbers of children in their classes, for example, have less time to work with children individually or to provide structure for children who require it. With greater economic challenges, families frequently have less time to oversee their children's activities and development. In my experience, children are commonly referred to clinics by schools with explicit directives to medicate them for "hyperactivity." It is not uncommon for alternative diagnoses or treatments to be rejected by the school. The treating therapist or physician may be faced with the dilemma that to not medicate may subject the child to punitive treatment in the school system.

STRENGTHS AND RESOURCES
ARE INSUFFICIENTLY ADDRESSED

The critique that the medical model is deficit-driven and ignores the child's strengths or resources is hardly new, but carries specific consequences for children and adolescents. Although prior to the 1980s mental health diagnosis was less important in the child mental health field than when working with adults (Lonigan et al., 1998), a shift toward pathology models has since occurred. A question that has become more heretical within child mental health systems is whether diagnostic models should focus on strengths rather than psychopathology, despite the lack of evidence that medical model diagnoses result in greater treatment efficacy. One counter-position has been articulated by Bill O'Hanlon in the following way: "What we need is a list of strengths as powerful and as validating as the florid vocabulary of diseases found in DSM-IV to combat our national obsession with pathology" (Selekman, 1997, p. 24).

As I have taught and supervised student therapists from a variety of disciplines and orientations over the years, I have been struck with the discomfort experienced by many student therapists when I have encouraged them to look for the positive aspects of their clients' problems and to redefine their negative problems by articulating the positive (reframing). Although clients clearly welcomed new understandings of their situations, the therapists often viewed this process as naive or, worse, as dishonest, the "sugar coating" of a negative behavior. The discomfort appeared stronger in therapists whose previous educational experiences were more grounded in theoretical models that emphasized pathology or deficits. Many students maintained this position despite my attempts to demonstrate that reframing allows the therapist to shed her or his biases to "see" more clearly the client's motivations or use of coping mechanisms. I began to realize that many clinicians are so well indoctrinated into a model of psychopathology that they have difficulty viewing negative behavior in a dialectic way. The fear they often articulate is that to ignore the negative is to accept it.

Folk wisdom is filled with sayings that suggest that children "grow out" of behaviors, including negative ones, as they move to new developmental stages. Developmental research supports this commonly held idea. We also recognize, particularly in developing children, that overattention to particular phenomena exacerbate rather than alleviate them. For example, attention to dysfluent speech at critical ages may result in stuttering; fretting over a child's insomnia produces more lack of sleep. Yet as therapists we frequently feel an "obligation" to attend to the symptoms rather than to the strengths. The deficit model is not only incongruent with the feminist perspective, as elaborated throughout this volume, it is also the antithesis of developmental paradigms in that it emphasizes taking away rather than adding behaviors, skills, coping mechanisms, or adaptations. Developmental perspectives focus on growth, flexibility, resilience, and implementing new strategies when old ones fail. Taking away behaviors before a child or adolescent has mastered other behaviors can be problematic. Psychological development requires the learning of new skills obtained by building on one's strengths and previous learning. Diagnostic schemas that assess and catalog strengths would foster growth and healthy development by high-lighting the paths to particular behavioral and psychological goals.

SEXISM, RACISM, AND HOMOPHOBIA CLEARLY CONTRIBUTE TO CHILDREN'S MENTAL HEALTH PROBLEMS BUT NOT TO DIAGNOSTIC FRAMEWORKS

Twenty years has made a difference in the ways gender-role expectations and stereotypes influence mental health practitioners' beliefs about what constitutes pathology in boys and girls. Twenty years ago, I witnessed more than a few practitioners across multiple mental health settings describe girls as young as 6 years of age or in adolescence as "seductive" and even diagnose them with "hysteria" because of their styles of dress, which usually was "standard American garb." I have also witnessed girls wearing another standard U.S. uniform, blue jeans, described as "masculine" and diagnosed with gender identity disorders, particularly if they were not sexually developed. Practitioners used the diagnosis of gender identity disorder on youth who disclosed a gay or lesbian sexual orientation. These disclosures, for the most part, were not thought to predict an adolescent's stable or healthy sexual orientation but rather to reflect a "phase" of experimentation that an adolescent would outgrow. These beliefs seemed impervious to the adolescents' accounts of their own sexual histories, experiences, feelings, or level of insight.

Although the events described above may still occur, their frequency has been greatly reduced over the past two decades, thanks to greater information and an attitude change pertaining to gender roles and gender orientation. For example, the American Psychological Association's Children and Youth Committee has recommended the removal of gender identity disorder as a diagnostic category for children and adolescents. Today, clothing styles and stereotypic gender-role behavior appear to be less associated with personality attributions or diagnostic labels.

Nevertheless, sexism, and homophobia are at the root of serious issues pertaining to the diagnosis and misdiagnosis of children and adolescents. Diagnoses of gender identity disorder continue to be made, with boys given this label four times as often as are girls, a phenomenon that is likely rooted in stereotypic expectations of boy's gender-role behavior. The socially constructed origins of many mental health problems are ignored in favor of medical diagnoses. For example, girls are predominantly diagnosed with eating disorders, and in spite of 20 years of research and analysis showing the relationship of eating disorders to societal expectations and reward structures, media pressure, and the profit motives of the diet industry, these diagnoses have become increasingly biologically and medically oriented. For both girls and boys, the relationship of severe eating disorders to sports and dance (e.g., gymnastics, wrestling, and ballet) has been established but not reflected in diagnostic schemas.

A second area that has been ignored is the impact of peer-related sexual and physical harassment and violence on children and youth. A previous section described the mental health and diagnostic ramifications of child sexual and physical abuse committed by adults. Reports of sexual harassment, rape, and physical intimidation and assault, primarily of boys targeting girls, have received increasing attention by the public and the press. However, even as these problems have been exposed (Pipher, 1994), few remedies have followed. For the most part, schools and other public institutions still appear reluctant to recognize the harmful effects of this behavior and initiate appropriate preventative and educational actions. The mental health consequences of these daily occurrences are not covered in diagnostic systems, and diagnostic interviews rarely explore these events to integrate them into diagnostic profiles or treatment plans. Inquiries about battering, although prevalent among adolescents, are made infrequently. Although the negative impact of gay bashing and overt homophobia on the mental, physical, and social well-being of gay, lesbian, bisexual, and transgendered adolescents has been documented, adolescent victims are rarely accorded diagnoses that reflect these experiences, and diagnostic interviewers rarely solicit this type of information from them.

Ethnic and racial stereotypes effect mental health diagnosis and outcomes in similarly negative ways. White adolescents who break the law are more likely to receive mental health diagnosis and treatment than are persons of color, who are more likely to be sent to juvenile correctional facilities (Valdez, 1996) even though youth of color manifest higher depression scores on scales (Emslie, Weinberg, Rush, Adams, & Rintelmann, 1990; Garrison, Jackson, Marsteller, McKewon, & Addy, 1990) than do white males. Societal stereotypes of youth of color tend to portray them as predatory; their vulnerability and introspection are rarely pictured. Given the anxiety that has been generated around children of color, it is not surprising that they are handed punishment rather than treatment. Even the 1990s rash of random attacks and killings in schools by white males has not appeared to change the image of youth of color. Nor have the suicide data that position adolescent males of color at the top of the list (United States Office of the Surgeon General, 1999). Given this well-documented phenomenon, one can confidently conclude that something is wrong. Youth of color are clearly not receiving the services and interventions they need, although more children of color are involved in mental health systems than ever before.

Porter, Garcia, Jackson, and Valdez (1997) previously addressed how the mental health issues of children and adolescents of color are misunderstood and misrepresented. Many of the reasons are similar to those addressed in previous sections. Additional reasons include lack of understanding of cultural identity development and its impact on development in general, minimizing and ignoring the impact of the severe stressors that permeate the lives of many children and adolescents in U.S. society, and "mistaking cultural stereotypes for actual manifestations of culture" (p. 65). The authors urged mental health professionals to incorporate more culturally responsive strategies in their work, in order to "understand the psychological consequences of colonialism and intergenerational oppression," [to] "see the relationship among having one's language demeaned; one's rituals forbidden, forgotten, stolen, or co-opted; one's communities annihilated (whether by economic neglect, boycott, or redlining, by putting highways through and toxic dumps next to them, or through forced relocations) to PTSD, depression, despair, hopelessness, and helplessness. . . . Understanding how persons from a particular culture have survived in positive, adaptive ways . . . is essential" (p. 66).

TOWARD A DEVELOPMENTAL–ECOLOGICAL DIAGNOSTIC SYSTEM

An effective mental health schema for children and adolescents would incorporate developmental, ecological, social constructivist, and feminist frameworks within an interactive process. The ecological perspective, as described by Koss-Chioino and Vargas (1999), is the interweaving and interaction of all aspects of one's environment with all experiences, both to form the person and to "be" the person.

The Preamble of the United Nations Convention on the Rights of the Child (United Nations, 1989), adopted in 1989, states that children should be prepared to live in the "spirit of peace, dignity, tolerance, freedom, equality, and solidarity" (Andrews & Freeman, 1997). Specific articles of the convention specifically address issues that pertain to children's mental health, particularly if one adopts a holistic view of child well-being. They include the child's rights to be heard, to have access to mental health and disability services, to developmentally appropriate autonomy and privacy, to family integrity, to recovery treatment following trauma, to the least restrictive environment, to protection from harm, and to protection in out-of-home placements (Prilleltensky, 1994). The ecological, multicultural, feminist perspective promotes the holistic well-being and empowerment described in the U.N. Convention. It represents a strength-based, non-stigmatizing, empowerment model where collaboration with the child, honoring of the child's goals, power analysis, inclusion, and social change are essential.

THE CANARY IN THE MINESHAFT: AS SOCIETY GOES, SO GO ITS CHILDREN

As a feminist, I must pose the question of whether children should receive mental health diagnoses at all. The more alienating a society, the more alienated are its children. The fewer the resources for children, the more predatory or exploitative the society, the more mental health problems one should expect. This reasoning suggests that it is the society and not its children that should be diagnosed. Although I agree that the problems we are facing in our children and adolescents reflect societal problems, I also believe that we would be ill treating children and families if we returned solely to sociological explanations of behavior. This solution would oversimplify as much as the medical models currently do. Children and adolescents benefit more from an assessment that provides a holistic understanding of their lives. A purely constructivist approach that does not take into account, at the very least, the interaction of sociocultural and biopsychological factors seem regressive in both theory and practice.

REFERENCES

Andrews, A. B., & Freeman, M. L. (1997). Congruence of international children's rights and feminist principles as a foundation for therapy with young people. *Women and Therapy, 20*, 7–27.

Angold, A., & Costello, E. J. (1993). Depressive comorbidity in children and adolescents: Empirical, theoretical, and methodological issues. *American Journal of Psychiatry, 150*, 1779–1791.

Apter, A., Bleich, A., Plutchik, R., & Mendelsohn, S. (1988). Suicidal behavior, depression, and conduct disorder in hospitalized adolescents. *Journal of the American Academy of Child and Adolescent Psychiatry, 27*, 696–699.

Ballou, M. (1995). Naming the issue. In E. J. Rave & C. C. Larsen (Eds.), *Ethical decision making in therapy: Feminist perspectives* (pp. 42–56). New York: Guilford Press.

Brumback, R. A., Dietz-Schmidt, S. G., & Weinberg, W. A. (1977). Depression in children referred to an educational diagnostic center: Diagnosis and treatment and analysis of criteria and literature review. *Diseases of the Nervous System, 38,* 529–535.

Cairns, B. B., Peterson, G., & Nickerman, H. (1988). Suicidal behavior in aggressive adolescents. *Journal of Clinical Child Psychology, 17,* 298–309.

Cohen, J. A., & Mannarino, A. P. (1993). Sexual abuse. In R. T. Ammerman, C. G. Last, & M. Hersen (Eds.), *Handbook of prescriptive treatments for children and adolescents* (pp. 347–366). Boston: Allyn & Bacon.

Conoley, J. C., & Larson, P. (1995). Conflicts in care: Early years of the lifespan. In E. J. Rave & C. C. Larsen (Eds.), *Ethical decision making in therapy: Feminist perspectives* (pp. 202–222). New York: Guilford Press.

Deykin, E. Y., Alpert, J. J., & McNamarra, J. J. (1985). A pilot study of the effect of exposure to child abuse or neglect on adolescent suicidal behavior. *American Journal of Psychiatry, 142,* 1299–1303.

Egeland, B., Sroufe, L. A., & Erickson, M. (1983). The developmental consequences of different patterns of maltreatment. *Child Abuse and Neglect, 7,* 45–69.

Einbender, A., & Friedrich, W. (1989). The psychological functioning and behavior of sexual abused girls. *Journal of Consulting and Clinical Psychology, 57,* 155–157.

Emslie, G. J., Weinberg, W. A., Rush, A. J., Adams, R. M., & Rintelmann, J. W. (1990). Depressive symptoms by self-report in adolescence: Phase I of the development of a questionnaire for depression by self-report. *Journal of Child Neurology, 5,* 114–121.

Finney, J. W., Riley, A. W., & Cataldo, M. F. (1991). Psychology in primary health care: Effects of brief targeted therapy on children's medical care utilization. *Journal of Pediatric Psychology, 16,* 447–461.

Forehand, R., Brody, G., Slotkin, J., Fauber, R., McCombs, A., & Long, N. (1988). Young adolescents and maternal depression: Assessment, interventions, and family predictors. *Journal of Consulting and Clinical Psychology, 56,* 422–426.

Friedrich, W. N., Beilke, R. L., & Urquiza, A. J. (1987). Children from sexually abusive families: A behavioral comparison. *Journal of Interpersonal Violence, 2,* 391–402.

Horne, A., Norsworthy, K., Forehand, R., & Frame, C. (1990). *A delinquency prevention program.* Unpublished manuscript, Department of Education, University of Georgia, Athens.

Horne, A. M., & Glaser, B. A. (1993). Conduct disorders. In R. T. Ammerman, C. G. Last, & M. Hersen (Eds.), *Handbook of prescriptive treatments for children and adolescents* (pp. 85–101). Boston: Allyn & Bacon.

Garrison, C. Z., Jackson, K. L., Marsteller, F., McKewon, R., & Addy, C. (1990). A longitudinal study of depressive symptomatology in young adolescents. *Journal of the American Academy of Adolescent Psychiatry, 29,* 580–585.

Jenson, P. A., Bhatara, V. S., Vitiello, B., Hoagwood, K., Feil, M., & Burke, L. B. (1999). Psychoactive medication prescribing practices for U.S. children: Gaps between research and clinical practice. *Journal of the American Academy of Child and Adolescent Psychiatry, 38,* 557–565.

Kaslow, N., Rehm, L., & Siegel, A. W. (1984). Social-cognitive and cognitive correlates of depression in children. *Journal of Abnormal Child Psychology, 12,* 605–
620.

Kazdin, A. E., Moser, J., Colbus, D., & Bell, R. (1985). Depressive symptoms among
physically abused and psychiatrically disturbed children. *Journal of Abnormal
Psychology, 94,* 298–307.

Koss-Chioino, J. D., & Vargas, L. A. (1999). *Working with Latino youth: Culture, development, and context.* San Francisco: Jossey-Bass.

Kovacs, M., Paulauskas, S., Gatsonis, C., & Richards, C. (1988). A longitudinal study
of comorbidity with and risk for conduct disorders. *Journal of Affective Disorders,
15,* 205–217.

Lakey, B. B., Hartdagen, S. E., Frick, P. J., & McBurnett, K. (1988). Parsing the con-
founded relationship to parental divorce and antisocial personality. *Journal of Abnormal Psychology, 97,* 334–337.

Liburd, R., & Rothblum, E. (1995). The medical model. In E. J. Rave & C. C. Larsen
(Eds.), *Ethical decision making in therapy: Feminist perspectives* (pp. 177–201).
New York: Guilford Press.

Livingston, R. (1987). Sexually and physically abused children. *Journal of the American Academy of Child Psychiatry, 26,* 413–415.

Lonigan, C. J., Elbert, J. C., & Johnson, S. B. (1998). Empirically supported psychosocial interventions for children: An overview. *Journal of Clinical Child Psychology, 27,* 138–145.

Mannarino, A. P., Cohen, J. A., & Gregor, M. (1989). Emotional and behavior difficulties in sexually abused girls. *Journal of Interpersonal Violence, 4,* 437–451.

Mannarino, A. P., Cohen, J. A., Smith, J. A., & Moore-Motily, S. (1990). *Six and twelve
month follow-up of sexually abused girls.* Unpublished manuscript, Department of
Psychology, University of Pittsburgh.

Melton, G. B. (1983). Toward personhood for adolescents: Autonomy and privacy as
values in public policy. *American Psychologist, 38,* 99–103.

Patterson, G., Reid, J., Jones, R., & Conger, R. (1975). *A social learning approach to
family intervention: Vol. I. Families with aggressive children.* Eugene, OR: Castalia.

Pipher, M. (1994). *Reviving Ophelia.* New York: Ballantine Books.

Porter, N., Garcia, M., Jackson, H., & Valdez, D. (1997). The rights of children and adolescents of color in mental health systems. *Women and Therapy, 20,* 57–74.

Prilleltensky, I. (1994). The United Nations Convention on the Rights of the Child:
Implications for children's mental health. *Canadian Journal of Mental Health, 13,*
77–93.

Reeves, J. C., Werry, J. S., Elkind, G. S., & Zametkin, A. (1987). Attention deficit, conduct, oppositional, and anxiety disorders in children: II. Clinical characteristics.
Journal of the American Academy of Child and Adolescent Psychiatry, 26, 144–155.

Selekman, M. D. (1997). *Solution-focused therapy with children: Harnessing family
strengths for systemic change.* New York: Guilford Press.

Sherwin, S. (1992). *No longer patient: Feminist ethics and health care.* Philadelphia:
Temple University Press.

Sirles, E. A., Smith, J. A., & Kusama, H. (1989). Psychiatric status of intrafamilial child
sexual abuse victims. *Journal of Child and Adolescent Psychiatry, 28,* 225–229.

Stark, K. D., Dempsey, M., & Christopher, J. (1993). Depressive disorders. In R. T.

Ammerman, C. G. Last, & M. Hersen (Eds.). *Handbook of prescriptive treatments for children and adolescents* (pp. 115–143). Boston: Allyn & Bacon.

United Nations General Assembly. (1989). *The convention on the rights of the child.* New York: United Nations.

U.S. Office of the Surgeon General. (1999). *Report of the Surgeon General on children's mental health.* Washington, DC: U.S. Government Printing Office.

Valdez, D. (1994, August). *Multicultural training and supervision for child and adolescent therapists.* Workshop at the annual meeting of Division 37 of the American Psychological Association, Los Angeles, CA.

White, M. (1988, Winter). The process of questioning: A therapy of literary merit? *Dulwich Centre Newsletter,* pp. 8–14.

Wishik, J., Bachman, D. L., & Bertch, L. M. (1989). A neurobehavioral perspective of aggressive behavior: Implications for pharmacological management. *Residential Treatment for Children and Youth, 6,* 101–109.

Chapter 11

Depression and Schizophrenia in Women

The Intersection of Gender, Race/Ethnicity, and Class

ELIZABETH SPARKS

The influence of gender on psychopathology has received significant research attention over the last three decades. Much of this work has focused on gender differences in depression. Major depression is one of the most common forms of psychopathology worldwide, and it is much more common in women than in men. The general consensus in the literature is that women experience depression at a rate that is at least twice that of men, although some studies report even higher ratios. There have been a number of comprehensive reviews of the literature on the role that gender plays in the etiology of depression (e.g., Culbertson, 1997; McGrath, Keita, Strickland, & Russo, 1990; Sprock & Yoder, 1997), and numerous theories have been proposed to explain these differences. The American Psychological Association's National Task Force on Women and Depression published an extensive review of this literature in 1990, focusing on risk factors and treatment issues for depression in women. A more recent review conducted by Sprock and Yoder (1997) updated the American Psychological Association's Task Force Report and highlighted research published during the intervening years. The work of Culbertson (1997) expanded the review of gender and depression to include international studies.

The examination of gender differences in schizophrenia and other chronic mental illnesses has not kept pace with the literature on depression; however, the existing research notes some differences in men and women that seem consistent across ethnic groups in the United States and cross-culturally (Bachrach, 1984; Forrest & Hay, 1971; Test & Berlin, 1981). This literature focuses on gender-related demographic differences among individuals diagnosed with schizophrenia, chiefly age at onset, course of illness, and response to treatment. The general conclusion is that gender identification, whether biologically or culturally derived, influences role expectations and behaviors, which in turn effect the expression of chronic mental illness.

Thus, the existing literature has drawn a number of conclusions with respect to the ways that gender affects the development and manifestation of psychiatric illness. The theories attempting to explain gender differences in depression and schizophrenia span biological, psychological, social, and cultural variables (Weissman & Klerman, 1985). Much of this literature, however, has not examined the role that race/ethnicity[1] and socioeconomic status play in the development, manifestation, and treatment of depression and schizophrenia in women. It is difficult, given the current state of the literature, to obtain a comprehensive picture of the etiology of these psychiatric disorders in *all* women since the bulk of the research has been conducted with white participants. The goal of the present chapter is to explore the influence of gender, race/ethnicity, and class on the etiology and manifestation of depression and schizophrenia in women. It is an attempt to understand these disorders within a sociocultural context, and to examine the ways in which the experience of psychopathology is shaped by a woman's status within the U.S. cultural context. The basic assumption underlying the thesis taken in this chapter is that individual experience is embedded in a social context where the influences of gender, race/ethnicity, and social class vary according to whether one is a member of a privileged or a disenfranchised group on these three variables. A woman's self-perception and the way she is perceived by society are determined by cultural stereotypes of her gender, race/ethnicity, and social class. Some researchers (e.g., Barbee, 1992; Poussaint, 1990) have suggested that mental health and mental illness exist in a sociopolitical context, such that historical, economic, and sociocultural factors influence who is labeled as mentally ill, the type of psychiatric label that is applied, the treatment approaches utilized, and the nature of prevention efforts. In order to develop a more comprehensive picture of depression and schizophrenia in women, it is important to examine the intersection of gender, race/ethnicity, and social class on these disorders.

In this chapter, I take what has been termed a *radical psychosocial perspective* (Brown, 1998) to review the literature. This perspective relates the findings from research on gender differences in depression and schizophrenia to broader cultural and societal issues. To describe this broader context, I review research on the existence of racism in the mental health system. I next focus on depression in women, and present a brief overview of the research on gender differences. I highlight those studies that have been published since the comprehensive review conducted by Sprock and Yoder (1997), with particular emphasis on research addressing depression in women of color. I examine the theories that have been posited in the literature to explain gender differences in depression, giving emphasis to those that seem most applicable to an analysis of race/ethnicity and class. I then review the literature on gender differences in schizophrenia, highlighting some of the explanations for these findings. I review studies that have found racial bias in the assessment and diagnosis of schizophrenia and discuss the role that social class seems to play in the development of these disorders. I conclude the chapter with recommendations for further research integrating gender, race/ethnicity, and class into the exploration of factors that influence the development and treatment of depression and schizophrenia in women.

RACISM AND MENTAL ILLNESS

Over the last 30 years several studies have supported the contention that racial bias exists in the assessment and diagnosis of mental illness (Wade, 1991). People of color experience disproportionately and unacceptably high rates of physical and mental illness and premature mortality, despite significant advances in medical science, improvements in access to health care, and the elimination of legal forms of race and gender discrimination (Lillie-Blanton, Bowie, & Ro, 1996). Research suggests that one of the factors that contribute to racial differences in mental health is therapist bias. Jenkins-Hall and Sacco (1991) found that therapists held more negative evaluations of depressed than nondepressed clients, and that the special combination of being African American and depressed led to the most negative evaluation. According to Jones (1982), white therapists generally rated their African American clients as more psychologically impaired than did African American therapists. A similar type of bias has been found in the diagnosis of Hispanic clients. White professionals have been found to misconstrue uncooperative behavior among Hispanics as evidence of psychosis (Rendon, 1974). Moreover, professionals' lack of knowledge of Puerto Rican culture can lead to misdiagnosis (Teichner, Cadden & Berry, 1981). Ethnic minority clients are also more likely to be labeled as having a chronic syndrome, as opposed to an acute episode, when diagnosed with psychosis or affective disorders (Sata, 1990). Results of a study by Pavkov, Lewis, and Lyons (1989) on psychiatric diagnoses and racial bias revealed that being African American is predictive of a diagnosis of schizophrenia. Both African Americans and Hispanics are more likely to be misdiagnosed as schizophrenic when they were, in fact, suffering from bipolar affective disorder (Mukherjee, Shukla, & Woodle, 1983). The same symptoms that would be labeled "emotional" or "affective" disorders among whites are labeled "schizophrenic" among African Americans (Solomon, 1992). Fernando (1988) reviewed the literature in England and found that a diagnosis of schizophrenia was given significantly more often to West Indians and West Africans than to other United Kingdom-born or migrant groups.

Thus, people of color in general and African Americans in particular are overdiagnosed in some categories and underdiagnosed in others (Gullattee, 1969; Thomas & Sillen, 1972). In a review of the existing literature in the early 1980s Adebimpe (1981) identified a number of possible causes for the misdiagnosis of African American psychiatric patients, including social and cultural distance between patient and clinicians; stereotypes of African American psychopathology; false-positive symptoms and biased diagnostic instruments; and the combined effects of various sources of diagnostic error. Despite the apparent societal changes with regards to race/ethnicity that have occurred over the last 20 years, Williams, Yu, Jackson, and Anderson (1997) found similar differences between people of color and whites. This study focused on the differential health status between African Americans and whites. African Americans reported lower levels of psychological well-being; higher rates of self-reported ill health; and more bed-days than whites did. Race-related stress, as well as general measures of stress, were generally adversely related to health and were more strongly related to indicators of mental health than to indicators of physical health. The mental health of African Americans tended to exceed that of whites once the researchers adjusted for race-related stress (Williams et al., 1997). They concluded that race matters in terms of health, and that the sources of racial disparities can be traced to inequalities created and maintained by the economic, legal, and political structures of society.

Fabrega (1990) drew similar conclusions in his review of Hispanic mental health research. The diagnosis and treatment of psychopathology for Hispanics is complicated by cultural biases inherent in traditional mental health practices. Often this research seems to exclude, disregard, or simply be insensitive to aspects of psychopathology that are reflective of behavior patterns shaped by Hispanic cultural traditions. Much of the existing research points to bias in diagnosis and to differences between traditional paradigms of disorders and Hispanic (and other ethnic minority) models of psychiatric illness and distress. Thus, research on gender differences in depression and schizophrenia is embedded within a larger mental health context where racial bias in assessment, diagnosis, and treatment exists. It is difficult to determine the extent to which this bias is operating in the diagnosis and treatment of depression and schizophrenia in women of color; however, we must assume that it has exerted some measure of influence on their experiences of these disorders, and we must therefore endeavor to keep this in mind as we review the literature.

BRIEF OVERVIEW OF THE RESEARCH ON GENDER AND DEPRESSION[2]

One of the most consistent findings in the literature on gender differences in depression is the greater prevalence of depressive disorders and symptoms of psychological distress in women than in men (Goldman & Ravid, 1980; Nolen-Hoeksema, 1987, 1990; Weissman & Klerman, 1977). In general, these gender differences hold for white, black, and Hispanic women (Potter, Rogler, & Moscicki, 1995; Russo, Amaro, & Winter, 1987; Russo & Sobel, 1981) and persist even when income level, education, and occupation are controlled (Ensel, 1982; Radloff, 1975). The common interpretation in the literature is that women are at higher risk for experiencing depression due to differences in socialization between women and men in our society, different learned styles of coping with emotional distress, and innate biological differences (Pumariega, Johnson, Sheridan, & Cuffe, 1996).

Although it is a general trend for women to experience higher rates of depression than men, it should be noted that not all of the research findings across cultures are the same in this regard (Culbertson, 1997). In developing countries, the depression and gender ratios are not the same. Findings from low-income nations, such as those in Africa, yield mixed gender–depression ratios. It has been found, however, that symptomatology for depression appears to be fairly similar across nations (Culbertson, 1997).

The number of national and international studies of depression that involve gender comparisons has increased for both developed and developing countries, clearly indicating that the cultural and biopsychosocial dimensions of depression are significant factors to be examined. Gender, therefore, is an important variable in cross-culturally conceptualizing, assessing, and treating depression (Culbertson, 1997). In general, there appears to be little doubt that there are significant gender differences in depression, with women developing the disorder at a rate that is at least twice that of men (Wetzel, 1994).

EXPLANATIONS FOR GENDER DIFFERENCES IN DEPRESSION

A number of theories have been proposed in the literature to explain gender differences in depression. These theories include biological, psychosocial, and environmental factors. The biological theory posits that changes or imbalances in levels of estrogen, progesterone, or other female hormones bring about depression in women (Harris, Johns, & Fung, 1989). This theory, however, has been severely challenged by empirical research. The hormonal explanations of gender differences in depression have not, thus far, been well supported (Nolen-Hoeksema, 1995).

A second theory suggested in the literature is that gender differences are due to developmental differences between men and women. Research exploring this theoretical perspective has examined the emergence of gender differences in depression during adolescence. Studies have found that preadolescent boys are much more likely to be depressed than preadolescent girls both in clinical samples (Kashani, Cantwell, Shakim, & Reid, 1982) and in the general population (Anderson, Williams, McGee, & Silva, 1987). It appears that the switch in gender differences emerges by age 14 to 15 (Nolen-Hoeksema, 1990; Petersen et al., 1993). Hankin and colleagues (1998) explored this finding in a carefully designed, 10-year longitudinal study. They found that gender differences begin to emerge between ages 13 and 15 for both the overall rates and new cases of depression. However, the 15- to 18-year age period seems to be the most critical because the rates of depression increase dramatically for both genders, with the female rate rising to double the prevalence rate for males.

In a recent study examining the age gap in depression, Wichstrom (1999) explored the role of intensified gender socialization to explain the emergence of gender differences in depression during adolescence. Structural equation modeling and regression analyses demonstrated that gender differences could be explained, in part, by increased developmental challenges for girls, including pubertal development, dissatisfaction with weight and attainment of a mature female body, and increased importance of feminine sex-role identification

It is interesting to note that the gender differences that are found between women and men during late adolescence and adulthood seem to dissipate by old age. Feinson (1987) reviewed the literature on the level of depressive symptoms among older persons and found inconsistent findings. Eleven studies showed higher rates for women than for men; however, four other studies had either higher rates for men or no gender differences. In a study of older African Americans, Brown, Milburn, and Gary (1992) found no gender differences in overall level of depressive symptomatology among individuals 65 years of age and older. In the elderly, stressful life events, which did not vary by gender, seemed to contribute more to depressive symptomatology than either social roles or socioeconomic status.

A third explanatory theory asserts that differential reactions to stress occur in men and women, which lead to differing levels of vulnerability to depression. Vulnerability–stress models of depression offer a framework to explain gender differences in adolescents by describing how cognitive and interpersonal vulnerability may interact with the increasing levels of stress experienced by youth as they progress through adolescence (Nolen-Hocksema & Girgus, 1994). One such model, the diathesis–stress model, posits that girls are more likely to posses certain preexisting risk factors that make them susceptible to the range of depressive symptoms when confronted with increasing social and physical challenges in adolescence. Broderick (1998) suggests that differences in the ways that boys and girls react to stressful situations may be due to such factors as emotional expressivity, socialization about appropriateness of coping strategies, or experience with a range of coping opportunities.

The diathesis–stress model has also been applied to explain gender differences in adults. Brown (1998) examined the relationship between experiences of loss and depression, focusing on the effect that negative life events have on an individual's vulnerability to depression. In this study, the presence of a severely threatening life event in the 6 months prior to the onset of depression was common among those with nonmelancholic/ nonpsychotic conditions, whether or not it was a first episode (Brown, 1998; Brown & Harris, 1989). Examining this explanatory theory further, Pianta and Egeland (1994) conducted a study that examined the relationship between stressful life events and depressive symptoms in a diverse group of low-income mothers. They found the relationship to be complex and bidirectional, depending, in part, on the type of stress experienced. Not only did health stress and family fights lead to depressive symptoms, but depressive symptoms predicted heath stress, family fights, marital/partner stress, financial stress, household changes, and stress due to substance abuse in the family. They concluded that there is a complex interaction between stressful life events and psychiatric symptoms that should be carefully explored.

The focus of much of the research on gender differences in depression has been on sex roles and the way in which men and women are socialized, which is the fourth explanatory theory (see Bassoff & Glass [1982], Marsh & Myers [1986], Nolen-Hoeksema & Girgus [1994], and Whitley [1984], for reviews of this literature). Research has found that gender-role orientation is a major personality factor that accounts for individual differences in susceptibility to depression (Cheng, 1999). Various researchers have stressed the importance of interactions between gender and social roles (such as marriage, parenting, and employment) in the etiology of psychological disorders. According to this perspective, depression is expected to differ for men and women because of differing societal expectations. Many of women's traditional roles, particularly homemaking, are given low societal value (Canino et al., 1987), and the ways that women are socialized to be nonassertive, self-sacrificing, and dependent on others have been associated with depression. The connection between self-esteem and depression also seems to disadvantage women. Their self-esteem is built largely around relatedness and emotional connections in their professional as well as their domestic lives, and they tend to become depressed as a result of cutoffs or disruptions in close relationships (Papp, 2000).

The gender gap in depression is thought to occur as a result of the unequal adult statuses for men and women in this culture (Mirowsky, 1996). Researchers have concluded that much of the gender difference seems to exist because women experience greater trade-offs and tensions from work and family than do men (Gore & Mangione, 1983; Lennon, 1998; Ross & Mirowsky, 1988). Support for this conclusion is seen in studies that find higher rates of depression and demoralization among married women compared with married men (Gove & Geerken, 1977; Radloff, 1975); among mothers of young children compared to mothers of older children and nonmothers (Gore & Mangione, 1983; McLanahan & Adams, 1987); and among full-time homemakers compared to employed women (Rosenfield, 1980). Women carry a greater burden of total housework and paid work hours, pay greater costs for caring for the problems of family and friends, face greater practical constraints on personal employment and advancement, and get less autonomy, authority, recognition, and pay when employed (Kessler & McLeod, 1984; Reskin & Padavic, 1994). Mirowsky's (1996) findings support the hypothesis that the gender gap in depression does not appear to arise solely from sexual differentiation, whether biological or social, but from emerging sexual stratification between women and men. However, there are a number of studies that fail to document these effects, suggesting that there may be a complex interaction between gender roles and psychological distress that requires further investigation.

Cheng (1999) examined the interaction between feminine sex-role orientation and social support to determine the extent to which femininity, as measured by the Bem Sex Role Inventory (Bem, 1974, 1981) may act as a mitigating factor in depression. Her thesis is that feminine individuals, because of their stronger affiliative needs, may be especially sensitive to features in their social environment. Their greater concern for harmonious relations with others can be potentially beneficial in alleviating depression when social support is available. However, when social support is needed but not available, these same personality traits may increase an individual's vulnerability to depression (Cheng, 1999). She concludes that feminine gender role orientation was inversely related to depression through its interaction with social support. This is a relatively novel finding and the author suggests that it should be regarded as tentative, requiring additional research to support the moderating role that social support and femininity jointly play in the alleviation of depression.

THE INTERSECTION OF GENDER AND RACE/ETHNICITY IN DEPRESSION

Little research specifically addresses racial differences in the mental health of women or attempts to explain the longevity of these differences (U.S. Department of Health and Human Services, 1985). As stated earlier, gender differences in the rates in depression in women seem to remain constant across ethnicity/race and social class (Lester & DeSimone, 1995; Munford, 1994). Kelly, Kelly, Brown, and Kelly (1999) examined gender differences in depression among a culturally diverse group of college students. They found that the prevalence of depression in females is higher than in males irrespective of ethnicity. Similarly, a study of body image and depression conducted by Grant and colleagues (1999) found that low-income African American girls reported higher rates of depressive symptoms than their male peers. There have, however, been studies that found differences be-tween ethnic groups in the incidence of depression. Brown (1990) identi-fied certain conditions that increase African American women's vulnerabil-ity for depression. These include being poor, between 19 and 45 years of age, unemployed, having less than a high school education, having minor children in the household, and being divorced or separated. Barbee (1992) concludes that much of the research on gender differences is acontextual, stating that it ignores the interactive effects of gender, race, and social class in the oppression of African American women. There have, however, been some studies that examined depression in African American women within context. Dressler (1985) found a positive relationship between extended kin support and depressive symptoms, where women who reported higher active coping strategies also reported fewer depressive symptoms. Barbee found that African American women make distinctions among types of de-pression, such that the type determined relief-seeking strategies. Dressler and Badger (1985) found that depressive symptoms in women were modi-fied by community and geographic region, although the trend for women to report significantly more symptoms than men was consistent with other re-search.

In addition to the racial differences in the prevalence of depressive symptoms and diagnoses, ethnicity has also been associated with differen-tial rates of depressive symptoms. For example, recent studies report rates of depressive symptomatology in Mexican American immigrant women as high as 41.5% (Vega, Kolodny, Valle, & Hough, 1986) and 64% (Salgado de Snyder, 1987). It has been suggested that disparities between women of color and white women reflect, in part, the former's greater exposure to adverse social environments (e.g., poverty, neighborhood pollutants, and unsafe working conditions) that place them at risk for illness and injury (Lillie-Blanton et al., 1996). These disparities also reflect inequities in ac-cess to health care. Research has documented the consequences of financial barriers to access to health care (Davis & Rowland, 1983) and the ways that race and/or socioeconomic status affects the quality of the provider–client encounter.

The literature on depression in women of color has also focused on their unique cultural experiences and how these seem to influence the ex-planatory theories. Several authors have suggested that the adoption of tra-ditional gender roles contribute to the higher rates of depression found in women. Since cultures differ in the extent to which traditional gender roles are normative for women, it is expected that sex-role explanations for gender differences may vary cross-culturally. Researchers have noted that the adoption of traditional gender roles is more common among Hispanics than among Anglo groups (Comas-Díaz, 1988; Vazquez-Nuttall, Romero-Garcia, & DeLeon, 1987), which places Hispanic women at even higher risk for depression (Canino et al., 1987; Frerichs, Aneshensel, & Clark, 1981; Potter et al., 1995; Vega, Warheit, Buhl-Auth, & Meinhardt, 1984).

Falik and Scott-Collins (1996) found that Latinas are more likely than women as a whole to agree with negative statements about themselves. They are significantly more likely to report feelings of depression (53% vs. 40% of women in general). These higher rates of depression may be associated with the material circumstances of Latinas' lives (i.e., lower income, less education, restricted opportunities), but they may also be affected by a cultural tendency toward downplaying self-worth and well-being (Falik & Scott-Collins, 1996). Within this cultural context, expressions of high self-worth may be seen as boastful and social rewards may accrue to those who report feeling less than happy. Moscicki, Rae, Regier, and Locke (1987) found that a significant proportion of Latinas report psychological distress. The explanation for this finding is unclear, but may be related to methodological artifact (Wrinkle, Andalzua, & Reed-Sanders, 1988), the need to access limited health care resources (Canino et al., 1987), or religious beliefs within the Latino culture (Monk, 1990).

African American women have different gender role experiences. They are socialized to be stronger, more independent, and more resourceful than are Anglo women. They appear to have more egalitarian male–female relationships, and thus adherence to gender roles may be moderated considerably by cultural differences (Bernstein, 1991–1992). In a review of the literature on African American women and depression, Barbee (1992) discussed many of the explanatory theories presented in the general literature in terms of their applicability to the experiences of African American women. She highlighted an area that is sometimes minimized, that of the role of violent victimization. Adult victims of violence are significantly more likely to qualify for psychiatric diagnoses like major depression than nonvictims (Koss, 1990). Women of color (in particular, African American women) experience high rates of victimization, and are disproportionately exposed to three types of criminal violence: aggravated assault, forcible rape, and homicide. Homicide is one of the 10 leading causes of death for African American women, while the other two types of violence have reported rates that are almost three times that of white women (U.S. Department of Justice, 1991). A similar trend is found for intimate violence (Coley

& Beckett, 1988; Katz & Mazur, 1979; Kercher & McShane, 1984). Although the interaction between violent victimization and depression in African American women is not clear from the literature, the differential impact of violence in the lives of African American women supports the need to examine depression within this context for women of color.

Thus, the limited research on depression in women of color suggests that they may be at higher risk for developing depression due to the socioenvironmental factors that they are exposed to. Cultural experience may influence the etiology of depression in these women, and they may also have unique ways of coping with depressive symptomatology that effect diagnosis of the disorder and response to treatment. There is clearly a need for additional research to explore these possibilities.

BRIEF OVERVIEW OF THE RESEARCH
ON GENDER AND SCHIZOPHRENIA

Prior to the 1980s there was little focus on gender differences in schizophrenia research. Wahl and Hunter (1992) in their review of the literature found that there was a predominance of male subjects used in sample populations, with males outnumbering females 2:1, and very little attention paid to exploring possible gender differences within mixed-sex samples. This trend has begun to shift, and currently there is more research on gender differences in schizophrenia (e.g., Angermeyer, Goldstein, & Kuehn, 1989; Brunette & Drake, 1997; Faraone, Chen, Goldstein, & Tsuang, 1994; Goldstein, 1988, 1995b; Lewine, 1981). This literature has primarily focused on age at onset, symptom presentation, and treatment outcomes. In general, it is assumed that age at onset and course of illness are determined by inherent or developmental differences between men and women (Angermeyer & Kuhn, 1988; Lewine, 1988; Lindamer, Loht, Harris, & Jeste, 1997; Seeman, 1995). With regards to age at onset, studies have found that men develop the illness earlier than do women, which can have negative effects on the initial severity of the illness and its longitudinal course (Faraone et al., 1994). The peak period of onset in men is age 18–25 years, and for women it is age 25 to mid-30s (Angermeyer et al., 1989; Goldstein, Tsuang, & Faraone, 1989; Hafner, Riecher, & Maurer, 1989). In addition to a delayed peak of onset of schizophrenia for women, some investigators have found that women additionally experience a smaller peak after ages 40 to 45 (Hafner, Maurer, Loffler, & Riecher-Rossler, 1993; Hafner, Riecher-

Rossler, Maurer, Fatkenheuer, & Loffler, 1992). Although the conditions that create these differences are not known, a number of possible explanations have been suggested, including (1) the elevation of female hormones during puberty (Seeman & Lang, 1990); (2) increased incidences of brain trauma in male infants; (3) differential immune systems; (4) heightened exposure of male adolescents to certain triggers such as alcohol and drug abuse or familial demand and criticism; and (5) young women's heightened social support (Goldstein, 1995a; Seeman, 1988). It has also been suggested by some that there may be different subtypes of schizophrenia for men and women (Lewine, 1981).

There has been some research support for the association between estrogen and psychosis (Hallonquist, Seeman, Lang, & Rector, 1993; Kendell, Chalmers, & Platz, 1987; Riecher-Rossler et al., 1990; Riecher-Rossler, Hafner, Stumbalum, Maurer, & Schmidt, 1994). Hafner and colleagues (1998) conducted a series of 12 substudies that explored in detail gender differences in age at onset of schizophrenia. They concluded that women had a lower threshold for developing schizophrenia until menopause, after which the rates and severity of the illness for women are comparable to those for men. In general, data from clinical studies provide indirect evidence that estrogen may confer a protective effect against developing schizophrenia, delaying its onset until menopause (Lindamer et al., 1997). For women, late-onset schizophrenia (i.e., postmenopausal) is more frequent, with a relative risk of 2 to 3, and comparatively more severe than in men who develop the disorder later in life. For men, late-onset schizophrenia is less frequent and milder on average than early-onset schizophrenia.

It has also been suggested that this finding may be influenced by differences in age at first admission, which seems to vary according to geographic region. The World Health Organization's (WHO) cross-cultural study of first episode patients with schizophrenia reported that women had a higher mean age at onset (as determined by first admission) than men in both developing and developed countries (Hambrecht, Maurer, & Sartorius, 1992). This difference may be caused by cultural differences in the elapsed time before parents bring children into treatment or related to sex-role expectations (Angermeyer & Kuhn, 1988; Lewine, 1981). Not only does the differential age at onset affect the early social course of the disorder in men and women, it also seems to influence treatment outcomes. Women have more favorable short-term outcomes than men. Although estrogens may explain some of the differences in treatment outcomes, it is also likely that differences in premorbid history are influential in treatment responsiveness. Men with schizophrenia experience poorer premorbid histories than women, with the later having better early childhood histories in terms of school achievement and social functioning (Goldstein, 1995b).

Gender differences are also found in symptomatology. Women express more positive symptoms (e.g., paranoia, persecutory delusions, and auditory hallucinations) and more affective symptoms, while negative symptoms (e.g., affective flattening and social withdrawal) tend to be more severe in men (Goldstein & Link, 1988; Lewine, 1981; Rector & Seeman, 1992). The consensus in the literature is that women with schizophrenia benefit more from psychosocial treatments and have a better response to neuroleptics than men (Seeman, 1995). In an acute episode of psychosis, women may require lower doses of neuroleptics to achieve remission (Kolakowska, Williams, & Arden, 1985; Seeman, 1983). One reason that has been suggested for this differential responsiveness is that female hormones increase the effectiveness of neuroleptics (Bellodi, Morabito, & Macciardi, 1982; Seeman, 1981). This difference, however, seems to dissipate, or even reverse, with age (Seeman, 1986). Other reasons that have been posited to explain the gender difference in response to neuroleptics include women's greater likelihood of continuing with prescribed medication doses (Kessler, Brown, & Broman, 1981) and their proportionally greater lipid stores, which makes it possible for women to continue free of relapse for a longer period of time after ceasing medication (Lehmann & Ban, 1974).

Studies have also found that women enter the hospital less often than do men following initial admission. Once women enter the hospital, however, they appear to have a better prognosis than men (Angermeyer et al., 1989; Salokangas, 1983). It has been suggested that social traits, psychosexual development, bonding ties with family of origin, and adjustment to working life are different for men and women with schizophrenia. As a result, men are admitted more frequently and for more prolonged hospitalizations than women (Goldstein, 1988). According to Salokangas (1983), the length of hospitalization for men is twice that for women. These findings cannot be completely explained by the social background characteristics of the patients (e.g., age, marital status, education, or employment status), by the diagnostic subtypes, age of first admission, or by illness behavior. Another factor that may affect the treatment course for schizophrenia is society's differential response to the disorder in women and men (Goldstein & Kreisman, 1988). There seems to be less societal tolerance of schizophrenia in men, as compared to the attitude toward women, which may contribute to the higher rates of hospitalizations for men (Tudor, Tudor, & Gove, 1977). Thus, the factors that may be important in understanding the relationship of gender to treatment outcome in schizophrenia include age at onset, family history, clinical expression, response to treatment, and illness behavior factors (e.g., compliance with treatment and tolerance of deviance by others) (Goldstein, 1988).

Finally, there are three additional psychosocial factors that may contribute to gender differences in schizophrenia, namely, motherhood, homelessness, and violent victimization. Motherhood encompasses a range of psychological, social, familial, and physiological factors that may vary greatly in women with schizophrenia. For many women with schizophrenia, this role is often associated with both anticipatory and actual loss, as they confront such issues as never becoming pregnant, choosing to abort, and/or being required to relinquish their children (Apfel & Handel, 1993). With regards to homelessness, it is important to note that the rate of mental illness among homeless women appears to be greater than that among homeless men, despite the fact that their actual numbers among the homeless population are less (Virgonia, Buhrich, & Teesn, 1993). Similarly, women with schizophrenia and other chronic psychiatric disorders have a lifetime risk for violent victimization that is disproportionately high (Goodman, Dutton, & Harris, 1995).

Thus, the literature suggests that women and men with schizophrenia manifest the illness differently. Women have better premorbid functioning and develop the illness later in life than do men. They also have distinct symptom profiles, and have a better response to neuroleptics, all of which contribute to their having more favorable treatment outcomes. Yet, even with their better responsiveness to medication and more positive response to psychosocial treatments, women with schizophrenia appear to be at increased risk for suicide, medical comorbidity, substance abuse, and violent victimization (Canuso, Goldstein, & Green, 1998).

THE INTERSECTION OF GENDER
AND RACE/ETHNICITY IN SCHIZOPHRENIA

The influence of race/ethnicity on schizophrenia in women has received very little attention in the literature; however, at least one author has suggested that schizophrenia is the diagnosis in psychiatry that is most likely to reflect political and social influences (Fernando, 1988). The judgments that have to be made by the clinician in differentiating schizophrenia from other illnesses, and from normal behavior, require a determination of people's thinking, beliefs, and emotional reactions. The clinician has to decide whether the patient's perceptions are true or imaginary, a decision that is largely determined by evaluating the patient's interactions with others (including the attending clinician), which can be influenced by social norms. Sartorius and colleagues (1986) explored early manifestations and first-contact incidence of schizophrenia in different cultures. The participants were drawn from 12 research centers in 10 different countries. A total of 1,379 individuals who met specified inclusion criteria for schizophrenia and other nonaffective disorders were examined using standardized instruments on entry into the study and on two consecutive follow-ups at annual intervals. The study found that individuals in different cultures who met the standardized criteria for schizophrenia were remarkably similar in their symptom profiles. However, the 2-year pattern of course was considerably more favorable in patients in developing countries compared with patients in developed countries, a finding that has been supported in other research.

Within the U.S. context, research has found that schizophrenia is often overdiagnosed in nonwhite patients with psychosis (Jones & Gray, 1986; Mukherjee et al., 1983; Neighbors, Jackson, & Campbell, 1989). Possible reasons for this situation include (1) racial bias in clinicians (Adebimpe, 1981; Lawson, 1986); (2) lack of cultural understanding between clinicians and nonwhite clients (Flaherty, Naidu, & Lawton, 1981; Lawson, Hepler, & Holiday, 1991); and (3) differing symptom presentations among ethnic groups (Adebimpe, Chu, & Klein, 1982; Fabrega, Mezzich, & Ulrich, 1988). A recent study by Strakowski, Shelton, and Kolbrenner (1993) examined charts of 173 patients with psychotic disorders discharged from a large state psychiatric hospital and found that African American patients were significantly more likely to be diagnosed with schizophrenia than white patients. This racial pattern was observed even in the group of patients that were hospitalized for the first time. Additionally, African American patients received higher doses of antipsychotic medication irrespective of diagnosis. Although the reasons for the overdiagnosis of African American patients in this study could not be determined, it was suggested that there may be some inherent bias in the application of diagnostic criteria to the symptom presentations in these clients. It is also possible that the diagnostic measures used to determine diagnosis might not be culturally sensitive. The problem with cultural relevancy in standardized psychological measurements has been noted in other studies (e.g., Callahan & Wolinsky, 1994; Goodman et al., 1995). This research suggests that race/ethnicity continues to affect clinical diagnoses of patients with psychotic symptomatology, which may lead to inaccurate assessment and, potentially, inadequate treatment for women of color.

THE ROLE OF SOCIAL CLASS
IN DEPRESSION AND SCHIZOPHRENIA

The results of epidemiological research on psychiatric disorders have documented that the highest overall prevalence rates of psychiatric disorders have been found among persons in the lowest socioeconomic status (Dohrenwend et al., 1998). The evidence suggests that the relationship between psychopathology and social class holds for a number of subtypes, including schizophrenia and major depression (at least in women). Two principle theories have been proposed to explain this finding: social causation and social selection (Kohn, 1972). The social causation explanation, proposed by environmentally oriented theorists, holds that the rates of some types of psychiatric disorders are higher in lower-class groups because their members are exposed to greater environmental adversity and stress. The social selection explanation argues that mental illness is higher in lower-class groups because persons with a psychiatric disorder or with other predisposing personal characteristics drift down into or fail to rise out of lower-class groups. Despite a large body of research that has examined this question, the controversy continues regarding which of these theories best explains the correlation between mental illness and social class (Dohrenwend et al., 1998). Proponents of both theoretical perspectives have presented evidence to support their positions; however, no one has demonstrated that one position is more compelling.

The social causation perspective on depression identifies poverty and marginalization as important factors in the etiology of depression in women. Women who are poor, belong to an ethnic minority, and who experience chronic mental illness are particularly marginalized in this society. They are at higher risk for receiving inadequate care in the medical and mental health arenas and have less access to insurance, preventive measures, and information concerning specific conditions (Falik & Scott-Collins, 1996). A similar correlation between poverty and schizophrenia in women seems to exist, although there has been very little research that specifically examines this interaction. One study that is relevant to this issue examines the experiences of violent victimization in homeless women with serious mental illness (Goodman et al., 1995). The researchers interviewed 99 women who were episodically homeless and had serious mental illnesses. A majority of these women were also ethnic minorities (80% African American; 2% Asian American; 2% other). Most of the respondents reported severe abuse at the hands of multiple perpetrators, usually beginning in childhood and extending through adulthood. The probability of adult victimization, given child physical or sexual abuse, was .97, making the likelihood of becoming a victim of violence an everyday occurrence for these women. Being seriously mentally ill, ethnic minority, poor, and homeless contributes to extreme marginalization and stigma, which in turn influences the course of illness and treatment options.

CONCLUSION

This chapter has explored the intersection of gender, race/ethnicity, and socioeconomic status on depression and schizophrenia in women. It seems clear from the existing literature that there are gender differences in both depression and schizophrenia that occur across ethnic groups and cultures. The explanations for these differences vary; however, a great deal of research interest has been focused on the influence of psychosocial factors (such as social roles and poverty) on the development and manifestation of depression and schizophrenia in women. Although relatively sparse, the literature on depression and schizophrenia in women of color suggests that these women fare worse than white women in the diagnosis and treatment of psychiatric disorders. Women of color are at higher risk for depression; if schizophrenic, they are more at risk for misdiagnosis and violent victimization.

It is apparent that there is a need for additional research on depression and schizophrenia in women of color. Particular attention should be paid to identifying the factors that contribute to their heightened risk and to developing treatment interventions that are culturally sensitive and effective. However, more is needed if there is to be a change in the differential prevalence rates for mental illness in women of color. As noted in the literature, altering the racial bias that is endemic to the mental health system requires macrolevel changes that address the inequities in income, housing, health care, and other related socioenvironmental factors that adversely impact the lives of women of color. The field of psychology can contribute to this effort by carefully attending to the ways in which problems are defined and research questions are conceptualized. It is imperative that studies examining psychiatric disorders in women be conceptualized, analyzed, and interpreted within context so that the intersection of gender, race/ethnicity, and social class can become the "norm" for future clinical research.

NOTES

1. Throughout this chapter, I use the term race/ethnicity. Race is defined as a socially constructed concept that refers to individuals who have been placed into a group based on physical characteristics. Ethnicity is defined as a cultural product that denotes the interaction between cultural reference groups that share the social context of a third culture. In the United States, race and ethnicity are often used interchangeably.
2. I refer the reader to McGrath, Keita, Strickland, and Russo (1990), Sprock and Yoder (1997), and Culbertson (1997) for comprehensive reviews of the literature on gender and depression.

REFERENCES

Adebimpe, V. R. (1981). Overview: White norms and psychiatric diagnosis of black patients. *American Journal of Psychiatry, 138*(3), 279–285.

Adebimpe, V. R., Chu, C., & Klein, H. E. (1982). Racial and geographic differences in the psychopathology of schizophrenia. *American Journal of Psychiatry, 139*, 888–891.

Anderson, J. C., Williams, S., McGee, R., & Silva, P. A. (1987). DSM-III disorders in preadolescent children: Prevalence in a large sample from the general population. *Archives of General Psychiatry, 44*, 69–76.

Angermeyer, M. C., Goldstein, J. M., & Kuehn, L. (1989). Gender differences in schizophrenia: Re-hospitalization and community survival. *Psychological Medicine, 19*, 365–382.

Angermeyer, M. C., & Kuehn, L. (1988). Gender differences in age at onset of schizophrenia: An overview. *European Archives of Psychiatry and Neurological Science, 237*, 351–364.

Apfel, R. J., & Handel, M. H. (1993). *Madness and loss of motherhood: Sexuality, reproduction, and long-term mental illness.* Washington, DC: American Psychological Press.

Bachrach, L. L. (1984). Deinstitutionalization and women. *American Psychologist, 39*, 1171–1177.

Barbee, E. L. (1992). African American women and depression: A review and critique of the literature. *Archives of Psychiatric Nursing, 6*(5), 257–265.

Bassoff, E. S., & Glass, G. V. (1982). The relationship between sex roles and mental health: A meta-analysis of twenty-six studies. *Counseling Psychologist, 10*, 105–112.

Bellodi, L., Morabito, A., & Macciardi, F. (1982). Analytic considerations about observed distribution of age of onset in schizophrenia. *Neuropsycholobiology, 8*, 93–101.

Bem, S. L. (1974). The measurement of psychological androgyny. *Journal of Consulting and Clinical Psychology, 42*, 155–162.

Bem, S. L. (1981). *Bem Sex-Role Inventory professional manual.* Palo Alto, CA: Consulting Psychologists Press.

Bernstein, B. L. (1991–1992). Central issue importance as a function of gender and ethnicity. *Current Psychology: Research and Reviews, 10*(4), 241–252.

Broderick, P. C. (1998). Early adolescent gender differences in the use of ruminative and distracting coping strategies. *Journal of Early Adolescence, 18*(2), 173–191.

Brown, D. R. (1990). Depression among blacks. In D. S. Ruiz (Ed.), *Handbook of mental health and mental disorders among black Americans* (pp. 71–93). New York: Greenwood Press.

Brown, D. R., Milburn, N. B., & Gary, L. E. (1992). Symptoms of depression among older African Americans: An analysis of gender differences. *Gerontologist, 32*(4), 789–795.

Brown, G. W. (1998). Loss and depressive disorder. In B. P. Dohrenwend (Ed.), *Adversity, stress, and psychopathology* (pp. 358–370). New York: Oxford University Press.

Brown, G. W., & Harris, T. O. (1989). *Life events and illness.* London: Unwin Hyman.

Brunette, J. F., & Drake, R. E. (1997). Gender differences in patients with schizophrenia and substance abuse. *Comprehensive Psychiatry, 38*(2), 109–116.

Callahan, C. M., & Wolinsky, F. D. (1994). The effect of gender and race on the measurement properties of the CES-D in older adults. *Medical Care, 32*(4), 341–356.

Canino, G. J., Rubio-Stipec, M., Shrout, P., Bravo, M., Stolberg, R., & Bird, H. R. (1987). Sex differences and depression in Puerto Rico. *Psychology of Women Quarterly, 11*, 443–459.

Canuso, C. M., Goldstein, J. M., & Green, A. I. (1998). The evaluation of women with schizophrenia. *Psychopharmacology Bulletin, 34*(3), 271–277.

Cheng, C. (1999). Gender-role differences in susceptibility to the influence of support availability on depression. *Journal of Personality, 67*(3), 439–467.

Coley, S. M., & Beckett, J. O. (1988). Black battered women: A review of the literature. *Journal of Counseling and Development, 66*, 266–270.

Comas-Díaz, L. (1988). Cross-cultural mental health treatment. In L. Comas-Díaz & E. H. Griffith (Eds.), *Clinical guidelines in cross-cultural mental health* (pp. 337–361). New York: Wiley.

Culbertson, F. M. (1997). Depression and gender: An international review. *American Psychologist, 52*(1), 25–31.

Davis, K., & Rowland, D. (1983). Uninsured and underserved: Inequities in health care in the United States. *Milbank Memorial Fund Quarterly, 61*, 149–176.

Dohrenwend, B. P., Levav, I., Shrout, P. E., Schwartz, S., Naveh, G., Link, B. G., Skodol, A. E., & Stueve, A. (1998). Ethnicity, socioeconomic status, and psychiatric disorders: A test of the social causation/social selection issue. In B. P. Dohrenwend (Ed.), *Adversity, stress, and psychopathology* (pp. 285–318). New York: Oxford University Press.

Dressler, W. W. (1985). Extended family relationships, social support, and mental health in a southern black community. *Journal of Health and Social Behavior, 26*, 39–48.

Dressler, W. W., & Badger, L. W. (1985). Epidemiology of depressive symptoms in black communities. *Journal of Nervous and Mental Disease, 173*, 639–645.

Ensel, W. M. (1982). The role of age and the relationship of gender and marital status to depression. *Journal of Nervous and Mental Disease, 170*, 536–548.

Fabrega, H. (1990). Hispanic mental health research: A case for cultural psychiatry. *Hispanic Journal of Behavioral Science, 12*(4), 339–365.

Fabrega, H., Mezzich, J., & Ulrich, R. F. (1988). Black–white differences in psychopathology in an urban psychiatric population. *Comprehensive Psychiatry, 29,* 285–297.

Falik, M. M., & Scott-Collins, K. (Eds.). (1996). *Women's health: The Commonwealth Fund Survey.* Baltimore: Johns Hopkins University Press.

Faraone, S. V., Chen, W. J., Goldstein, J. M., & Tsuang, M. T. (1994). Gender differences in age at onset of schizophrenia. *British Journal of Psychiatry, 164,* 625–629.

Feinson, M. C. (1987). Mental health and aging: Are there gender differences? *Gerontologist, 27,* 703–711.

Fernando, S. (1988). *Race and culture in psychiatry.* London: Croom Helm.

Flaherty, J. A., Naidu, J., & Lawton, R. (1981). Racial differences in perception of ward atmosphere. *American Journal of Psychiatry, 128,* 815–817.

Forrest, A. D., & Hay, A. J. (1971). Sex differences and the schizophrenic experience. *Acta Psychiatrica Scandinavica, 47,* 137–149.

Frerichs, R. R., Aneshensel, C. S., & Clark, V. A. (1981). Prevalence of depression in Los Angeles County. *Journal of Epidemiology, 113,* 691–699.

Goldman, N., & Ravid, R. (1980). Community surveys: Sex differences in mental illness. In M. Guttentag, S. Salasin, & D. Belle (Eds.), *The mental health of women* (pp. 31–51). New York: Academic Press.

Goldstein, J. M. (1988). Gender differences in the course of schizophrenia. *American Journal of Psychiatry, 145*(6), 684–689.

Goldstein, J. M. (1995a). Gender and the familial transmission of schizophrenia. In M. V. Seeman (Ed.), *Gender and psychopathology* (pp. 201–226). Washington, DC: American Psychiatric Press.

Goldstein, J. M. (1995b). The impact of gender on understanding the epidemiology of schizophrenia. In M. V. Seeman (Ed.), *Gender and psychopathology* (pp. 159–199). Washington, DC: American Psychiatric Press.

Goldstein, J. M., & Kreisman, D. (1988). Gender, family environment, and schizophrenia. *Psychological Medicine, 18,* 861–872.

Goldstein, J. M., & Link, B. (1988). Gender and the expression of schizophrenia. *Journal of Psychiatric Research, 22*(2), 141–155.

Goldstein, J. M., Tsuang, M. T., & Faraone, S. V. (1989). Gender and schizophrenia: Implications for understanding the nature of the disorder. *Psychiatry Research, 28,* 243–253.

Goodman, L. A., Dutton, M. A., & Harris, M. (1995). Episodically homeless women with serious mental illness: Prevalence of physical and sexual assault. *American Journal of Orthopsychiatry, 65*(4), 468–478.

Gore, S., & Mangione, T. W. (1983). Social roles, sex roles, and psychological distress. *Journal of Health and Social Behavior, 24,* 300–312.

Gove, W. B., & Geerken, M. R. (1977). The effect of children and employment on the mental health of married men and women. *Social Forces, 56,* 66–79.

Grant, K., Lyons, A., Landis, D., Cho, M. H., Scudiero, M., Reynolds, L., Murphy, J., & Bryant, H. (1999). Gender, body image, and depressive symptoms among low-income African American adolescents. *Journal of Social Issues, 55*(2), 299–316.

Gullattee, A. C. (1969). The Negro psyche: Fact, fiction and fantasy. *Journal of the National Medical Association, 61*, 119–129.

Hafner, H., Heiden, W., Behrens, S., Gattaz, W. F., Hambrecht, M., Loffler, W., Maurer, K., Munk-Jorgensen, P., Nowotny, B., Riecher-Rossler, A. N., & Stein, A. (1998). Causes and consequences of the gender difference in age at onset of schizophrenia. *Schizophrenia Bulletin, 24*(1), 99–113.

Hafner, H., Maurer, K., Loffler, W., & Riecher-Rossler, A. (1993). The influence of age and sex on the onset and early course of schizophrenia. *British Journal of Psychiatry, 16*, 80–86.

Hafner, H., Riecher, A., & Maurer, K. (1989). How does gender influence age at first hospitalization for schizophrenia?: A transnational case register study. *Psychological Medicine, 19*, 903–918.

Hafner, H., Riecher-Rossler, A., Maurer, K., Fatkenheuer, B., & Loffler, W. (1992). First onset and early symptomatology of schizophrenia: A chapter of epidemiological and neurobiological research into age and sex differences. *European Archives of Psychiatry and Neurological Science, 242*, 109–116.

Hallonquist, J. D., Seeman, M. V., Lang, M., & Rector, N. A. (1993). Variation in symptom severity over the menstrual cycle of schizophrenics. *Biological Psychiatry, 33*, 207–209.

Hambrecht, M., Maurer, K., & Sartorius, N. (1992). Transnational stability of gender differences in schizophrenia?: An analysis based on the WHO study on determinants of outcome of severe mental disorders. *European Archives of Psychiatry and Clinical Neuroscience, 242*, 6–12.

Hankin, B. L., Abramson, L. Y., Moffitt, T. E., Silva, P. A., McGee, R., & Angell, K. E. (1998). Development of depression from preadolescence to young adulthood: Emerging gender differences in a 10–year longitudinal study. *Journal of Abnormal Psychology, 107*(1), 128–140.

Harris, B., Johns, S., & Fung, H. (1989). The hormonal environment of post-natal depression. *British Journal of Psychiatry, 154*, 660–667.

Jenkins-Hall, K., & Sacco, W. P. (1991). Effect of client race and depression on evaluations by white therapists. *Journal of Social and Clinical Psychology, 10*, 322–333.

Jones, B. E., & Gray, B. A. (1986). Problems in diagnosing schizophrenia and affective disorders among blacks. *Hospital Community Psychiatry, 37*, 61–65.

Jones, E. E. (1982). Psychotherapists' impressions of treatment outcome as a function of race. *Journal of Clinical Psychology, 38*, 722–731.

Kashani, J. H., Cantwell, D. P., Shakim, W. O., & Reid, J. C. (1982). Major depressive disorder in children admitted to an inpatient community mental health center. *American Journal of Psychiatry, 139*, 671–672.

Katz, S., & Mazur, M. (1979). *Understanding the rape victim: A synthesis of research findings.* New York: Wiley.

Kelly, W. E., Kelly, K. E., Brown, F. C., & Kelly, H. B. (1999). Gender differences in depression among college students: A multi-cultural perspective. *College Student Journal, 33*, 72–76.

Kendell, R. E., Chalmers, J. C., & Platz, C. (1987). Epidemiology of puerperal psychoses. *British Journal of Psychiatry, 150*, 662–673.

Kercher, G., & McShane, M. (1984). The prevalence of child sexual abuse victimization in an adult sample of Texas residents. *Child Abuse and Neglect, 8,* 495–502.

Kessler, R. C., Brown, R. L., & Broman, C. L. (1981). Sex differences in psychiatric help-seeking evidence from four large scale surveys. *Journal of Health and Social Behavior, 22,* 49–64.

Kessler, R. C., & McLeod, J. (1984). Sex differences in vulnerability to undesirable life events. *American Sociological Review, 49,* 620–631.

Kohn, M. L. (1972). Class, family, and schizophrenia: A formulation. *Social Forces, 50,* 295–304.

Kolakowska, T., Williams, A. O., & Arden, M. (1985). Schizophrenia with good and poor outcome: Early clinical features, response to neuroleptics and signs of organic dysfunction. *British Journal of Psychiatry, 146,* 229–246.

Koss, M. P. (1990). The women's mental health agenda: Violence against women. *American Psychologist, 45,* 374–380.

Lawson, W. B. (1986). Racial and ethnic factors in psychiatric research. *Hospital Community Psychiatry, 37,* 50–54.

Lawson, W. B., Hepler, N., & Holiday, J. (1991). Diagnosis of blacks in a state system. *Schizophrenia Research, 4,* 263–267.

Lehmann, H. E., & Ban, I. A. (1974). Sex differences in long-term adverse effects of phenothiazines. In I. S. Forest, C. J. Carr, & E. Usdin (Eds.), *Phenothiazines and structurally related drugs* (pp. 249–254). New York: Raven Press.

Lennon, M. C. (1998). Domestic arrangements and depressive symptoms: An examination of housework conditions. In B. P. Dohrenwend (Ed.), *Adversity, stress and psychopathology* (pp. 409–421). New York: Oxford University Press.

Lester, D., & DeSimone, A. (1995). Depression and suicidal ideation in African American and Caucasian students. *Psychological Reports, 77*(1), 18.

Lewine, R. J. (1981). Sex differences in schizophrenia: Timing of subtype? *Psychological Bulletin, 90,* 432–444.

Lewine, R. J. (1988). Gender and schizophrenia. In M. T. Tsuang & J. C. Simpson (Eds.), *Handbook of schizophrenia* (Vol. 3, pp. 379–397). Amsterdam: Elsevier.

Lillie-Blanton, M., Bowie, J., & Ro, M. (1996). African American women: Social forces and the use of preventive health services. In M. M. Falik & K. S. Collins (Eds.), *Women's health: The Commonwealth Fund Survey* (pp. 99–122). Baltimore: Johns Hopkins University Press.

Lindamer, L. A., Lohr, J. B., Harris, M. J., & Jeste, D. V. (1997). Gender, estrogen and schizophrenia. *Psychopharmacology Bulletin, 33*(2), 221–228.

Link, B. G., Lennon, M. C., & Dohrenwend, B. P. (1998). Some characteristics of occupations as risk or protective factors for episodes of major depression and nonaffective psychotic disorders. In B. P. Dohrenwend (Ed.), *Adversity, stress and psychopathology* (pp. 398–408). New York: Oxford University Press.

Marsh, H. W., & Myers, M. (1986). Masculinity, femininity, and androgyny: A methodological and theoretical critique. *Sex Roles, 14,* 397–430.

McGrath, E., Keita, G. P., Strickland, B. R., & Russo, N. F. (Eds.). (1990). *Women and depression: Risk factors and treatment issues: Final report of the American Psychological Association Task Force on Women and Depression.* Washington, DC: American Psychological Association Press.

McLanahan, S. S., & Adams, J. (1987). Parenthood and psychological well-being. *Annual Review of Sociology*, *13*, 237–257.

Mirowsky, J. (1996). Age and gender gap in depression. *Journal of Health and Social Behavior*, *37*, 362–380.

Monk, A. (1990). Health care for the aged: The pursuit of equity and comprehensiveness [Special issue: Health care of the aged: Needs, policies, and services]. *Journal of Gerontological Social Work*, *15*(3–4), 1–20.

Moscicki, E. K., Rae, D. S., Reiger, D. A., & Locke, B. Z. (1987). The Hispanic Health and Nutrition Examination Survey: Depression among Mexican Americans, Cuban Americans, and Puerto Ricans. In M. Gaviria & J. Arana (Eds.), *Health and behavior: Research agenda for Hispanics* (pp. 145–159). Chicago: University of Illinois at Chicago.

Mukherjee, S., Shukla, S., & Woodle, J. (1983). Misdiagnosis of schizophrenia in bipolar patients: A multiethnic comparison. *American Journal of Psychiatry*, *140*, 1571–1574.

Munford, M. B. (1994). Relationship of gender, self-esteem, social class, and racial identity to depression in blacks. *Journal of Black Psychology*, *20*, 157–174.

Neighbors, H. W., Jackson, J. S., & Campbell, L. (1989). The influence of racial factors on psychiatric diagnosis: A review and suggestions for research. *Community Mental Health Journal*, *25*, 301–311.

Nolen-Hoeksema, S. (1987). Sex differences in unipolar depression: Violence and theory. In J. M. Hooley, J. M. Neale, & G. C. Davison (Eds.), *Readings in abnormal psychology* (pp. 209–248). New York: Wiley.

Nolen-Hoeksema, S. (1990). *Sex differences in depression*. Stanford, CA: Stanford University Press.

Nolen-Hoeksema, S. (1995). Epidemiology and theories of gender differences in unipolar depression. In M. V. Seeman (Ed.), *Gender and psychopathology* (pp. 63–87). Washington, DC: American Psychiatric Press.

Nolen-Hoeksema, S., & Girgus, J. S. (1994). The emergence of gender differences in depression during adolescence. *Psychological Bulletin*, *115*, 424–443.

Papp, P. (2000). Gender differences in depression: His and her depression. In P. Papp (Ed.), *Couples on the fault line: New directions for therapists* (pp. 130–151). New York: Guilford Press.

Pavkov, T. W., Lewis, D. A., & Lyons, J. S. (1989). Psychiatric diagnosis and racial bias: An empirical investigation. *Professional Psychology: Research and Practice*, *20*, 365–388.

Petersen, A. C., Compas, B. E., Brooks-Gunn, J., Stemmiere, M., Ey, S., & Grant, K. E. (1993). Depression in adolescence. *American Psychologist*, *48*, 155–168.

Pianta, R. C., & Egeland, B. (1994). Relation between depressive symptoms and stressful life events in a sample of disadvantaged mothers. *Journal of Counseling and Clinical Psychology*, *42*(6), 1229–1234.

Potter, L. B., Rogler, L. H., & Moscicki, E. K. (1995). Depression among Puerto Ricans in New York City: The Hispanic Health and Nutrition Examination Survey. *Social Psychiatry and Psychiatric Epidemiology*, *30*, 185–193.

Poussaint, A. F. (1990). The mental health status of black Americans. In D. S. Ruiz (Ed.), *Handbook of mental health and mental disorder among black Americans* (pp. 17–52). New York: Greenwood Press.

Pumariega, A. J., Johnson, N. P., Sheridan, D., & Cuffe, S. P. (1996). The influence of race and gender on depressive and substance abuse symptoms in high-risk adolescents. *Cultural Diversity and Mental Health, 2*(2), 115–123.

Radloff, L. S. (1975). Sex differences in depression: The effects of occupation and marital status. *Sex Roles, 1,* 243–255.

Ramirez de Arellano, A. B. (1996). Latino women: Health status and access to heath care. In M. M. Falik & K. Scott Collins (Eds.), *Women's health: The Commonwealth Fund Survey* (pp. 123–144). Baltimore: Johns Hopkins University Press.

Rector, N. A., & Seeman, M. V. (1992). Auditory hallucinations in women and men. *Schizophrenia Research, 7,* 233–236.

Rendon, M. (1974). Transcultural aspects of Puerto Rican mental illness. *International Journal of Social Psychiatry, 20,* 18–24.

Reicher-Rossler, A., Maurer, K., Loffler, W., Fatkenheuer, B., van der Heiden, W., Munk-Jorgenson, P., van Gulick-Bailer, M., & Loffler, W. (1990). Gender differences in age at onset and course of schizophrenic disorders. In H. Hafner, W. F. Gattaz, & W. Janzarik (Eds.), *Search for the causes of schizophrenia* (pp. 14–33). Berlin: Springer-Verlag .

Reicher-Rossler, A., Hafner, H., Stumbalum, M., Maurer, K., & Schmidt, R. (1994). Can estradiol modulate schizophrenic symptomatology? *Schizophrenic Bulletin, 20,* 203–213.

Reskin, B. F., & Pedavic, I. (1994). *Women and men at work.* Thousand Oaks, CA: Pine Forge Press.

Rosenfield, S. L. (1980). Sex differences in depression: Do women always have higher rates? *Journal of Health and Social Behavior, 21,* 33–42.

Ross, C. E., & Mirowsky, J. (1988). Components of depressed mood in married men and women: The Center for Epidemiologic Studies Depression Scale. *American Journal of Epidemiology, 119,* 997–1004.

Russo, N. F., Amaro, H., & Winter, M. (1987). The use of inpatient mental health services by Hispanic women. *Psychology of Women Quarterly, 11,* 427–442.

Russo, N. F., & Sobel, S. B. (1981). Sex differences in the utilization of mental health facilities. *Professional Psychology, 12,* 7–19.

Salgado de Snyder, V. N. (1987). Factors associated with acculturative stress and depressive symptomatology among married Mexican immigrant women. *Psychology of Women Quarterly, 11,* 475–488.

Salokangas, R. K. (1983). Prognostic implications of the sex of schizophrenic patients. *British Journal of Psychiatry, 142,* 145–151.

Sartorius, N., Jablensky, A., Korten, A., Emberg, G., Anker, M., Cooper, J. E., & Day, R. (1986). Early manifestations and first-contact incidence of schizophrenia in different cultures. *Psychological Medicine, 16,* 909–928.

Sata, L. (1990, April). *Working with persons from Asian backgrounds.* Paper presented at the Cross-Cultural Psychotherapy Conference, Hahnemann University, Philadelphia.

Seeman, M. V. (1981). Gender and the onset of schizophrenia: Neurohumoral influences. *Psychiatric Journal of the University of Ottawa, 6,* 136–138.

Seeman, M. V. (1983). Interaction of sex, age, and neuroleptic dose. *Comprehensive Psychiatry, 24,* 125–128.

Seeman, M. V. (1986). Current outcome in schizophrenia: Women vs. men. *Acta Psychiatrica Scandinavica, 73*, 607–617.

Seeman, M. V. (1988). Schizophrenia in women and men. In L. L. Bachrach & C. C. Nadelson (Eds.), *Treating chronically mentally ill women* (pp. 21–28). Washington, DC: American Psychiatric Press.

Seeman, M. V. (1995). Gender differences in treatment response in schizophrenia. In M. V. Seeman (Ed.), *Gender and psychopathology* (pp. 227–251). Washington, DC: American Psychiatric Press.

Seeman, M. V., & Lang, M. (1990). The role of estrogens in schizophrenia gender differences. *Schizophrenia Bulletin, 16*(2), 185–194.

Solomon, A. (1992). Clinical diagnosis among diverse populations: A multicultural perspective. *Families in Society, 73*, 371–377.

Sprock, J., & Yoder, C. Y. (1997). Women and depression: An update on the report of the APA task force. *Sex Roles, 36*(6), 269–303.

Strakowski, S. M., Shelton, R. C., & Kolbrenner, M. L. (1993). The effects of race and comorbidity on clinical diagnosis in patients with psychosis. *Journal of Clinical Psychiatry, 54*, 96–102.

Teichner, V., Cadden, J. J., & Berry, G. W. (1981). The Puerto Rican patient: Some historical, cultural and psychological aspects. *Journal of the American Academy of Psychoanalysis, 9*, 277–290.

Test, M. A., & Berlin, S. B. (1981). Issues of special concern to chronically mentally ill women. *Professional Psychology, 12*, 136–145.

Thomas, A., & Sillen, S. (1972). *Racism and psychiatry.* New York: Brunner/Mazel.

Tudor, W., Tudor, J. F., & Gove, W. R. (1977). The effect of sex role differences on the social control of mental illness. *Journal of Health and Social Behavior, 18*, 98–112.

U.S. Department of Health and Human Services. (1985). *Report of the secretary's task force on black and minority health.* Washington, DC: U.S. Government Printing Office.

U.S. Department of Justice, Office of Justice Programs, Bureau of Justice Statistics. (1991). *Criminal victimization in the United States: 1973–1988 trends.* Washington, DC: U.S. Government Printing Office.

Vazquez-Nuttall, E., Romero-Garcia, L., & DeLeon, B. (1987). Sex roles and perceptions of femininity and masculinity of Hispanic women: A review of the literature. *Psychology of Women Quarterly, 11*, 409–425.

Vega, W. A., Kolodny, B., Valle, R., & Hough, R. (1986). Depressive symptoms and their correlates among immigrant Mexican women in the United States. *Social Science Medicine, 22*, 645–652.

Vega, W. A., Warheit, G. J., Buhl-Auth, J., & Meinhardt, K. (1984). The prevalence of depressive symptoms among Mexican Americans and Anglos. *American Journal of Epidemiology, 120*, 592–607.

Virgonia, A., Buhrich, N., & Teesn, M. (1993). Prevalence of schizophrenia among women in refuges for the homeless. *Australlian and New Zealand Journal of Psychiatry, 27*(3), 405–410.

Wade, J. C. (1991). Institutional racism: An analysis of the mental health system. *American Journal of Orthopsychiatry, 63*(4), 536–544.

Wahl, O. F., & Hunter, J. (1992). Are gender effects being neglected in schizophrenia research? *Schizophrenia Bulletin, 16*(2), 313–317.

Weissman, M. M., & Klerman, G. L. (1977). Sex differences and the epidemiology of depression. *Journal of Health and Social Behavior, 26,* 156–162.

Weissman, M. M., & Klerman, G. L. (1985). Gender and depression. *Trends in Neuroscience, 8,* 416–420.

Weissman, M. M., & Klerman, G. L. (1987). Gender and depression. In R. Formanek & A. Gurian (Eds.), *Women and depression: A lifespan perspective* (pp. 3–15). New York: Springer-Verlag.

Wetzel, J. W. (1994). Depression: Women at risk. *Social Work in Health Care, 19*(3–4), 85–108.

Whitley, B. E. (1984). Sex-role orientation and psychological well-being: Two meta-analyses. *Sex Roles, 12,* 207–222.

Wichstrom, L. (1999). The emergence of gender difference in depressed mood during adolescence: The role of intensified gender socialization. *Developmental Psychology, 35*(1), 232–245.

Williams, D. R., Yu, Y., Jackson, S. J., & Anderson, N. B. (1997). Racial differences in physical and mental health: Socioeconomic status, stress and discrimination. *Journal of Health Psychology, 2*(3), 335–351.

Wrinkle, R. D., Andalzua, H., & Reed-Sanders, D. (1988). Analysis of scales measuring self-esteem, life satisfaction, and mastery for Hispanic elderly populations. In M. Sotomayor & H. Curiel (Eds.), *Hispanic elderly: A cultural signature* (pp. 185–200). Edinburg, TX: Pan American University Press.

Index

Page numbers followed by "f" indicate figure, "t" indicate table

Body Image group
  description of, 251–252
  See also Chrysalis Program; Eating disorders
Borderline personality disorder
  diagnosis, 154
  treatment of, 233–234
  See also Chrysalis Program; Personality disorders
Both-and theories, 15–16
Boundaries
  group, 91
  Relational-Cultural Theory, 52–53
  spirituality and, 94n
Briquet's syndrome, 145

C

Capitalism, 105–106
Categoricalism, 17–18. *See also* research
Central relational paradox, 49–50. *See also* Relational–Cultural Theory
Children and poverty, 128, 132–134
Children, diagnosing
  addressing strengths and resources, 270–272
  developmental-ecology system, 274–275
  developmental issues, 263
  health care costs, 269–270
  ignoring content, 268–269
  issues of abuse, 266–268
  power and control issues, 264–265
  role of stereotypes in, 272–274
  See also Diagnosis
Chrysalis Program
  assessment of treatment, 244–248
  classism, 243–244
  contradictions of, 256–259
  description of, 232, 239–241
  diagnosis, 234–237
  disordered eating, 250–252
  ethics and spirituality, 252–255, 254f
  patient treatment history, 237–238
  socialization, 250
  therapeutic community, 241–243
  treatment of dissociative disorders, 248–249
  treatment outcomes, 255–256t
  See also Personality disorders
Classism
  affects on relationships, 53–54
  challenging in treatment, 243–244
  concept of difference, 114
  feminist ecological theory, 127–128, 132–134
  Relational–Cultural Theory, 55
  resilience research, 58
Climate, 129–130. *See also* Feminist ecological model
Cognitive-behavioral approaches, 148–149
Collective Kitchen
  description of, 251
  See also Chrysalis Program; Eating disorders
Conduct disorder, 265–266, 267
Conflict between the sexes, 37
Connection
  alcohol use and, 207
  associated with resilience, 64–66

fostered through relationships, 49–50
psychology's responsibility in, 107
resilience, 60, 66
Consciousness
  critical, 110, 126–127
  discourse and, 6
Constructivism
  description of, 72–74
  identity, 76–79, 79–83, 92–93
  social, 104
  See also Postmodernism
Control
  hardiness, 58
  premenstrual syndrome and postpartum depression, 185
  socialization, 204–205
Convergence hypothesis
  explanation of, 202–203
  See also Addiction; Gender roles
Conversion disorder
  definition of, 145
  diagnosis, 154–155
  See also Dissociative disorder
Critical consciousness
  feminist ecological theory, 126–127
  liberation psychology, 110
Critical discourse analysis, 22–23
Critical perspective, 110
Critical theory
  description of, 104–108
  feminist ecological theory, 138
  liberation psychology, 110
Cultural bias
  attachment theory, 32–33
  See also Bias
Cultural determinism, 15–16
Culture
  biases in diagnosis, 281–283
  definition of, 111
  diagnosing children and adolescents, 273–274
  evolutionary psychology, 35
  feminist ecological theory, 123–124
  integration with gender, 114
  premenstrual syndrome and postpartum depression, 184–189
  See also Multiculturalism

D

Delusions, 164
Depression
  abuse and, 266
  diagnosing in children and adolescents, 264
  diagnosis, 265
  evolutionary psychology, 39
  gender differences, 279–280, 283–284, 284–287
  postpartum depression and, 183
  premenstrual syndrome and, 183
  race/ethnicity, 287–290
  research, 296
  role of power in, 43
  role of social class, 295–296
  substance use and, 207–208, 208–209
  See also Postpartum depression

Ethnicity
definition of, 297n
depression and, 287–290
schizophrenia, 293–295
See also Race; Women of color; Youth of color
Evolutionary psychology
critiques of, 38–43
description of, 34–37
Executive function
development of identity, 81, 82
identity creation, 77–79
Experiences
culture's role in, 124–125
excluding of at the institutional level, 125–126
feminist ecological theory, 137–138
feminist standpoint epistemologies, 104
identity, 76–77
liberation psychology, 109
understanding, 114
Exploitation
addiction and, 219–220
critical theory, 106
Eye movement desensitization and reprocessing, 9. *See also* Trauma theory

F

Factitious disorder
definition of, 146
See also Somatoform disorders
Family
dysfunction, 266–267
feminist ecological theory, 123
traditional views of, 134
Family therapy, 148–149
Feminism backlash, 21–23
Feminist ecological model
concepts of time and history, 130–131
coordinates of, 131–134
critique of traditional personality theories, 134–135
description of, 117–119, 120f
exosystem, 125–127
inner circle, 119, 121–122
integration of theories, 135–136
macrosystem, 127–128
microsystem, 122–125
planetary/climatic conditions, 128–130
summarized, 135–139
Feminist empiricism
Psychology of Women Quarterly, 7–8
See also Empiricism
Feminist psychology
description of, 101–102
evolutionary psychology and, 42–43
postmodernism, 6–8
Feminist therapy theory
addiction, 221–222
contributions to feminist ecological theory, 136
description of, 102–108
social change, 107
Fight/flight response, 65
Forgiveness, 10

Functional somatic disorders
definition of, 146
diagnosis, 153
See also Somatoform disorders

G

Gender
diagnosis of identity disorder, 272–273
division of parenting, 134
feminist ecological theory, 123–124
integration with culture, 114
oppression, 102
organization of psychology, 8
rethinking, 13–14
See also Gender differences; Gender roles
Gender differences
depression, 279–280, 283–284, 284–287
diagnosis of illness, 155–156
schizophrenia, 279–280, 290–293
See also Gender
Gender roles
addiction and, 210–211
addiction behaviors, 209–210
challenging within the Chrysalis Program, 250
depression and, 286–287, 288–289
diagnosis issues, 272–274
evolutionary psychology, 39–40
postpartum depression, 184
premenstrual syndrome, 182–183
research on addiction, 220–221
substance use, 201–202, 202–204, 206
See also Gender
Genetic predisposition, 149–150. *See also* Somatoform disorders
Group-referenced identity
description of, 84–92
therapy implications, 93
See also Identity
Growth-fostering relationships
outcomes, 49–50
See also Relational–Cultural Theory
Growth through relationships, 49–50

H

Hallucinations postpartum, 180
Happiness
barriers to, 36–37
evolutionary theory, 40–41
Hardiness, 58
Health care costs
diagnosing of children and adolescents, 268–269, 269–270
somatoform disorders, 156–157
Health care system
feminist ecological theory, 126
See also Health care costs
Helplessness, 43. *See also* Power
Heterosexism
affects on relationships, 53–54
internal locus of control, 63
resilience research, 58

S

Schizophrenia
  gender differences, 280, 290–293
  race/ethnicity, 293–295
  research, 296
  role of social class, 295–296
Self-awareness
  Chrysalis Program, 240
  cultural competence and, 93
  reflexive, 77–79
Self-esteem
  addiction and, 207–208
  associated with resilience, 62
  role of power in, 43
Self-in-relation theory. *See* Relational–Cultural
    Theory
Self-worth and addiction, 207–208. *See also*
    Addiction
Separation, 50–51. *See also* Development
Sex differences
  evolutionary psychology, 39–40, 42
  evolutionary theory, 35–37
  Relational–Cultural Theory, 54
  research, 11–12
  See also Difference
Sex trade market and addiction, 214–215. *See also*
    Addiction
Sexism
  affects on relationships, 53–54
  co-construed meanings, 93
  concept of difference, 114
  diagnosing children and adolescents, 272–274
  internal locus of control, 63
  language of somatoform diagnosis, 164
  resilience research, 58
Sexist biases
  evolutionary psychology, 41–42
  See also Bias
Sexual abuse
  diagnosing in children and adolescents, 267
  peer related, 273
  premenstrual syndrome and, 183
  somatoform disorders, 152
Sexuality
  challenging within the Chrysalis Program, 250
  development, 41–42
  rethinking, 13–14
Sick role, 162
Social activism
  liberation psychology, 110
  See also Activism; Social change
Social causation, 295–296
Social change
  addiction recovery, 222
  critical theory, 104–108
  feminist ecological theory, 127, 137–138
  feminist therapy, 103
  institutions and, 125–126
  liberation psychology, 108
  transformative multiculturalism, 113
Social context
  feminist psychology, 16–17
  identity and, 77–79, 83–89
Social esteem, 62. *See also* Resilience

Social justice
  critical theory and, 106–108
  liberation psychology, 110
Social selection, 295–296
Social structural theory, 39–40
Social support
  addiction, 217–218
  associated with resilience, 64–66
Socialization
  challenging within the Chrysalis Program, 250
  gender differences in depression, 286
  positive aspects, 204–207
  women's subordinate status, 212
Somatoform disorders
  clinical implications, 165–166
  definition of, 145
  diagnosis, 152–153, 153–157
  experience of women, 162–163
  explanatory models, 147–152
  language of diagnosis, 163–165
  risk of diagnosis, 157–158
  stigmatization of, 161–162
Spirituality, 252–255, 254f. *See also* Chrysalis Pro-
    gram
Standardized assessment instruments, 17. *See also*
    research
Standpoint epistemologies, 104
Stereotypes
  addiction and, 210–211
  diagnosing children and adolescents, 273–274
  premenstrual syndrome as, 175–176
  sexist biases, 41–42
  via popular culture, 187–189
  women of color, 202
  See also Bias
Stigmatization
  diagnosis and, 269–270
  somatoform disorders, 161–162
Stone Center
  description of, 48–49
  models of development, 50–51
Strange Situation
  description of, 30
  problems with, 32
  See also Attachment theory
Strategies of disconnection, 49–50. *See also*
    Relational–Cultural Theory
Stress
  disorders of, 236
  evolutionary psychology, 43
  gender differences, 285
  postpartum depression, 184, 187
  premenstrual syndrome, 183
  resilience, 58–59
  responses to, 65–66
Stress–diathesis models
  gender differences in depression, 285–
    286
  treatment of somatoform disorders, 149–
    150
Structured psychodynamic treatment, 233
Subjectivity, 19
Substance use
  gender differences, 202–204
  See also Addiction